Chemical Carcinogens and DNA

Volume II

Editor

Philip L. Grover

Chester Beatty Research Institute
Institute of Cancer Research
Royal Cancer Hospital
London, England

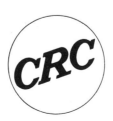

CRC PRESS, INC.
Boca Raton, Florida 33431

Library of Congress Cataloging in Publication Data

Main entry under title:

Chemical carcinogens and DNA.

   Bibliography: p.
   Includes index.
   1. Carcinogens.
   2. Deoxyribonucleic acid.
3. Chemical mutagenesis. I. Grover, Philip L.
RC268.6.C49   616.9'94'071   78-13255

This book represents information obtained from authentic and highly regarded sources. Reprinted material is quoted with permission, and sources are indicated. A wide variety of references are listed. Every reasonable effort has been made to give reliable data and information, but the author and the publisher cannot assume responsibility for the validity of all materials or for the consequences of their use.

International Standard Book Number 0-8493-5303-3(Volume I)
International Standard Book Number 0-8493-5304-1(Volume II)

Library of Congress Card Number 78-13255
Printed in the United States

PREFACE

Since so little is known in molecular terms about the organization of eukaryotic cells and the homeostatic mechanisms that control them, it is not very surprising that the changes that are involved in the acquisition of malignancy are not understood either. It is, however, generally accepted that chemical carcinogens exert their effects through initial reactions with specific targets within the cell. The nature of these targets also remains unknown but, partly because of correlations between mutagenicity and carcinogenicity and partly because of the simplistic appeal of the somatic mutation hypothesis, reactions of chemical carcinogens with nucleic acids, particularly DNA, continue to receive much attention.

These two volumes represent an attempt to make an up-to-date appraisal of chemical carcinogens from the point of view of their effects on DNA and the subject matter is arranged in a sequence. The opening contributions deal with extents to which carcinogens react with DNA and with the formation and detection of DNA-carcinogen adducts and these are followed by more specialized chapters dealing with the activation of particular types of chemical carcinogens and their reactions with DNA. The later contributions cover the conformational changes induced in nucleic acids by chemical carcinogens and deal with the mechanisms by which these chemical reactions may be translated, either directly or indirectly, into biological effects that include mutagenesis and carcinogenesis.

P. L. Grover
March 1978

THE EDITOR

Philip L. Grover, D.Sc., is a Senior Scientist on the staff of the Chester Beatty Research Institute, Institute of Cancer Research, London, England.

Dr. Grover graduated from the University of London in 1956 and subsequently obained M.Sc. and Ph.D. degrees for research on detoxication reactions. He joined the scientific staff of the Chester Beatty Research Institute in 1959 where he has worked, largely in collaboration with Dr. Peter Sims, on the metabolic activation of the carcinogenic polycyclic hydrocarbons. He was awarded a D.Sc. by the University of London in 1977.

CONTRIBUTORS

W. M. Baird, Ph.D.
Associate Professor
The Wistar Institute
Philadelphia, Pennsylvania

C. C. Chang, Ph.D.
Assistant Professor
Department of Human Development
College of Human Medicine
Michigan State University
East Lansing, Michigan

C. C. J. Culvenor, Ph.D., D.Sc.
Chief Research Scientist
CSIRO
Division of Animal Health
Animal Health Research Laboratory
Victoria, Australia

M. Duquesne, Ph.D.
Professor
Department of Physics
University of Paris and Institut Curie
Paris, France

R. C. Garner, Ph.D.
Senior Lecturer
Cancer Research Unit
University of York
York, United Kingdom

M. H. L. Green, Ph.D.
Scientist
MRC Cell Mutation Unit
University of Sussex
Brighton, United Kingdom

D. Grunberger, Ph.D.
Associate Professsor
College of Physicians and Surgeons
Institute of Cancer Research
Columbia University
New York, New York

M. V. Jago, Ph.D.
Principal Research Scientist
CSIRO
Division of Animal Health
Animal Health Research Laboratory
Victoria, Australia

E. Kriek, Ph.D.
Research Biochemist and Chief
Division of Chemical Carcinogenesis
The Netherlands Cancer Institute
Amsterdam, The Netherlands

P. D. Lawley, D.Sc.
Senior Lecturer
Pollards Wood Research Station
Institute of Cancer Research
Bucks, United Kingdom

V. M. Maher, Ph.D.
Associate Professor
Department of Microbiology and
  Public Health and Department of
  Biochemistry
  and
Co-Director
Carcinogenesis Laboratory-Fee Hall
Michigan State University
East Lansing, Michigan

G. P. Margison, Ph.D.
Scientific Officer
Paterson Laboratories
Christie Hospital and Holt Radium
  Institute
Manchester, United Kingdom

H. W. J. Marquardt, M.D.
Associate Member
Sloan-Kettering Institute for Cancer
  Research
New York, New York
  and
Associate Professor
Department of Pharmacology
Sloan-Kettering Division
Graduate School of Medical Sciences
Cornell University
New York, New York

C. N. Martin, Ph.D.
Research Fellow
Cancer Research Unit
University of York
York, United Kingdom

J. J. McCormick, Ph.D.
Associate Professor
Department of Microbiology and
  Public Health and Department of
  Biochemistry
  and
Co-Director
Carcinogenesis Laboratory-Fee Hall
Michigan State University
East Lansing, Michigan

P. J. O'Connor, Ph.D.
Senior Research Officer
Paterson Laboratories
Christie Hospital and Holt Radium
  Institute
Manchester, United Kingdom

D. H. Phillips, Ph.D.
Post-doctoral Fellow
McArdle Laboratory For Cancer
  Research
University of Wisconsin
Madison, Wisconsin

P. Sims, Ph.D., D.Sc.
Reader in Biochemistry
Institute of Cancer Research
Chester Beatty Research Institute
London, United Kingdom

J. E. Trosko, Ph.D.
Professor
Department of Human Development
College of Human Medicine
Michigan State University
East Lansing, Michigan

P. Vigny, Ph.D.
Associate Professor
Department of Physics
University of Paris and Institut Curie
Paris, France

I. B. Weinstein, M.D.
Professor
College of Physicians and Surgeons
Division of Environmental Sciences and
  Institute of Cancer Research
Columbia University
New York, New York

J. G. Westra, Ph.D.
Research Chemist
Division of Chemical Carcinogenesis
The Netherlands Cancer Institute
Amsterdam, The Netherlands

TABLE OF CONTENTS

VOLUME I

VOLUME II

Chapter 1

METABOLIC ACTIVATION OF AROMATIC AMINES AND AMIDES AND INTERACTIONS WITH NUCLEIC ACIDS

E. Kriek and J. G. Westra

TABLE OF CONTENTS

I. INTRODUCTION*

Aromatic amines are valuable chemicals in many areas of industry and research that are particularly important as intermediates in the dyestuff and pharmaceutical industries. A number of these compounds are well-known cancer producing agents that are active both in experimental animals and in humans. According to the International Agency for Research on Cancer (IARC) monographs[1] and a recent review,[2] the epidemiology of aromatic amine carcinogenesis is essentially the epidemiology of human bladder cancer of industrial origin. In the U.S., 14 different compounds have recently been listed as subject to an Emergency Standard[3] issued by the Occupational Safety and Health Administration (OSHA), Department of Labor. These compounds are either already accepted as being, or are currently under suspicion of being, important industrial carcinogens. Of these 14 chemicals, 7 are aromatic amines and a zero tolerance for these compounds has been proposed.[4] A number of aromatic amines and their corresponding nitro derivatives that were not covered in previous IARC monographs[1] have been considered recently by an IARC working group,[5] because a number of them are still widely used as colorants in hair dyes, as dye intermediates, and in the manufacture of plastics and other synthetic polymers. Not all aromatic amines are potent carcinogens. They form a class of compounds with great diversity in species and tissue specificity that is partly dependent on their chemical structure. In so far as the carcinogenicity of aromatic amines is governed by their chemical structure, two factors are important: (1) the type of aromatic ring system and (2) the presence of other substituents. The carcinogenic potential of aromatic amines in relation to their chemical structure has been discussed recently by Clayson and Garner,[6] and an article on the same subject by Arcos and Argus has also appeared.[7]

In common with the polycyclic aromatic hydrocarbons, the majority of the administered dose of an aromatic amine or amide is converted in vivo to ring-hydroxy or phenolic metabolites. This process occurs primarily in the liver and is catalyzed by the microsomal mixed-function oxidase system involving pyridine nucleotide, flavoprotein, cytochrome P-450, and oxygen. The phenolic metabolites are excreted in the urine as O-glucuronides and O-sulfates. Originally, among these metabolites, the *ortho*-hydroxyamines were proposed by Clayson[8] as proximate carcinogens, i.e., as metabolites that are closer to the ultimate reactant than the parent carcinogen. The ultimate reactant is the metabolite capable of reacting nonenzymically with critical cellular components to initiate carcinogenesis. This hypothesis was based on the ability of some o-hydroxyamines to produce tumors of the mouse bladder epithelium upon implantation into the lumen of this organ.[8] However, the carcinogenicity of o-hydroxyamines has proved to be very limited; many o-hydroxyamines appeared to be inactive in the mouse

---

* Abbreviations used: AF, 2-aminofluorene; N-hydroxy-AF, N-hydroxy-2-aminofluorene; AAF, 2-acetylaminofluorene; N-hydroxy-AAF, N-hydroxy-2-acetylaminofluorene; N-acetoxy-AAF, N-acetoxy-2-acetylaminofluorene; N-GlO-AAF, glucuronide of N-hydroxy-2-acetylaminofluorene; N-GlO-AF, glucuronide of N-hydroxy-2-aminofluorene; N-hydroxy-1-AAF, N-hydroxy-1-acetylaminofluorene; N-hydroxy-3-AAF, N-hydroxy-3-acetylaminofluorene; N-hydroxy-4-AAF, N-hydroxy-4-acetylaminofluorene; N-acetoxy-3-AAF, N-acetoxy-3-acetylaminofluorene; N-acetoxy-4-AAF, N-acetoxy-4-acetylaminofluorene; AB, 4-amionazobenzene; N-hydroxy-AB, N-hydroxy-4-aminoazobenzene; MAB, N-methyl-4-aminoazobenzene; N-hydroxy-MAB, N-hydroxy-N-methyl-4-aminoazobenzene; N-benzoyloxy-MAB, N-benzoyloxy-N-methyl-4-aminoazobenzene; DAB, N,N-dimethyl-4-aminoazobenzene; AABP, 4-acetylaminobiphenyl; N-hydroxy-AABP, N-hydroxy-4-acetylaminobiphenyl; AABP4'F, 4-acetylamino(4'-fluoro)biphenyl; N-hydroxy-AABP4'F, N-hydroxy-4-acetylamino(4'-fluoro)biphenyl; AAS, 4-acetylaminostilbene; N-hydroxy-AAS, N-hydroxy-4-acetylaminostilbene; N-acetoxy-AAS, N-acetoxy-4-acetylaminostilbene; AAP, 2-acetylaminophenanthrene; N-hydroxy-AAP, N-hydroxy-2-acetylaminophenanthrene; DPEA, 2-([2,4-dichloro-6-phenyl]phenoxy)ethylamine.

bladder and disagreement existed even on the validity of the test itself. Therefore, *o*-hydroxyamine formation cannot be considered as a general activation route for aromatic amines and will not be discussed in this chapter.

Gradually, through the discovery of specific metabolic reactions, and through the detection of protein- and nucleic acid-bound derivatives of aromatic amines in the target tissues, definite proof was obtained that the parent compounds were not carcinogenic per se. Rather, it was evident that they are carcinogenic as a consequence of the formation of certain reactive intermediates (ultimate carcinogens), which are capable of reacting with cellular constituents. Although quantitatively a minor reaction, *N*-oxidation has become of unique importance in studies on the mechanism of action of carcinogenic aromatic amines and amides. Derivatives of the *N*-hydroxy compounds are the only type of enzymically formed metabolites with sufficient chemical reactivity to react nonenzymically, with the formation of covalent bonds, with cell constituents. Under certain conditions, some *N*-hydroxy amines have sufficient chemical reactivity themselves to react without further activation. The aims of the present chapter are the following: (1) to discuss briefly the formation of *N*-hydroxy derivatives of aromatic amines and amides: (2) to summarize known pathways by which *N*-hydroxy compounds can be further metabolized in vivo, and (3) to describe what is known at present of the properties of reactive metabolites of aromatic amines, particularly the products that are formed in reactions with nucleic acids. A number of relevant reviews has appeared during recent years.[9-12]

The aminoazo dyes, a group of compounds related to the aromatic amines, have long been considered as a separate class of carcinogens. However, it was recently established in the Millers' laboratory that they undergo metabolic activation in rat liver in essentially the same manner as the aromatic amines. Therefore, the aminoazo dyes will not be considered as a separate class of carcinogens in this chapter.

II. METABOLIC ACTIVATION REACTIONS OF AROMATIC AMINES AND AMIDES

A. *N*-Oxidation to Hydroxamic Acids

The presence of nitrogen in a multiplicity of chemicals possessing physiological activity, together with the realization that oxidation of this nitrogen can modify the physiological activity, has led to an enormous increase in the interest shown in this metabolic pathway. A monograph on this subject, edited by Bridges et al.,[13] is available. The modifications of pharmacological activity observed, due to *N*-oxidation of the compounds, may vary considerably; sometimes enhancing pharmacological activity and in other instances reducing this activity to very low levels. Differentiation of various types of biological *N*-oxidation in organic compounds has been outlined recently by Gorrod.[14] In this chapter, only the *N*-oxidations leading to activation will be discussed.

Definitive demonstration that aromatic amines are oxidized on the nitrogen under physiological conditions was provided in 1960 by Cramer et al.[15] *N*-Hydroxy-2-acetylaminofluorene (*N*-hydroxy-AAF) was found in the urine of rats almost entirely as the glucuronic acid conjugate after continuous feeding of the versatile carcinogen 2-acetylaminofluorene (AAF). A similar formation of *N*-hydroxy-AAF from AAF by rabbit liver microsomes in vitro was described 2 years later by Irving.[16] The *N*-oxidation of aromatic amines and amides is also carried out by the mixed-function oxidase system located in the endoplasmic reticulum. The role of cytochrome P-450 in the *N*-oxidation of individual amines has been discussed by Uehleke,[17] and Kiese[18] has compiled a list of aromatic amines and amides which are *N*-oxidized in vitro by liver microsomes of various species. In most of these species, including cat, chicken, dog, hamster, guinea pig, rabbit, and rat, N-hydroxy derivatives are excreted in the urine either in free or conjugated form. Enomoto and Sato[19] demonstrated that microsomes from human liver are also capable of carrying out the N-oxidation of AAF. The general reaction is illustrated in Figure 1. Some controversy exists in the earlier literature on the question of whether the guinea pig is capable of N-oxidation reactions. This species is refractory to liver carcinogenesis by AAF, an observation that was attributed by Miller et al.[20] to the apparent inability of this animal to N-oxidize AAF. However, Kiese et al.[21] showed that 2-aminofluorene (AF) was N-oxidized at least as rapidly as aniline by guinea pig liver microsomes, with rates comparable to those found with rabbit liver microsomes (Appel et al.[22]). The apparent discrepancy between the positive data on the N-oxidation of AF in opposition to the negative results with the N-acetyl derivative is due to the low rate of N-oxidation of the latter compound and to the much higher rate of deacetylation of N-hydroxy-AAF by guinea pig liver as compared to other species.[23]

Following the original studies with AAF, similar results with other carcinogenic aromatic amines and amides supported the requirement for N-oxidation as a first activation step for these compounds. Thus, 4-acetylaminobiphenyl (AABP),[24] 4-acetylaminostilbene (AAS),[25] 2-acetylaminophenanthrene (AAP),[26] and N-methyl-4-aminoazobenzene[10] are all N-oxidized in rat liver, and each of the N-hydroxy derivatives is more carcinogenic than the parent amide.

Another property reflecting the activation of aromatic amines and their N-acetyl derivatives by N-oxidation was the higher level of binding to proteins and nucleic acids that occurred in vivo following administration of the N-hydroxy compounds as compared to the parent carcinogens. In vitro, however, little or no reactivity of the N-hydroxy arylamides towards proteins of nucleic acids or towards their constituents could be detected in model reactions under physiological conditions. With the exception of some arylhydroxylamines (Section II.C), which showed reactivity in vitro under special conditions, other activation reactions of the N-hydroxy arylamides were implicated in order to account for the observed binding of arylamide residues to proteins and to nucleic acids in vivo.

B. Esterification Reactions of Arylhydroxamic Acids
1. O-Glucuronides

Like the aromatic ring hydroxy compounds (phenols), N-hydroxy derivatives are readily conjugated with glucuronic acid through a reaction catalyzed by the liver enzyme, glucuronyl transferase. This type of conjugation is quantitatively the most important type of reaction involved in the excretion of N-hydroxy compounds and has been reviewed by Irving.[27] The reaction predominates in all species investigated with the exception of cats.[28] The first O-glucuronide obtained by biosynthesis was that of the carcinogen N-hydroxy-AAF, and its chemical properties have been studied in detail by Hill and Irving.[29] Sensitivity to alkali appeared to be a general property of this type of glucuronides, which is due to an intramolecular migration of the N-acetyl group.[29] This O-glucuronide reacts in vitro at neutral pH with methionine, guanosine, and nucleic acids, and the reactions were similar in some respects as those reported earlier for the synthetic ester N-acetoxy-AAF (Section II.B.2), but differed considerably in

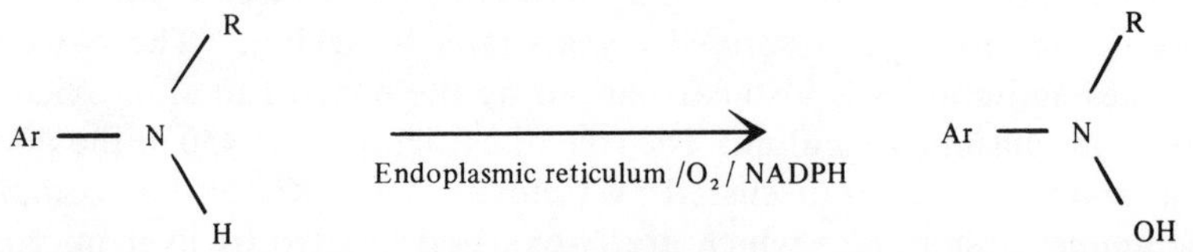

$$Ar - N \overset{\displaystyle R}{\underset{\displaystyle H}{<}} \quad \xrightarrow{\text{Endoplasmic reticulum } /O_2/ \text{ NADPH}} \quad Ar - N \overset{\displaystyle R}{\underset{\displaystyle OH}{<}}$$

FIGURE 1.   General activation reaction of aromatic amines and amides by N-oxidation. Ar, aromatic hydrocarbon; R, H, acetyl, alkyl.

rate and in the nature of the end products formed. The reaction products formed with methionine and with guanosine are presented in the general reaction scheme illustrated in Figure 2. In the reaction of N-G1O-AAF with methionine, guanosine, and nucleic acids, the proportionate yield of the deacetylated products increased with rising pH and a higher reaction rate. Hill[30] suggested that the more reactive N-G1O-AF could be formed by deacetylation. In a recent study, Cardona and King[31] confirmed that N-G1O-AAF is activated by enzymic deacetylation in vitro, which was reflected in the formation of AF-tRNA adducts. The reactive O-glucuronide of N-hydroxy-AF has been synthesized by Irving and Russel.[32]

Glucuronidation as a metabolic pathway relevant for aromatic amine carcinogeneis has been subjected to criticism in the past.[33] However, it is now felt that glucuronides of N-hydroxy amines and amides are important metabolites, because they represent transport forms of these carcinogens. After their formation in the liver, the glucuronides are transported to other organs where they may be sujected to various enzymic reactions. Williams et al.[34] demonstrated that N-G1O-AAF is hydrolyzed readily by the bacterial flora in the gut and the N-hydroxy compound liberated undergoes further substantial changes (Sections II.C to E). Reduction of N-hydroxy-AAF and resorption in the lower portion of the gastrointestinal tract may lead to further metabolism. A similar situation can be envisaged in the urine bladder (Section II.D.2). In addition, O-glucuronides, and more particularly N-glucuronides, of arylhydroxylamines may be responsible for the covalent binding of arylamine residues to nucleic acids in various tissues, including the liver (Section III). Studies by Malejka-Giganti et al.[35] suggest that N-hydroxy-AAF is also involved as a proximate carcinogen in mammary gland carcinogenesis induced in the rat by AAF.

2. O-Acetates

Despite numerous examples of the biological N-acetylation of aromatic amines and sulfonamides (reviewed by Parke[36]), the enzymic O-acetylation of N-hydroxy amides has never been demonstrated. In a comparative study by Lotlikar and Luha[37] on the

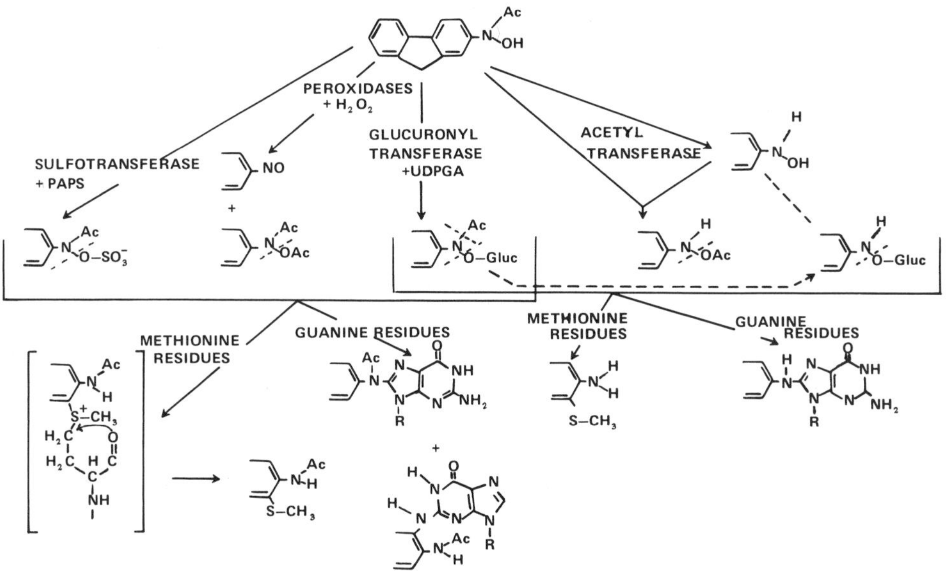

FIGURE 2. Metabolic activation reactions of N-hydroxy-2-acetyl-aminofluorene and formation of reaction products with methionine and guanine residues. (From Miller, E. C. and Miller, J. A., *Proc. 11th Int. Cancer Congress, Vol. 2, Chemical and Viral Oncogenesis*, Bucalossi, P., Veronesi, U., and Cascinelli, N., Eds., Excerpta Medica, Amsterdam, 1975, 8. With permission).

nonenzymic acylation of N-hydroxy-AAF by acetyl-CoA, carbamoyl phosphate, or acetyl phosphate, acetyl-CoA was by far the best acylating agent. The products of the reaction indicated that the intermediate formed was N-acetoxy-AAF. However, the reaction appeared to be strongly dependent on the pH of the medium and exhibited a rather high pH optimum at pH 10. At neutrality, only 10 to 20% of the optimal amount of acetylation was observed. Other N-hydroxy amides derived from naphthalene, phenanthrene, or stilbene reacted several times faster with carbamoyl phosphate than with acetyl-CoA.[37] Because acetyl-CoA is present in most mammalian tissues, the possibility that arylhydroxamic acids are O-acetylated nonenzymically in vivo cannot be excluded at present. Nevertheless, synthetic esters like N-acetoxy-AAF have proven to be extremely useful as model for studies of the reactivity of this type of compounds with various tissue nucleophiles. As a typical example, N-acetoxy-AAF reacts readily at neutral pH with proteins and nucleic acids and certain of their constituents, such as methionine, tryptophan, tyrosine, guanosine, and deoxyguanosine.[38] The reaction products formed with nucleic acids by several aromatic amides have been chemically identified in this manner and will be described in Section III of this chapter.

Acetyl esters of arylhydroxamic acids can be prepared easily in analytically pure form by acetylation of the N-hydroxy compounds in a mixture of acetic anhydride and pyridine according to a procedure described by Irving and Veazey.[39]

3. O-Sulfates

Studies by Miller and co-workers[40,41] on the reactivities of a number of reactive esters of N-hydroxy-AAF showed a wide range in stability of these compounds in aqueous solvents. Whereas the weakly reactive ester N-G1O-AAF has a half-life of several days,[40] the more reactive ester N-acetoxy-AAF and N-benzoyloxy-AAF have half-lives of a few hours.[41] The ionic and highly unstable sulfuric acid ester (potassium salt) has a half-life in water of less than 1 min and showed, as expected, greater reactivity than the other esters.[41] Because of their short lifespans and high reactivity, the isolation of sulfate esters from tissues, bile or from the urine from animals receiving aromatic amines has not been possible. Evidence for the formation of AAF-N-sulfate in rat liver as an ultimate carcinogenic metabolite has been obtained indirectly by several investigators. Its formation in liver preparations has been demonstrated by employing in vitro assays dependent upon the presence of 3'-phosphoadenosine 5'-phosphosulfate (PAPS). Assays of this type have been developed independently by DeBaun et al.[42] and by King and Philips.[43] In this first, the sulfotransferase activity of liver was measured by estimating the amounts of 1- and 3-methylmercapto-AAF formed in reactions of enzymically-generated AAF-N-sulfate with excess methionine[42] (see general reaction scheme in Figure 2). In the second assay, tRNA was used as the trapping agent for the reactive AAF-N-sulfate.[43] In later studies, the presence and level of sulfotransferase activity in liver correlated quite well with the susceptibility to hepatic carcinogenesis by N-hydroxy-AAF under a variety of conditions.[44] Additional evidence that AAF-N-sulfate is the reactive ultimate carcinogen derived from AAF or its N-hydroxy metabolite was provided by Weisburger et al.[45] based on the inhibition of AAF carcinogenesis by acetanilide. Acetanilide is metabolized mainly to the p-hydroxy derivative, although N-oxidation occurs to a small extent. Buch et al.[46] reported that in rats p-hydroxyacetanilide is excreted as a glucuronic and sulfuric acid ester. With increasing dosage the glucuronide production remained relatively constant, but the sulfate ester formation increased and was limited only by the availability of inorganic sulfate. It was postulated by Miller that one reason for the inhibition of AAF carcinogenicity by large amounts of acetanilde was the unavailability of sulfate. DeBaun et al.[42] indeed noted that the amount of AAF residues bound to proteins and nucleic acids depended heavily on the presence of inorganic sulfate, but not of other inorganic ions. This finding was further substantiated by Weisburger et al,[45] who showed that addition of sulfate restored the carcinogenicity in rats given N-hydroxy-AAF and acetanilide.

The activation pathway through O-esterification by sulfuric acids seems to be restricted exclusively to liver. DeBaun et al.[44] were unable to detect sulfotransferase activity in kidney, mammary gland, and s.c. tissue. Similarly, Irving et al.[47] did not detect this enzymic activity in the sebaceous ear duct gland. However, in each of these tissues N-hydroxy-AAF has strong carcinogenic activity so that other activation reactions must be involved in these organs.

Unlike AAF-N-sulfate, which is too unstable to obtain in a pure form, the sulfuric acid esters (potassium salts) of N-hydroxy-4-acetylaminobiphenyl,[44] N-hydroxy-4-acetylamino-4'-fluorobiphenyl[48] and N-hydroxy-2-acetylaminophenanthrene[49] have been prepared by direct chemical synthesis in an analytically pure form. The interaction of these N-sulfates with nucleic acids and their constituents have been studied in detail (Section III).

An anomalous carcinogenic N-hydroxy amide is N-hydroxy-3-acetylaminofluorene. Although it is carcinogenic to the mammary glands and ear duct glands of the rat, none of its esters has shown electrophilic reactivity towards the nucleophiles described in this section.[50,51] This finding suggests that other activation reactions are required for this compound to exhibit carcinogenic activity.

Phosphorylation of N-hydroxy amides is at most a minor pathway in rat liver. Evidence has been obtained by Tada and Tada[52] for an ATP-dependent phosphorylation of the carcinogen 4-hydroxylaminoquinoline-1-oxide in rat liver.

C. Pathways of Formation of Arylhydroxylamines

1. Enzymatic Deacetylation of Arylhydroxamic acids

Enzymic removal of the N-acetyl group, a known metabolic pathway for arylamides, has also been observed for the N-hydroxy derivatives. Two types of deacetylase have been detected; one is a soluble enzyme,[53] the other is located in the endoplasmic reticulum of the liver.[23] The microsomal enzyme activity was very high in the liver of guinea pig and hamster, but was low in rat liver when N-hydroxy-AAF was used as substrate. Irving[23] found that the product formed, N-hydroxy-AF could be trapped in situ using trisodium pentacyanoamineferrate. The latter compound forms a stable colored complex with hydroxylamines which can be used as a quantitative measure for deacetylation activity. Kriek[54] demonstrated that N-hydroxy-AF was able to react with guanine in nucleic acids in an acid-catalyzed reaction in vitro (see also Section III). A similar type of reaction at neutral pH was employed by King and Phillips[55] to measure the reaction products formed from N-hydroxy-AF generated in situ upon incubation of N-hydroxy-AAF together with guanosine or tRNA and soluble rat-liver enzymes in a system favoring deacetylation. However, the possibility exists that this interaction occurs via intramolecular transacetylation, followed by electrophilic attack of the O-acetyl derivative (see also Section II.D.1 and References 75 and 76).

Whether arylhydroxylamines are actually involved as reactive intermediates in the binding of aromatic amines to cellular constituents in vivo is not clear. Available data, discussed in Section II.D, support the view that the more reactive O- and N-glucuronides are involved as ultimate carcinogenic reactants.

2. N-Oxidation of Arylamines

Whereas the carcinogenicity of primary aromatic amines in rodents depends on their N-acetylation and subsequent activation reactions, other pathways must be involved in species which do not have the capacity to N-acetylate aromatic amines. Thus, as was shown by Radomski et al.,[56-58] the carcinogenicities of 1- and 2-aminonaphthalene and 4-aminobiphenyl for the urinary bladder of the dog depend on the N-oxidation of the amines. In a recent study, Radomski et al.[59] reported the isolation of the glucuronic acid conjugate of *N*-hydroxy-4-aminobiphenyl from dog urine. The available evidence indicated that the urinary conjugate was the *N*-glucuronide rather than the *O*-glucuronide.

A well-documented example of *N*-oxidation of an arylamine as a first activation step is the hepatocarcinogen *N*-methyl-4-aminoazobenzene. Nucleoside derivatives isolated from hydrolysates of hepatic RNA and DNA from rats to which MAB has been administered have been characterized in Miller's laboratory by using the guanosine derivatives prepared by reaction with the synthetic ester *N*-benzoyloxy-MAB.[60-62] The recent chemical synthesis of *N*-hydroxy-MAB by Kadlubar et al.[63] enabled a study of metabolic formation and subsequent esterification to be made. Incubation of MAB with rat-liver microsomes and a NADPH-generating system yielded both 4-aminoazobenzene (AB) and *N*-hydroxy-AB, as illustrated in Figure 3. The microsomal demethylation by the mixed-function oxidase system is a well-established reaction.[64] *N*-oxidation of the primary amine (AB) is consistent with the detection of a conjugate of *N*-acetyl-*N*-hydroxy-AB as an urinary metabolite of AB, MAB, and DAB.[65] In a recent study, Kadlubar et al.[63] demonstrated the formation of *N*-hydroxy-MAB in the microsomal oxidation of MAB by isolating the nitrone (Figure 3) through extraction with an organic solvent. The nitrone decomposes nonenzymically, in an acid-catalyzed reaction, to *N*-hydroxy-MAB. In addition, Kadlubar et al.[63] showed that *N*-hydroxy-MAB is activated in a PAPS-dependent reaction by rat-liver cytosol in a similar manner to *N*-hydroxy-AAF.

3. Reduction of Nitro Compounds

One of the acute toxic effects of aromatic nitro compounds, as well as of the corresponding amines, is a disturbance of hematopoiesis in man and animals. Available experimental evidence, reviewed by Weisburger,[66] points to arylhydroxylamines as the

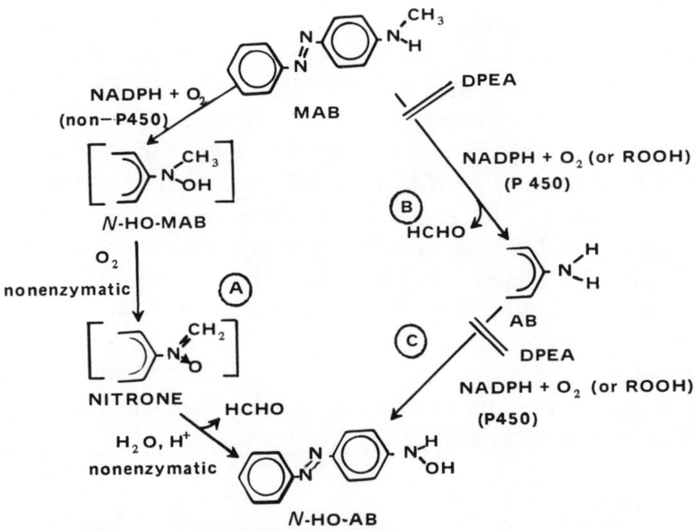

FIGURE 3. The metabolism of *N*-methyl-4-aminoazobenzene (MAB) by rat-liver microsomes by two pathways, both of which yield *N*-hydroxy-4-aminoazobenzene (*N*-HO-AB). (From Miller, J. A. and Miller, E. C., *Screening Tests in Chemical Carcinogenesis*, Montesano, R., Bartsch, H., and Tomatis, L., Eds., IARC Scientific Publications No. 12, International Agency for Research on Cancer, Lyon, France, 1976, 153. With permission).

active intermediate. All known sequential steps in the reduction of aromatic nitro compounds to arylamines via nitroso and hydroxylamine derivatives have also been shown to occur in vivo. The nitro analogs of aromatic amines are also carcinogens, often exhibiting the same organotropic effects as the amines. Moreover, a number of nitro compounds induce tumors of the forestomach upon feeding to rodents, suggesting that reduction to reactive intermediates can occur in the gastric mucosa. The early work on the in vivo reduction of aromatic nitro compounds, reviewed by Williams,[67] suggested that nitro reductase was present only in the soluble fraction of rodent liver. Later work by Gillette et al.[68] and Kato et al.[69] revealed that a sequence of at least two steps is involved. In model systems, rat-liver microsomes reduced p-nitrobenzoic acid to p-hydroxylaminobenzoic acid and also to p-aminobenzoic acid.[69] The time course of the reaction clearly indicated that the N-hydroxy derivative was the intermediate. The reaction was strongly stimulated by addition of flavine mononucleotide and required appreciable amounts of NADPH. In the presence of oxygen the reaction was severely inhibited. Rat-liver cytosol also reduced p-nitrobenzoic acid to the N-hydroxy derivative, but little p-aminobenzoic acid was formed. In contrast to the microsomal reduction, oxygen was not inhibitory in the cytosol reduction. An additional difference was found following pretreatment with phenobarbital or methylcholanthrene. The microsomal NADPH-mediated reduction of both nitro and hydroxylamine derivative was significantly enhanced by such pretreatment, but the reduction effected by the soluble fraction was not influenced. Gillette and Gram[70] provided evidence that cytochrome P-450 is also involved in the reduction of nitro compounds, since carbon monoxide inhibited the reduction with microsomes from mouse, rat, and rabbit. Nitroreductase has been demonstrated by Juchau[71] in human and rodent placental homogenates, and by Adamson et al.[72] in different strains of mice and a variety of other species.

A typical example of activation of a carcinogenic nitro compound through reduction is 4-nitroquinoline-1-oxide (4-NQO). This compound is reduced to 4-hydroxylaminoquinoline-1-oxide, a strong carcinogen for s.c. tissue and for the skin. A summary of chemical, metabolic, and various biological studies with 4-NQO and related compounds has been made by Endo et al.[73]

D. Esterification Reactions of Arylhydroxylamines
1. O-Acetates

Substantial evidence has accumulated during recent years showing that other electrophilic metabolites of N-hydroxy-AAF are also formed by various tissues and must be considered as potential ultimate carcinogenic reactants. The various possibilities have been summarized in the reaction scheme depicted in Figure 2. As outlined in Section II.C.1., N-hydroxy-AF was held responsible for the observed binding of AF residues to nucleic acids in vivo. As shown by King and Phillips,[57] this form of activation of N-hydroxy-AAF is effected by rat-liver cytosol, without the need for cofactors, and involves enzymic deacetylation. Bartsch et al.[74] were the first to show that the actual activation took place by enzymic transfer of the N-acetyl group of N-hydroxy-AAF to the oxygen of the hydroxylamine. This result was further substantiated by King and co-workers[75-76] in a series of studies. The enzymic transacetylation is of particular importance in the activation of N-hydroxyamides for the following reasons: (1) several other carcinogenic arylhydroxylamines are acetylated in a similar manner and (2) transacetylase activity was also detected in other tissues. Considerable activity was found in kidney, stomach, and small intestine, whereas lung and spleen possessed less activity. Blood, brain, and muscle were essentially without activity. Considerable difference was observed between hepatic and mammary transacetylase with respect to their stability, pH-activity curves, and substrate specificity, suggesting the possibility that they are isoenzymes.[74] In a recent study, King et al.[77] showed that human liver, small intestine, and colon also have enzymes capable of activating arylhydroxamic acids by transacetylation. Evidence for two species of arylhydroxamic acid acetyltransferase was presented recently by Olive and King.[78] These authors showed that the small intestine of the Sprague-Dawley rat contained two species of acetyltransferase, which were separable by gel filtration on Sephadex® G-100. These enzymes differed in their relative abilities to utilize N-hydroxy-AAF and N-hydroxy-AABP as substrates. The resulting N-acetoxy-arylamines are highly reactive and may be responsible for the observed binding of AF residues to nucleic acids (Section III). Because of their reactivity, it has not been possible to prepare N-acetoxy-arylamines by direct chemical synthesis.

2. N-Glucuronides

The O-glucuronidation of N-hydroxy arylamides in vitro by UDPGA-supplemented rat-liver microsomes is now well documented and O-glucuronides are found as major metabolites of the N-oxidation pathway and are present in urine. Initially, Irving[27] suggested that these urinary O-glucuronides were sufficiently electrophilic to react directly with cellular constituents of the bladder epithelium and in this way initiate the carcinogenic process. Alternatively, hydrolysis of the glucuronide by bacterial glucuronidase to N-hydroxy arylamide (or amine) could provide precursors for metabolic activation. Kriek[54] showed that arylhydroxylamines have reactivity with guanine in nucleic acids, in particular at low pH values. He suggested that arylnitrenium ions, Ar-N$^+$-H, are formed as reactive intermediates, responsible for the observed binding to guanine in RNA and DNA. Recent studies by Kadlubar et al.[79] showed that UDPGA-supplemented liver microsomes from dogs, rats, and humans metabolized the N-hydroxy derivatives of 2-aminonaphthalene (and presumably also those of 4-aminobiphenyl, 2-aminofluorene, and 4-aminoazobenzene) to the corresponding N-glucuronides. The metabolite from N-hydroxy-2-aminonaphthalene was identified by means of UV, IR, and mass spectral analysis of the glucuronide and its nitrone derivative as N-(β-1-glucosiduronyl)-N-hydroxy-2-aminonaphthalene. The N-glucuronides appeared to be relatively stable at neutral pH, but at pH 5 they rapidly hydrolyzed back to the corresponding hydroxylamines. The latter compounds are subsequently converted to reactive intermediates, probably arylnitrenium ions, capable of reaction with nucleic acids and proteins. Direct evidence for the H$^+$-dependent arylnitrenium ion formation from N-hydroxy-1-amino-naphthalene was presented recently by Kadlubar et al.[80] using solvolysis in (^{18}O)H$_2$O and H$_2$O-ethanol mixtures. Radomski et al.[59] provided additional evidence that the N-glucuronide of N-hydroxy-4-aminobiphenyl is the water-soluble transport form of this carcinogen that delivers the active metabolite to the bladder. The hydrolysis of the glucuronides to N-hydroxy arylamines and the conversion of the latter derivatives to highly reactive arylnitrenium ions in the normally acidic urine of dogs and humans may be important reactions for tumor induction in the urinary bladder.

E. Peroxidase or Free Radical Activation

A route of activation for arylhydroxamic acids, which has received relatively little attention as compared to esterification reactions, is peroxidase or free radical activation. Free radical activation of N-hydroxy-AAF was first studied almost simultaneously by Forrester et al.[81] and by Bartsch et al.[82-84] These authors demonstrated that the chemical or enzymic one-electron oxidation of N-hydroxy-AAF gives a nitroxide free radical which easily dismutates to yield 2-nitrosofluorene and N-acetoxy-AAF (Figure 4). A similar reaction occurred when bovine lactoperoxidase or human myeloperoxidase and H$_2$O$_2$ were used. Other N-hydroxy arylamides behaved in a similar manner. Stier et al.[85] claim that free radical formation from AF or AAF occurs with liver microsomes from phenobarbital-treated rabbits, but the radicals have not been characterized. The original observations[81-84] have been confirmed by Floyd et al.,[86] who also observed that the addition of ascorbate inhibited the activation of *N*-hydroxy-AAF in this system. In a more recent study, Floyd et al.[87] discovered that linoleic acid hydroperoxide, in the presence of hematin or methemoglobin, also activates *N*-hydroxy-AAF with the formation of 2-nitrosofluorene and *N*-acetoxy-AAF. This finding is of interest, because linoleic acid, and also linoleic acid hydroperoxide are lipid components of the microsomal membranes. The recent communication of Yang[88] that the type and amount of dietary fat has a significant effect upon the carcinogenic potency of AAF in rats may be related to radical activation of *N*-hydroxy-AAF. Generally, rats fed a diet high in corn oil, which is relatively unsaturated, were more susceptible to AAF than rats fed a diet high in tallow, which is more highly saturated. It was recently demonstrated by Floyd and Soong[89] that the nitroxyl free radical is an obligatory intermediate in the cumene hydroperoxide-hematin-induced oxidative activation of *N*-hydroxy AAF into 2-nitrosofluorene and *N*-acetoxy-AAF. The theoretically predicted linear relationship between the rate of *N*-hydroxy-AAF oxidation and the square of the free radical concentration was found to be true experimentally. The dismutation rate constant of the nitroxyl free radical was found to be $2.7 \times 10^{-5} M^{-1} \text{sec}^{-1}$.

III. INTERACTION WITH NUCLEIC ACIDS

The covalent binding of a number of carcinogens, including aromatic amines, to DNA in vivo is now well documented. The older available experimental material was

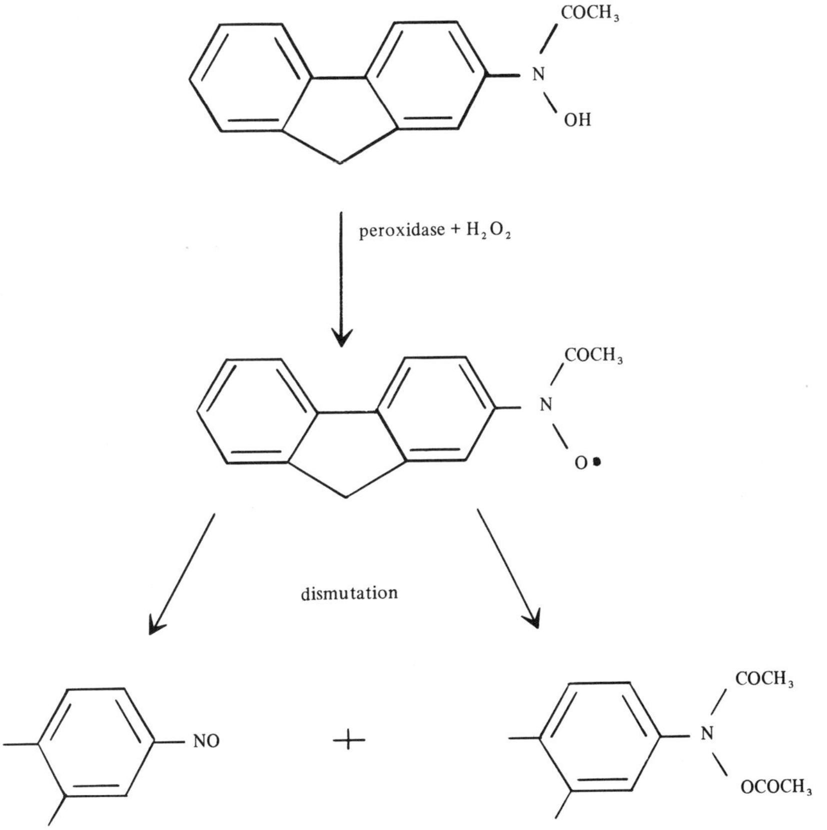

FIGURE 4. The one-electron oxidation of *N*-hydroxy-AAF to a nitroxide free radical and the subsequent dismutation of two nitroxide free radicals to *N*-acetoxy-AAF and 2-nitrosofluorene.

reviewed some years ago by Irving.[90] More recent data on this subject that is relevant to the aromatic amines will be discussed in this section.

Although in the process of carcinogenesis, the role of the binding of chemical carcinogens to DNA in the target organs is not understood in detail, it is difficult to believe that covalently bound carcinogens do not have consequences for the biochemical and biological properties of the DNA molecule, especially during replication or repair. Recent research on the mechanism of action of carcinogens has been directed more towards the role of DNA repair, particularly error-prone repair, in the carcinogenic process. This trend has been paralleled by studies on the interaction of carcinogens with DNA. Identification of the various reaction products in DNA is required for these studies, partly in order to exclude binding artifacts.

A. Sites of Covalent Reaction

1. 2-Acetylaminofluorene

At least three types of binding to DNA in rat liver occur simultaneously following administration of 2-acetylaminofluorene (AAF) or its *N*-hydroxy metabolite.[39,91,92] As has been pointed out in Section II, the actual reactive form responsible for the binding of AAF and of AF groups to DNA is not known at present. Because the reactive metabolites of AAF were among the first available by direct chemical synthesis, three derivatives have been used extensively in model studies on the interaction AAF with nucleic acids and proteins (see References 11 and 38 for recent reviews). Similarly, the reactive esters of *N*-hydroxy-AAF have been used to prepare the nucleoside derivatives employed as marker compounds for identification of the products formed in vivo. Whereas *N*-guanosin-8-yl-AAF was the major bound form present in rRNA and tRNA, 70% of the material bound to DNA was found to be deacetylated. Formation of product B, illustrated in Figure 5, by deacetylation of product A is not likely, because no deacetylase activity could be detected in isolated rat-liver nuclei. Approximately 80% of the AAF residues bound to rat-liver DNA have been identified as *N*-deoxyguanosin-8-yl-AAF (Figure 5A) (Kriek,[91,92] Irving and Veazey[39]). This derivative is removed from DNA in vivo with a biological half-life of 7 days, obviously by a DNA repair mechanism. The remaining fraction of the AAF residues (20%) was identified by Westra et al.[93] as 3-deoxyguanosin-*N*²-yl-AAF. The latter product, detected exclusively in DNA, was found to be persistent.[92] (Figure 5C). A product with similar chemical and chromatographic properties can be isolated from DNA reacted in vitro with *N*-acetoxy-AAF or AAF-*N*-sulfate.[92,93] As was demonstrated by Weinstein and co-workers,[94] substitution at the C^8 position in guanine causes appreciable local distortion of the double-helical structure of DNA. Although there are no physicochemical measurements available on the conformation of 3-deoxyguanosin-*N*²-yl-AAF, Corey-Pauling-Koltun space-filling molecular models constructed by Kriek[12] indicate that AAF bound to the 2 amino group of guanine may fit into the narrow groove of the DNA helix without much distortion. Differences in conformation may form the basis for the observed selectivity in repair of both AAF products (see also Weinstein and Grunberger in Volume II, Chapter 3). It is not clear at present whether the deacetylated moiety in DNA is always in the form of structure B (Figure 5) or if other forms are also present. Deacetylated products in DNA have been studied less extensively than the corresponding *N*-acetyl derivatives, because *N*-(guanin-8-yl)-arylamines are unstable in aqueous solution. This has obstructed the structural identification and quantitative analysis of these derivatives in DNA preparations. Theoretically, the decomposition of *N*-(guanin-8-yl)-arylamine products in DNA may result in the formation of apurinic sites.

As opposed to the binding of AAF to guanine, which is now well documented, the reaction with adenine is less well understood. Earlier studies by Miller et al.[95] had failed to show any reaction with adenine after treatment of DNA with *N*-acetoxy-AAF.

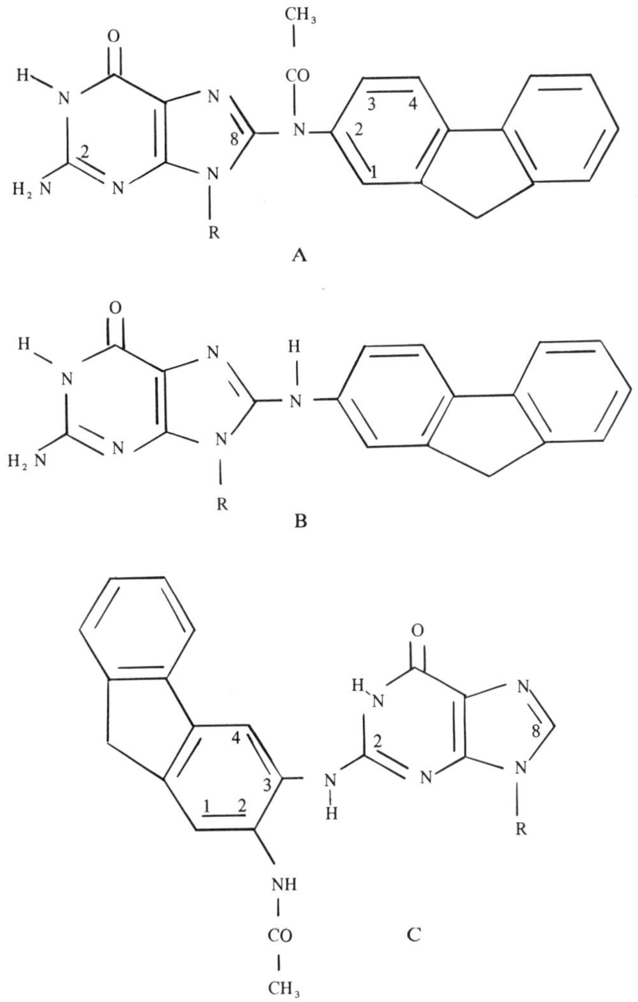

FIGURE 5. Products of nonenzymatic reaction of derivatives of *N*-hydroxy-AAF with deoxyguanosine and DNA. *N*-(deoxyguanosin-8-yl)-AAF (A) and 3-(deoxyguanosin-N²-yl)-AAf (C) are formed upon reaction of DNA with *N*-acetoxy-AAF or AAF-N-sulfate at neutral pH. Both products have been identified in rat-liver DNA in vivo after administration of *N*-hydroxy-AAF.[92,93] *N*-(deoxyguanosin-8-yl)-AF (B) is formed upon alkaline deacetylation of A, or by treatment of DNA with *N*-hydroxy-AF at pH 5. Compound B has not been identified in rat-liver DNA in vivo.

Similar efforts in our laboratory (Kriek, unpublished data) and by Fuchs and Daune[96] did not result in substantial amounts of modified adenine. Although Kapuler and Michelson[97] claim that appreciable amounts of dAMP residues had reacted upon treatment of DNA with *N*-acetoxy-AAF, these results were not substantiated by isolation and identification of the reaction products. It was demonstrated by Kriek and Reitsema[98] that adenine, when present in poly A in a single-stranded helical conformation reacts well with *N*-acetoxy-AAF. However, the significance of this reaction for the in vivo situation is not clear. At present no reaction products of AAF with adenine have been detected in in vivo studies.

No experimental evidence exists for the interaction of AAF and its derivatives with the phosphate groups in DNA. This type of reaction has been described for some alkylating agents[99] (see Volume I, Chapter 1). Although King et al.[100] claim that ary-lhydroxylamines react at pH 5 with the phosphate groups of RNA to form phosphate esters that lead to cleavage of the nucleic acid chain, their results were not substantiated by isolation and identification of reaction products. Moreover, the observed chain fission is not necessarily due to reaction with the phosphate groups. As pointed out above, guaninyl-arylamine reaction products are unstable in aqueous solution and may lead to the formation of apurinic sites. These sites are susceptible to hydrolysis under certain conditions leading to fission of the RNA chain.

Although binding of radioactively labeled AAF to DNA of parenchymal cells in the mammary gland of the rat[101] and to nucleic acids from the gastrointestinal tract[102] has been reported, the reaction products have not been characterized.

2. 4-Acetylaminobiphenyl

There exists a striking difference in organ specificity between the structurally related carcinogens 2-acetylaminofluorene and 4-acetylaminobiphenyl. Whereas the first compound is one of the most potent hepatocarcinogens, AABP has only very weak carcinogenic activity in the liver.[6,7] Although there are quantitative differences, simple correlations between the extent of binding, or the site of reaction, and carcinogenicity do not exist. As was demonstrated by Kriek,[103] the binding of aminobiphenyl residues to rat-liver nucleic acids following a single injection of N-hydroxy-AABP was lower than with the fluorene derivative. The major share of the aminobiphenyl residues bound to DNA were deacetylated, but a structural analysis of these products is not available. On the other hand, N-deoxyguanosin-8-yl-AABP has been identified in rat liver DNA in vivo, but the amount was at least 20 times lower than in the case of N-hydroxy-AAF. Persistently bound 3-deoxyguanosin-N^2-yl-AABP was also detected.[104]

A striking difference in reactivity between the sulfate esters (potassium salts) of N-hydroxy-AAF and N-hydroxy-AABP was detected by Kriek.[105] In reactions with native calf thymus DNA in vitro, both N-deoxyguanosin-8-yl-AABP and 3-deoxyguanosin-N^2-yl-AABP are formed, but the total binding is much lower and the ratio of the products is reversed as compared with the fluorene derivative.

In contrast to the values obtained with N-hydroxy-AAF in male rats, only 12% of the biphenyl residues bound to rRNA was identified as N-guanosin-8-yl-AABP following the injection of N-hydroxy-AABP.[103] This result was in good agreement with the very small amounts of 3-methylmercapto-AABP which could be released from liver proteins of male rats by DeBaun et al.[42] Recently, King et al.[112] showed that, in isolated liver parenchymal cells, N-hydroxy-AABP was bound to RNA mainly in the deacetylated form. The reaction was not influenced by addition of inorganic sulfate. King et al.[106] suggested that the observed binding is due to transacetylation of the hydroxamic acid (see Section II.D.1). These results indicate that other activation routes are required for the carcinogenic activity of AABP or its N-hydroxy derivative in extrahepatic tissues.

3. 4-Acetylamino4'-fluorobiphenyl

Rats ingesting 4-acetylamino-4'-fluorobiphenyl (AABP4'F) develop renal carcinomas in addition to hepatic and mammary gland carcinomas.[107-109] The binding of this compound to rat liver and kidney DNA was studied recently by Driek and Hengeveld[48] following administration of (G-³H)N-hydroxy-AABP4'F. The total binding levels in liver DNA and in kidney DNA were comparable to that observed with N-hydroxy-AAF in rat liver. Both N-deoxyguanosin-8-yl-AABP4'F and 3-deoxyguanosin-N^2-yl-AABP4'F were identified in DNA from liver and kidney, and each comprised approximately 10% of the total. The first product was removed rapidly from DNA in both organs with a biological half-life of 2 days; the other compound was persistent. Again, the major fraction of the material bound to DNA was found to be deacetylated. The interesting observation was made that the deacetylated products were removed in vivo at a much slower rate ($t_{1/2}$ = 10 days) from liver DNA as well as from kidney DNA. This result raises the possibility that arylamine reaction products in DNA are more important for the initiation of the carcinogenic process than the N-guanin-8-yl-arylamide derivatives, because of their low excision rate. The structure of the deacetylated reaction products of AABP4'F in DNA has not yet been characterized.

4. 2-Acetylaminophenanthrene

The interaction of the sulfate ester of N-hydroxy-2-acetylaminophenanthrene with nucleic acid in vitro was studied mainly by Scribner and Naimy.[49,110] These authors reported a remarkable difference in chemical reactivity between the sulfates of N-hydroxy-AAF and of N-hydroxy-AAP. As shown in Table 1, the phenanthryl derivative completely lacks the preference shown by the fluorene compound for substitution in guanine. The nitrogen at the 6 position of adenine had similar susceptibility for reaction with AAP-N-sulfate as the carbon-8 of guanine. The reaction products obtained after reaction of AAP-N-sulfate with DNA, followed by enzymic hydrolysis and Sephadex® LH-20 chromatography, are illustrated in Figure 6. Scribner and Naimy explain their results on the basis of the mechanism of substitution (discussed in Section III.B). To what extent these results reflect the in vivo situation is not known at present.

5. N-Methyl-4-aminoazobenzene

This compound represents one of the best studied examples of the group of carcinogenic azo dyes. Its reaction products with nucleic acids and proteins in vivo have been characterized by Miller and associates. Interaction products with nucleic acids have been elusive for a long time, because suitable, activated derivatives of this dye were not available. The synthetic ester N-benzoyloxy-MAB was used by Lin et al.[111] as a reactive derivative to prepare products of reaction with guanosine and deoxyguanosine (Figure 7). A similar type of substitution to that observed with N-acetoxy-AAF occurred at carbon-8 of guanine. The presence of these products was established by Lin et al.[112] in hydrolysates of RNA and DNA obtained from the livers of rats that had been given MAB. Lin and Fok[113] showed that in an oxidative medium, employing iodine or persulfate as oxidants, MAB becomes covalently bound to DNA or to polynucleotides. In a recent study, Kadlubar et al.[63] showed that N-hydroxy-MAB is activated by rat-liver microsomes, in a similar manner to N-hydroxy-AAF, by formation of the sulfate. When guanosine was used as reactant, N-guanosin-8-yl-MAB was isolated from the reaction mixture.

TABLE 1

Reactions of Esters of N-Arylacetohydroxamic Acids with
Nucleosides

Ester	Adenosine	Guanosine	Thymidine
N-OSO₃K-AAP	5	5	Trace
N-AcO-AAP	0.7	1	0
N-AcO-AAF	1.5	57	0

Note: The figures given is % reaction based on limiting reagent (nucleoside) and is calculated for material with an R_F of $\geq$ 0.90. Trace levels of reaction were found between all esters and cytidine or uridine.

From Scribner, J. D. and Naimy, N. K., *Cancer Res.*, 33, 1159, 1973. With permission.

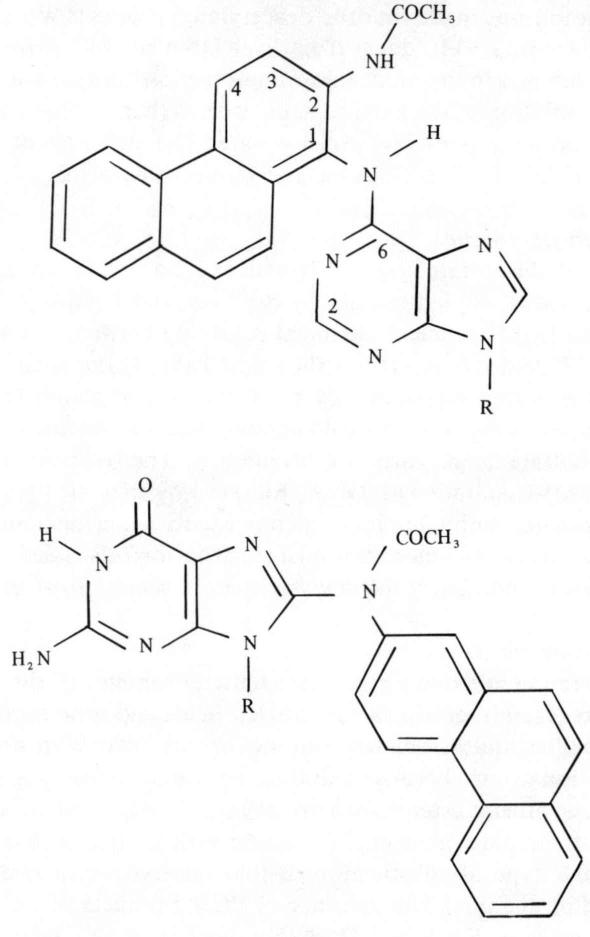

FIGURE 6.   Products of nonenzymatic reaction, at neutral pH, of AAP-*N*-sulfate with DNA.

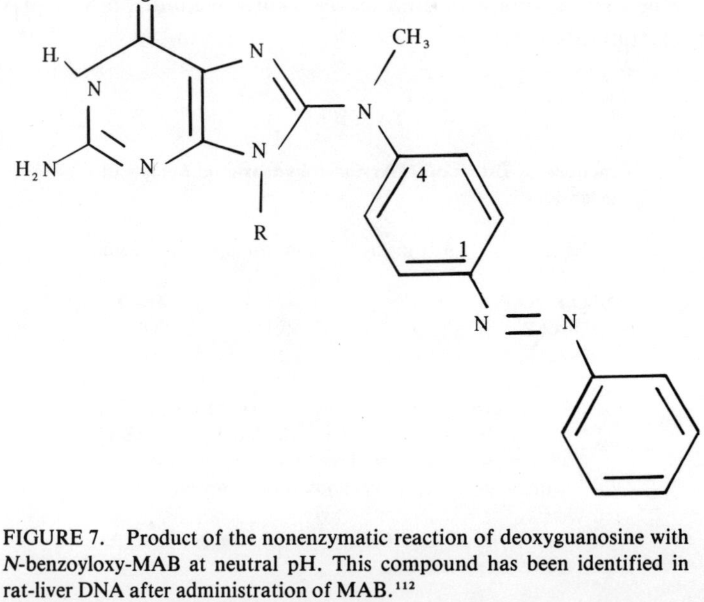

FIGURE 7.   Product of the nonenzymatic reaction of deoxyguanosine with *N*-benzoyloxy-MAB at neutral pH. This compound has been identified in rat-liver DNA after administration of MAB.[112]

Reaction products of azo dyes with nucleic acids in other organs have not been characterized. Persistent carcinogen-DNA adducts have been reported by Warwick and Roberts[114] for DAB in rat liver, but the type of binding was not identified.

6. Other Aromatic Amines and Amides

Relatively few studies have been carried out on the metabolism and reactions of other aromatic amines. The authors are aware of the fact that studies are in progress on a number of aromatic amines that have shown carcinogenic activity. These compounds will be included in this section.

Aminonaphthalenes — As pointed out already in Section II.D.2, the activation of N-hydroxy arylamines under acidic conditions may be a critical reaction in the initiation of bladder carcinogenesis by aromatic amines. Kadlubar et al.[80] report the reaction of (G-^{3}H)N-hydroxy-1-aminonaphthalene with nucleic acids at pH 5 to form bound derivatives. The degree of binding decreased in the order: DNA > poly G > rRNA > tRNA > poly A. Enzymic hydrolysis of DNA-containing aminonaphthalene residues yielded two different products. The major product was identified as an O^6-substituted deoxyguanosine derivative by chemical, UV, IR, NMR, and mass spectral analysis.

2-Aminoanthracene — 2-Aminoanthracene or 2-anthramine is of interest, because it is one of the few aromatic amines which leads to the formation of skin tumors when painted on the skin of rats or hamsters (Shubik et al.[115]). However, no data have been reported on the metabolic activation of 2-aminoanthracene in the skin. N-Hydroxy-2-aminoanthracene has been prepared by Scribner and Miller[116] by ammonium hydrosulfide reduction of 2-nitro-anthracene.

4-Acetylaminostilbene — Synthetic esters of N-hydroxy-4-acetylaminostilbene (N-hydroxy-AAS) react, like the esters of N-hydroxy-AAF, with nucleophiles such as guanosine, methionine, and tryptophan.[95,117] Quantitatively, however, the reactions with these nucleophiles are less extensive than the corresponding reactions with esters of N-hydroxy-AAF. Scribner and Naimy[118] studied the interaction of N-acetoxy-AAS with various nucleosides. Unlike reported in this study, the major reaction occurred at the N^1 nitrogen of cytidine (Figure 8).[138] The major adducts formed with guanosine and with adenosine involved similar reactions on the ethylene bridge of the carcinogen and the N^1 nitrogens. Two minor adducts were O^6 derivatives of guanosine. In addition, evidence was obtained that N-hydroxy-4-aminostilbene reacts with the C^8 of guanosine in dilute acid. The relevance of these substitution products for the in vivo situation is not known at present. Recent evidence obtained by Watabe and Akamatsu[119] indicates that epoxidation of the ethylenic bond of stilbene occurs and this reaction may complicate studies on the in vivo interactions of aminostilbenes.

3- and 4-Acetylaminofluorene — A detailed study on the carcinogenicity of fluorenyl hydroxamic acids and their N-acetoxy derivatives for the rat in relation to the reactivities of the esters towards nucleophiles was carried out by Yost et al.[120] and Zieve et al.[51] Previous studies by Gutmann et al.[121] had shown that the isomeric fluorenyl hydroxamic acids, N-hydroxy-2-AAF, N-hydroxy-3-AAF and N-hydroxy-1-AAF, exhibited differences in the degree of carcinogenicity and in tissue specificity when they were administered by i.p. injection. It was concluded by these authors that the site of substitution of the amino group in the fluorene system was a major factor in determining the carcinogenicity of the isomeric fluorenyl hydroxamic acids. N-Hydroxy-3-AAF appeared to be a specific mammary carcinogen, while N-hydroxy-4-AAF was only marginally carcinogenic when tested by several routes of administration in male and female Sprague-Dawley rats. The order of carcinogenicity of the isomeric esters paralleled that of the N-hydroxy compounds. In order to correlate the carcinogenicity of the N-acetoxy derivatives with their reactivities towards nucleophiles, the esters were reacted with methionine, guanosine, adenosine, and tRNA. The reactivity of N-acetoxy-4-

AAF was only one tenth of that of N-acetoxy-AAF in the reaction with methionine. It gave only minor amounts of adenosine adducts and failed to react with guanosine. N-Acetoxy-3-AAF did not react with either nucleoside or with methionine. The weak electrophilicity of N-acetoxy-4-AAF correlated with its marginal carcinogenicity, but N-hydroxy-3-AAF behaved anomalously in this respect. As has been discussed in Section II.B.3 of this chapter, other activation routes must be involved for 3-AAF or its N-hydroxy derivative.

B. Mechanistic Aspects of the Formation of Covalent Bonds

Almost all of the available data on chemical carcinogens now indicate that they are either electrophilic agents or that they are metabolized into such species. In the case of aromatic amines and amides, this electrophilic character is obtained by N-oxidation followed by one or more of the activation reactions described in Section II. In the case of AAF, correlative studies have shown that the N-sulfate is the major precursor of rRNA- and tRNA-bound AAF residues in rat liver. However, this reaction seems to be restricted to AAF, because other aromatic amides have been shown to be poor substrates for the liver sulfotransferase. In particular, the precursor of the DNA-bound AAF residues is uncertain, because of the extremely short half-life of the sulfate ester formed in the cytoplasm. Other forms of stabilization, for example, through noncovalent bonding to a carrier protein, may be possible, but at present there is no experimental evidence for the existence of a carrier protein of this type.

Similarly, the occurrence of acetyl esters of N-hydroxy amides in vivo has not been described. The mechanism of substitution by carcinogenic N-acetoxy-arylamides was studied in detail by Scribner et al.[117] and by Scribner and Naimy.[49,110] In the presence of nucleophiles less basic than acetate ion, the 2-fluorenyl and 4-stilbenyl N-acetoxy amides showed unimolecular ionization, whereas the corresponding 4-biphenyl and 3-phenanthryl derivatives appeared to form acetate ions by bimolecular displacement. In the presence of the more basic citrate trianion, all four esters showed increased rates of decomposition, and these approached maximal levels with increasing concentrations of the nucleophile. These observations were explained by the authors by postulating the formation of an intermediate ion pair in which the unshared pair of electrons of the nitrogen of the nitrenium ion is in a nonbinding sp^2-orbital and the nitrogen p-orbital is vacant. The extent to which this ion pair reacts further or returns to the ground state would be determined by the stabilization provided by the aromatic system. The relative differences in chemical properties were further interpreted by Scribner and Naimy[110] on the basis of Hückel molecular orbital calculations for the nitrenium ion. As opposed to the biphenyl derivative, a triplet state was postulated for the fluorenyl acetylnitrenium ion as illustrated in Figure 9. Experimental support for the triplet state was obtained from the reactivity of various N-acetoxy-arylacetamides towards the stable free radical 2,2-diphenyl-1-picrylhydrazyl. The fluorenyl derivative is much more reactive than the phenanthryl derivative, whereas the biphenyl and stilbenyl compounds did not react at all with this free radical. However, the rate of loss of the N-acetoxy group did not always correspond to the extent of substitution by methionine or guanosine. Similarly, the rates of decomposition of the N-acetoxy-arylamides did not correspond with the carcinogenic activities of these compounds or of their parent N-hydroxy derivatives. This lack of correlation is not unexpected in view of other important factors which are operative in vivo, such as penetration of the carcinogen into the target cell and the different rates of activation and deactivation occurring within the target cells.

A study of similar nature has been reported recently by Irving[122] on the reactivity of O-glucuronides of N-hydroxy amides towards polynucleotides. In this series, the fluorenyl derivative also appeared to be the most reactive. The relative order of reactivity of these glucuronides with polynucleotides, as measured by the covalent binding of the aryl moiety labeled with ^{3}H or ^{14}C, was glucuronide of N-hydroxy-AAF > glucuronide of N-hydroxy-AAS > glucuronide of N-hydroxy-AABP > glucuronide of N-hydroxy-AAP. This order of reactivity is the same as the relative order of reactivity reported by Scribner et al.[117] for the reaction of N-acetoxy arylamides with methionine and guanosine. As noted previously by Hill and Irving,[29] the reaction of the glucuronide of N-hydroxy-AAF was associated with significant loss of the N-acetyl group due to intramolecular transacetylation. At present, the O-glucuronides and O-sulfates of arylhydroxamic acids are the most likely candidates for the attachment of arylamide moieties to nucleic acids in vivo.

C. Distribution of Covalently Bound Aromatic Amine Residues in DNA

Little information is available on the distribution of covalently bound arylamines and amides in the DNA molecule. The question as to whether there is a preference for attack on DNA at certain localities is difficult to answer at present, but we would like to add a few comments on this subject. The available evidence shows that the reactivity of the ultimate carcinogenic metabolite is an important factor in determining the extent

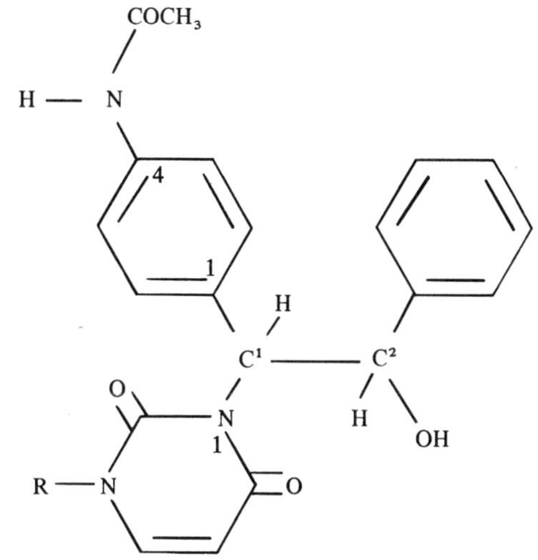

FIGURE 8. Product of the nonenzymatic reaction of N-acetoxy-AAS with cytidine at neutral pH.

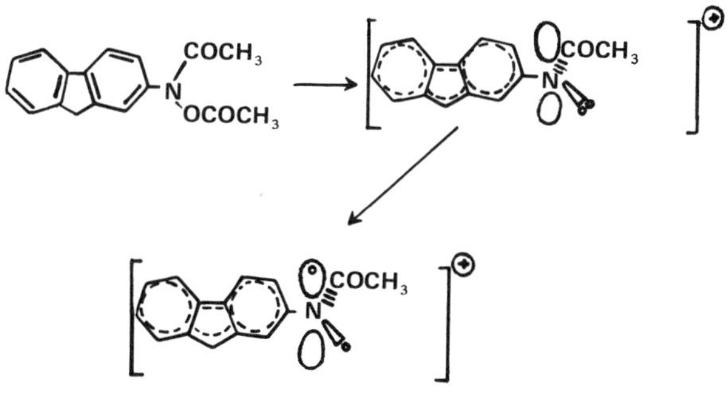

FIGURE 9. Electronic configurations postulated to exist during the ionization of N-acetoxy-AAF in aqueous media. (From Scribner, J. D. and Naimy, N. K., Cancer Res., 33, 1159, 1973. With permission).

and site of interaction, but that the environment of the nucleic acid base under attack is also important. The reaction of *N*-acetoxy-AAF or AAF-*N*-sulfate with deoxyguanosine in aqueous solution of pH 7 leads only to the formation of *N*-deoxyguanosin-8-yl-AAF (Product A in Figure 5), but, with DNA under similar conditions, 3-deoxyguanosin-*N²*-yl-AAF is formed as well. The ratio of the two products is dependent on temperature, pH, and salt concentration.[136] The amount of Product C (Figure 5) that is formed in vivo is higher than in native DNA that has been reacted in vitro with *N*-acetoxy-AAF. In RNA, both in vivo as well as in vitro, Product C was completely absent. Thus, in addition to the fact that the site of substitution in guanine is affected by the secondary structure of the DNA helix, the electrophilic center of the intermediate formed from *N*-acetoxy-AAF is shifted to some extent from the nitrogen to the ortho position. An opposite result might have been expected if only steric effects were involved. Steric effects generally lead to higher reactivity of nucleic acid bases in denatured DNA as compared to the native polymer. In fact, the extent of *N*-deoxyguanosin-8-yl-AAF is increased in denatured DNA, but the other product is not formed. These considerations have led to the general supposition that, in the reaction of DNA with reactive metabolites of aromatic amines and amides, adjacent bases cause a "neighboring group" effect by stacking interactions. Experimental evidence for this effect has been obtained in the case of AAF by Weinstein and associates (see Volume II, Chapter 3).

The identified sites of attack in DNA by aromatic amides have been summarized in Table 2. Although some compounds, particularly the fluorenyl and biphenyl derivatives, exhibit a specificity towards guanine, this effect is not shown by other aromatic amides. In other examples, such as AAS, both adenine and cytosine react equally well. It is to be expected that additional sites of attack will be identified in the near future.

Studies of Weinstein et al.[94] and by Fuchs and Daune[123] have shown that the arylamide substitution at carbon-8 of guanine is associated with appreciable distortion of the nucleotide. The conformation of the latter is changed from *anti* to *syn*. It was demonstrated by the same authors that this type of conformational change in DNA causes appreciable local denaturation of the DNA double helix. As a consequence, attachment of additional carcinogen residues would be expected preferentially in these regions. However, no experimental evidence has been reported to show that this effect really occurs.

The high selectivity of AAF derivatives towards guanine suggests that, in guanine-rich regions of the DNA molecule, a relatively high concentration of this carcinogen can be expected. The experiments of Harvan et al.[124] show that the synthetic polymer poly dG·dC is much more reactive than poly dA·dT. In addition, they found that the

TABLE 2

Identified Sites of Interaction of Aromatic Amines and Amides with Bases of DNA

Carcinogen	A	G	C	Ref.
2-Acetylaminofluorene	—	C^8, NH_2	—	91—93
4-Acetylaminobiphenyl	—	C^8, NH_2	—	103—105
4-Acetylamino-4′-fluorobiphenyl	—	C^8, NH_2	—	48
2-Acetylaminophenanthrene	NH_2	C^8	—	110
4-Acetylaminostilbene	N^1	O^6	NH_1	118
N-Methyl-4-aminoazobenzene	—	C^8	—	111, 112
1-Aminonaphthalene	—	O^6	—	80

Note: Reactions with thymine and at other sites have not been reported.

copolymer poly dGdC·polydCdG was more reactive towards N-acetoxy-AAF than the homopolymer poly dG·poly dC. The authors explained this effect by differences in stacking interaction of the bound fluorene moiety and subsequent differences in sensitivity for further attack. At present there is no evidence that this kind of preferential attack occurs in vivo and other aromatic amines might not show this preference. As shown in Table 1, AAP-N-sulfate reacts equally well with adenine and with guanine.

Some reports have appeared concerning the question as to whether there are different regions in chromatin which have different susceptibilities towards attack by carcinogens. Metzger et al.[125] reacted chromatin of duck erythrocytes with N-acetoxy-AAF in vitro and separated the DNA into staphylococcal nuclease-sensitive and nuclease-insensitive fractions. They observed that N-acetoxy-AAF reacted preferentially at the nuclease sensitive sites of the chromatin. These results are in opposition to those obtained by Ramanathan et al.[126] These authors isolated rat-liver chromatin after i.p. injection of N-hydroxy-AAF and treated the isolated chromatin with pancreatic nuclease. The carcinogen appeared to be attached preferentially to the nuclease insensitive sites. This result is also in opposition to the finding that interaction with alkylating agents took place mainly in the nuclease-sensitive regions. A possible explanation for the results with N-hydroxy-AAF may be based upon the assumption that the action of the nuclease is inhibited in AAF-substituted sites. The observations of Kriek[127] and of Scribner and Naimy[128] that DNA modified by N-acetoxy-AAF is less sensitive to degradation with snake venom phosphodiesterase, point in this direction. Moyer et al.[135] studied the in vivo binding of (9-^{14}C)N-hydroxy-AAF to rat-liver DNA in hetero- and euchromatin fractions. They observed that N-hydroxy-AAF was bound in four- to five-fold greater amounts to euchromatic DNA than to heterochromatic DNA 2 hr after a single injection of the compound. The bound carcinogen appeared to be eliminated more rapidly from euchromatin than from heterochromatin by repair processes. These results indicate that euchromatin DNA is more susceptible to electrophilic attack and subsequent repair processes than heterochromatin. The DNA repair may be associated with the greater transcriptional capacity of euchromatin as compared with heterochromatin. Unfortunately, no differentiation was made by Moyer et al.[135] between the excision rates of the various substitution products of AAF in DNA as described in Section III.A.1 of this chapter. The interaction of carcinogens with various sites of chromatin requires further study.

D. Other Modes of Interaction

In addition to the formation of covalent bonds between aromatic amines and amides and DNA, there are some indications that physical interaction can occur between these carcinogens, or their metabolites, and DNA. This possibility cannot be excluded and this type of interaction may play a role in carcinogenesis. Mutagenicity tests by Ames et al.[129] suggest that the combination of intercalation and covalent binding causes a strong mutagenic effect as, for example, in the case of 2-nitrosofluorene. This compound appeared to be an effective frame-shift mutagen. However, more recent findings do not support the intercalation hypothesis. The mutagenicity exhibited by 2-nitrosofluorene could be caused by the ability of the *Salmonella typhimurium* strain to reduce the compound to N-hydroxy-AF, since nitroreductase has been shown to be present in this group of bacteria by Fukuda and Yamamoto[130] and since Durston and Ames[131] showed that N-hydroxy-AF is a strong mutagen in their test system. These findings are supported by the results of Stout et al.,[132] who demonstrated that, upon incubation of N-hydroxy-AAF with liver cytosol, N-hydroxy-AF is the major mutagenic metabolite formed. An additional difficulty in the interpretation of the results from Durston and Ames[131] is the fact that on incubation of N-hydroxy-AF, the compound is rapidly transformed to 2-nitrosofluorene and 2,2′-azoxyfluorene.

Intercalation in vivo will be difficult to demonstrate experimentally, because the intercalation complexes are not expected to survive the common procedures employed to isolate DNA from the tissues. The available data on intercalation so far have been obtained from studies in vitro. It was demonstrated by Weinstein et al. (see Volume II, Chapter 3) and also by Fuchs et al.[123] that AAF bound to carbon-8 of guanine is intercalated between the adjacent bases in polynucleotides, but this result is an example of intercalation occurring after covalent binding. It is likely that this type of interaction is responsible for the observed frameshift mutations in the *S. typhimurium* test system.

Hong and Piette[133] showed that the physical behavior of spin-labeled aromatic amines towards DNA paralleled that of ethidium bromide, a well-known intercalating agent. By means of electron spin resonance measurements, these authors observed a similar type of interaction for 2-aminofluorene, 2-aminoanthracene and 6-aminochrysene as for ethidium bromide. Data of similar nature on metabolites of these aromatic amines are not available.

In addition to the arylamidating capacity, esters of arylhydroxamic acids can act as acylating agents. Thus, considerable acetylation of guanosine was observed when it was incubated with N-acetoxy-AABP (Miller and Miller,[95] Kriek,[137]). It was shown by Barry and Gutmann[134] that the acetyl group of N-acetoxy-AAF is transferred to the ε-amino group of lysine and, to a lesser extent, to the hydroxyl group of serine and threonine residues in RNAse, in calf thymus histones, and in nuclear proteins in rat liver. N-acetoxy-3-AAF, which did not show any arylamidating reactivity[120] was an even better acetyl donor than the 2 isomer, and RNAse was extensively modified by this compound. The possible effects of the acetylation of nuclear proteins by N-acetoxy-arylamides on the function of these proteins has been discussed by Barry and Gutmann.[134] However, no evidence is available yet for the occurrence of these reactions in vivo.

ACKNOWLEDGMENTS

The authors wish to thank Professor P. Emmelot for valuable suggestions and critical reading of the manuscript. They are indebted to Mr. A. Heerschap (Free University, Amsterdam), who provided a literature survey on chemical carcinogenesis.

The dedicated secretarial assistance of Miss I. H. Haighton in the preparation of the manuscrpt is gratefully acknowledged.

REFERENCES

1. *IARC Monographs on the Evaluation of the Carcinogenic Risk of Chemicals to Man,* Vol. 1 and 8, International Agency for Research on Cancer, Lyon, France, 1972, 1975.

2. **Parkes, H. G.,** The epidemiology of aromatic amine cancers, in *Chemical Carcinogens,* Searle, C. E., Ed., ACS Monograph 173, American Chemical Society, Washington, D.C., 1976, 462.

3. U.S. Government, Department of Labor, Occupational Safety and Health Standards, *Fed. Regist.,* 39, 20, 1974.

4. Health Research Group and Oil, Chemical and Atomic Workers, International Union, petition requesting a zero tolerance for ten carcinogens through an emergency temporary standard issued under authority of the Occupational Safety and Health Act, Washington, D.C., 1973.

5. *IARC Monographs on the Evaluation of the Carcinogenic Risk of Chemicals to Man,* Vol. 16, Some aromatic amines and related nitro compounds, International Agency for Research on Cancer, Lyon, France, 1978.

6. **Clayson, D. B. and Garner, R. C.,** Carcinogenic aromatic amines and related compounds, in *Chemical Carcinogens,* Searle, C. E., Ed., ACS Monograph 173, American Chemical Society, Washington, D.C., 1976, 366.

7. **Arcos, J. C. and Argus, M. F.,** *Chemical Induction of Cancer,* Vol. 2 A-B, Academic Press, New York, 1974.

8. **Clayson, D. B.,** *Chemical Carcinogenesis,* Little, Brown, Boston, 1962.

9. **Miller, E. C. and Miller, J. A.,** The metabolism of chemical carcinogens to reactive electrophiles and their possible mechanisms of action in carcinogenesis, in *Chemical Carcinogens,* Searle, C. E., Ed., ACS Monograph 173, American Chemical Society, Washington, D.C., 1976, 737.

10. **Miller, J. A. and Miller, E. C.,** The metabolic activation of chemical carcinogens — recent results with aromatic amines, safrole and aflatoxin B_1, in *Screening Tests in Chemical Carcinogenesis,* Montesano, R., Bartsch, H., and Tomatis, L., Eds., IARC Scientific Publications No. 12, International Agency for Research on Cancer, Lyon, France, 1976, 153.

11. **Miller, E. C. and Miller, J. A.,** The metabolic activation and reactivity of carcinogenic aromatic amines and amides, in *Proc. 11th Int. Cancer Congress,* Vol. 2, *Chemical and Viral Oncogenesis,* Bucalossi, P., Veronesi, U., and Cascinelli, N., Eds., Excerpta Medica, Amsterdam, 1975, 3.

12. **Kriek, E.,** Carcinogenesis by aromatic amines, *Biochim. Biophys. Acta,* 355, 177, 1974.

13. **Bridges, J. W., Gorrod, J. W., and Parke, D. V.,** *The Biological Oxidation of Nitrogen in Organic Molecules,* Taylor and Francis, London, 1972.

14. **Gorrod, J. W.,** Differentiation of various types of biological oxidation of nitrogen in organic compounds, *Chem. Biol. Interact.,* 7, 289, 1973.

15. **Cramer, J. W., Miller, J. A., and Miller, E. D.,** N-hydroxylation: a new metabolic reaction observed in the rat with the carcinogen 2-acetylaminofluorene, *J. Biol. Chem.,* 235, 885, 1960.

16. **Irving, C. C.,** N-hydroxylation of the carcinogen 2-acetylaminofluorene by rabbit liver microsomes, *Biochim. Biophys. Acta,* 65, 564, 1962.

17. **Uehleke, H.,** The role of cytochrome P-450 in the N-oxidation of individual amines, in *Microsomes and Drug Oxidations,* Estabrook, R. W., Gillette, J. R., and Leibman, K. C., Eds., Williams and Wilkins, Baltimore, 1973, 299.

18. **Kiese, M.,** The biochemical production of ferrihemoglobin-forming derivatives from aromatic amines, and mechanisms of ferrihemoglobin formation, *Pharmacol. Rev.,* 18, 1091, 1966.

19. **Enomoto, M. and Sato, K.,** N-Hydroxylation of the carcinogen 2-acetylaminofluorene by human liver tissue *in vitro, Life Sci.,* 6, 881, 1967.

20. **Miller, E. C., Miller, J. A., and Enomoto, M.,** The comparative carcinogenicities of 2-acetylaminofluorene and its N-hydroxy metabolite in mice, hamsters and guinea pigs, *Cancer Res.,* 24, 2018, 1964.

21. **Kiese, M., Reuner, G., and Wiedermann, I.,** N-hydroxylation of 2-aminofluorene in the guinea pig and by guinea pig liver microsomes *in vitro, Naunyn Schmiedebergs Arch. Pharmakol. Exp. Pathol.* 252, 418, 1966.

22. **Appel, W., Graffe, W., Kampffmeyer, H., and Kiese, M.,** Species differences in the hydroxylation of aniline and N-ethylaniline by liver microsomes, *Naunyn Schmiedebergs Arch. Pharmakol. Exp. Pathol.,* 251, 88, 1965.

23. **Irving, C. C.,** Enzymatic deacetylation of N-hydroxy-2-acetylaminofluorene by liver microsomes, *Cancer Res.,* 26, 1390, 1966.

24. **Miller, J. A., Wyatt, C. S., Miller, E. C., and Hartmann, H. A.,** The N-hydroxylation of 4-acetamidobiphenyl by the rat and dog and the strong carcinogenicity of N-hydroxy-4-acetylaminobiphenyl in the rat, *Cancer Res.,* 21, 1465, 1961.

25. **Andersen, R. A., Enomoto, M., Miller, E. C., and Miller, J. A.,** Carcinogenesis and inhibition of the Walker 256 tumor in the rat by trans-4-acetylaminostilbene, its N-hydroxy metabolite, and related compounds, *Cancer Res.,* 24, 128, 1964.

26. Miller, E. C., Lotlikar, P. D., Pitot, H. C., Fletcher, T. L., and Miller, J. A., N-hydroxy metabolites of acetylaminophenanthrene and 7-fluoro-2-acetylaminofluorene as proximate carcinogens in the rat, *Cancer Res.*, 26, 2239, 1966.

27. Irving, C. C., Conjugates of N-hydroxy compounds, in *Metabolic Conjugation and Metabolic Hydroylsis*, Vol. 1, Fishman, W. H., Ed., Academic Press, New York, 1970, 53.

28. Weisburger, J. H., Grantham, P. H., and Weisburger, E. K., The metabolism of N-2-fluorenylacetamide in the cat. Evidence for glucuronic acid conjugates, *Biochem. Pharmacol.*, 13, 469, 1964.

29. Hill, J. T. and Irving, C. C., Biosynthesis and studies of the alkaline sensitivity of the NO-glucuronide of the carcinogen N-2-fluorenyl acetohydroxamic acid, *Biochemistry*, 6, 3816, 1967.

30. Hill, J. T., Biosynthesis and Studies of the Alkaline Sensitivity of the Glucuronide of the Carcinogen N-2-Fluorenylacethydroxamic Acid, Ph. D. thesis, University of Tennessee, Memphis, 1968.

31. Cardona, R. A. and King, C. M., Activation of the O-glucuronide of the carcinogen N-hydroxy-2-fluorenylacetamide by enzymatic deacetylation *in vitro*: formation of fluorenylamine-tRNA adducts, *Biochem. Pharmacol.*, 25, 1051, 1976.

32. Irving, C. C. and Russell L. T., Synthesis of the O-glucuronide of N-2-fluorenylhydroxylamine. Reaction with nucleic acids and with guanosine 5′-monophosphate, *Biochemistry*, 9, 2471, 1969.

33. Miller, E. C., Smith, J. Y., and Miller, J. A., Lack of correlation between the formation of the glucuronide of N-hydroxy-2-acetylaminofluorene and susceptibility to hepatic carcinogenesis, *Proc. Am. Assoc. Cancer Res.*, 11, 56, 1970.

34. Williams, J. R., Jr., Grantham, P. H., Marsh, H. H., III, Weisburger, J. H., and Weisburger, E. K., The participation of liver fractions and of intestinal bacteria in the metabolism of N-hydroxy-2-fluorenylacetamide in the rat, *Biochem. Pharmacol.*, 19, 173, 1970.

35. Malejka-Giganti, D., Gutmann, H., and Rydell, R.. E., Mammary carcinogenesis in the rat by topical application of fluorenylhydroxamic acids, *Cancer Res.*, 33, 2489, 1973.

36. Parke, D. V., *The Biochemistry of Foreign Compounds*, Macmillan (Pergamon), New York, 1968.

37. Lotlikar, P. D. and Luha, L., Acetylation of the carcinogen N-hydroxy-2-acetylaminofluorene by acetyl coenzyme A to form a reactive ester, *Mol. Pharmacol.*, 7, 381, 1971.

38. Miller, J. A., Carcinogenesis by chemicals — an overview, *Cancer Res.*, 30, 559, 1970.

39. Irving, C. C. and Veazey, R. R., Persistent binding of 2-acetylaminofluorene to rat liver DNA *in vivo* and consideration of the mechanism of binding of N-hydroxy-2-acetylaminofluorene to rat liver nucleic acids, *Cancer Res.*, 29, 1799, 1969.

40. Miller, E. C., Lotlikar, P. D., Miller, J. A., Butler, B. W., Irving, C. C., and Hill, J. T., Reactions *in vitro* of some tissue nucleophiles with the glucuronide of the carcinogen N-hydroxy-2-acetylaminofluorene, *Mol. Pharmacol.*, 4, 147, 1968.

41. Maher, V. M., Miller, J. A., Miller, E. C., and Szybalski, W., Mutations and decreases in density of transforming DNA produced by derivatives of the carcinogens 2-acetylaminofluorene and N-methyl-4-aminoazobenzene, *Mol. Pharmacol.*, 4, 411, 1968.

42. DeBaun, J. R., Rowly, J. Y., Miller, E. C., and Miller, J. A., Sulfotransferase activation of N-hydroxy-2-acetylaminofluorene in rodent livers susceptible and resistant to this carcinogen, *Proc. Soc. Exp. Biol. Med.*, 129, 268, 1968.

43. King, C. M. and Phillips, B., Enzyme-catalyzed reactions of the carcinogen N-hydroxy-2-fluorenylacetamide with nucleic acid, *Science*, 159, 1351, 1968.

44. DeBaun, J. R., Miller, E. C., and Miller, J. A., N-hydroxy-2-acetylaminofluorene sulfotransferase: its probable role in carcinogenesis and in protein-(methion-S-yl) binding in rat liver, *Cancer Res.*, 30, 577, 1970.

45. Weisburger, J. H., Yamamoto, R. S., Williams, G. M., Grantham, P. H., Matsushima, T., and Weisburger, E. K., On the sulfate ester of N-hydroxy-N-2-fluorenylacetamide as a key ultimate hepatocarcinogen in the rat, *Cancer Res.*, 32, 491, 1972.

46. Büch, H., Rummel, W., Pfleger, K., Eschrich, C., and Texter, N., Ausscheidung freien und konjugierten Sulfates bei Ratte und Menschen nach Verabreichung von N-acetyl-p-aminophenol, *Naunyn Schmiedebergs Arch. Pharmakol. Exp. Pathol.*, 259, 276, 1968.

47. Irving, C. C., Janss, D. H., and Russell, L. T., Lack of N-hydroxy-2-acetylaminofluorene sulfotransferase activity in the mammary gland and Zymbal's gland of the rat, *Cancer Res.*, 31, 387, 1971.

48. Kriek, E. and Hengeveld, G. M., Reaction products of the carcinogen N-hydroxy-4-acetylamino-4′-fluorobiphenyl with DNA in liver and kidney of the rat, *Chem. Biol. Interact.*, 21, 179, 1978.

49. Scribner, J. D. and Naimy, N. K., Reaction of esters of N-hydroxy-2-acetamideophenanthrene with cellular nucleophiles and the formation of free radicals upon decomposition of N-acetoxy-N-arylacetamides, *Cancer Res.*, 33, 1159, 1973.

50. Bartsch, H., Dworkin, M., Miller, J. A., and Miller, E. C., Electrophilic N-acetoxyaminoarenes derived from carcinogenic N-hydroxy-N-acetylaminoarenes by enzymatic deacetylation and transacetylation, *Biochim. Biophys. Acta*, 286, 272, 1972.

51. Zieve, F. J. and Gutmann, H. R., Reactivities of the carcinogens N-hydroxy-2-fluorenylacetamide and N-hydroxy-3-fluorenylacetamide with tissue nucleophiles, *Cancer Res.*, 31, 471, 1971.

52. **Tada, M. and Tada, M.,** Enzymatic activation of the carcinogen 4-hydroxyaminoquinoline-1-oxide and its interaction with cellular macromolecules, *Biochem. Biophys. Res. Commun.,* 46, 1025, 1972.

53. **Grantham, P. H., Weisburger, E. K., and Weisburger, J. H.,** Dehydroxylation and deacetylation of N-hydroxy-N-2-fluorenylacetamide by rat liver and brain homogenates, *Biochim. Biophys. Acta,* 107, 414, 1965.

54. **Kriek, E.,** On the interaction of N-2-fluorenylhydroxylamine with nucleic acids *in vitro, Biochem. Biophys. Res. Commun.,* 20, 793, 1965.

55. **King, C. M. and Phillips, B.,** N-hydroxy-2-fluorenylacetamide. Reaction of the carcinogen with guanosine, ribonucleic acid, deoxyribonucleic acid and protein following enzymatic deacetylation or esterification, *J. Biol. Chem.,* 244, 6209. 1969.

56. **Radomsky, J. L. and Brill, E.,** Bladder cancer induction by aromatic amines: role of N-hydroxy metabolites, *Science,* 167, 992, 1970.

57. **Radomsky, J. L. and Brill, E.,** The role of N-oxidation products of aromatic amines in the induction of bladder cancer in the dog, *Arch. Toxicol.,* 28, 159, 1971.

58. **Radomsky, J. L., Rey, A. A., and Brill, E.,** Evidence for a glucuronic acid conjugate of N-hydroxy-4-aminobiphenyl in the urine of dogs given 4-aminobiphenyl, *Cancer Res.,* 33, 1284, 1973.

59. **Radomsky, J. L., Hearn, W. L., Radomski, T., Moreno, H., and Scott, W. E.,** Isolation of the glucuronic acid conjugate of N-hydroxy-4-aminobiphenyl from dog urine and its mutagenic activity, *Cancer Res.,* 37, 1757, 1977.

60. **Poirier, L. A., Miller, J. A., Miller, E. C., and Sato, K.,** N-benzoyloxy-N-methyl-4-aminoazobenzene: its carcinogenic activity in the rat and its reactions with proteins and nucleic acids and their constituents *in vitro, Cancer Res.,* 27, 1600, 1967.

61. **Lin, J.-K., Schmall, B., Sharpe, I. D., Miura, I., Miller, J. A., and Miller, E. C.,** N-substitution of carbon 8 in guanosine and deoxyguanosine by the carcinogen N-benzoyloxy-N-methyl-4-aminoazobenzene, *Cancer Res.,* 35, 832, 1975.

62. **Lin, J.-K., Miller, J. A., and Miller, E. C.,** Structures of hepatic nucleic acid-bound dyes in rats given the carcinogen N-methyl-4-aminoazobenzene, *Cancer Res.,* 35, 844, 1975.

63. **Kadlubar, F. F., Miller, J. A., and Miller, E. C.,** Hepatic metabolism of N-hydroxy-N-methyl-4-aminoazobenzene and othe N-hydroxy-arylamines to reactive sulfuric acid esters, *Cancer Res.,* 36, 2350, 1976.

64. **Mueller, G. C. and Miller, J. A.,** The metabolism of methylated aminoazo dyes. II. Oxidative demethylation by rat liver homogenates, *J. Biol. Chem.,* 202, 579, 1953.

65. **Sato, K., Poirier, L. A., Miller, J. A., and Miller, E. C.,** Studies on the N-hydroxylation and carcinogenicity of 4-aminoazobenzene and related compounds, *Cancer Res.,* 26, 1678, 1966.

66. **Weisburger, H. J. and Weisburger, E. K.,** N-oxidation enzymes, in *Handbook of Experimental Pharmacology,* Part 2, Brodie, B. B. and Gillette, J. R., Eds., Springer-Verlag, New York, 1971, 312.

67. **Williams, R. T.,** *Detoxication Mechanisms,* Wiley and Sons, New York, 1959, 428.

68. **Gillette, J. R., Kamm, J. J., and Sasame, H. A.,** Mechanisms of p-nitrobenzoate reduction in liver; the possible role of cytochrome P-450 in liver microsomes, *Mol. Pharmacol.,* 4, 541, 1968.

69. **Kato, R., Oshima, T., and Takanaka, A.,** Studies on the mechanism of nitro reduction by rat liver, *Mol. Pharmacol.,* 5, 487, 1969.

70. **Gillette, J. R. and Gram, T. E.,** Cytochrome P-450 reduction in liver microsomes and its relationship to drug metabolism, in *Microsomes and Drug Oxidations,* Academic Press, New York, 1969, 133.

71. **Juchau, M. R.,** Studies on the reduction of aromatic nitro groups in human and rodent placental homogenates, *J. Pharmacol. Exp. Ther.,* 165, 1, 1969.

72. **Adamson, R. H., Dixon, R. L., Francis, F. L., and Rall, D. P.,** Comparative biochemistry of drug metabolism by azo and nitro reductase, *Proc. Natl. Acad. Sci. U.S.A.,* 54, 1386, 1965.

73. **Endo, H., Ono, T., and Sugimura, T.,** Chemistry and biological actions of 4-nitroquinoline-1-oxide, *Recent Results Cancer Res.,* 34, 1, 1971.

74. **Bartsch, H., Dworkin, D., Miller, E. C., and Miller, J. A.,** Formation of electrophilic N-acetoxyarylamines in cytosols from rat mammary gland and other tissues by transacetylation from the carcinogen N-hydroxy-4-acetylaminobiphenyl, *Biochim. Biophys. Acta,* 304, 42, 1973.

75. **King, C. M.,** Mechanism of reaction, tissue distribution and inhibition of arylhydroxamic acid acryltransferase, *Cancer Res.,* 34, 1503, 1974.

76. **King, C. M. and Olive, C. W.,** Comparative effects of strain, species and sex on the acyltransferase and sulfotransferase-catalyzed activations of N-hydroxy-N-2-fluorenylacetamide, *Cancer Res.,* 35, 906, 1975.

77. **King, C. M., Olive, C. W., and Cardona, R. A.,** Activation of carcinogenic arylhydroxamic acids by human tissues, *J. Natl. Cancer Inst.,* 55, 285, 1975.

78. **Olive, C. W. and King, C. M.,** Evidence for a second arylhydroxamic acid acyltransferase species in the small intestine of the rat, *Chem. Biol. Interact.,* 11, 599, 1976.

79. **Kadlubar, F. F., Miller, J. A., and Miller, E. C.,** Hepatic microsomal N-glucuronidation and nucleic acid binding of N-hydroxy arylamines in relation to urinary bladder carcinogenesis, *Cancer Res.,* 37, 805, 1977.

80. **Kadlubar, F. F., Miller, J. A., and Miller, E. C.,** Reactivity of the carcinogen *N*-hydroxy-1-naphthylamine with nucleic acids, *Proc. Am. Assoc. Cancer Res.,* 18, 115, 1977.
81. **Forrester, A. M., Ogilvy, M. M., and Thompson, R. H.,** Mode of actions of carcinogenic amines. I. Oxidation of *N*-arylhydroxamic acids, *J. Chem. Soc.,* 1081, 1970.
82. **Bartsch, H., Traut, M., and Hecker, E.,** On the metabolic activation of *N*-hydroxy-*N*-2-acetylaminofluorene. II. Simultaneous formation of 2-nitrosofluorene and *N*-acetoxy-*N*-2-acetylaminofluorene from *N*-hydroxy-*N*-2-acetylaminofluorene via a free radical intermediate, *Biochim. Biophys. Acta,* 237, 556, 1971.
83. **Bartsch, H. and Hecker, E.,** On the metabolic activation of the carcinogen *N*-hydroxy-*N*-2-acetylaminofluorene. III. Oxidation with horse-radish peroxidase to yield 2-nitrosofluorene and *N'*-acetoxy-*N*-2-acetylaminofluorene, *Biochim. Biophys. Acta,* 237, 567, 1971.
84. **Bartsch, H., Miller, J. A., and Miller, E. C.,** *N*-acetoxy-*N*-acetylaminoarenes and nitrosoarenes. One-electron non-enzymatic and enzymatic products of various carcinogenic aromatic acethydroxamic acids, *Biochim Biophys. Acta,* 273, 40, 1972.
85. **Stier, A., Reitz, I., and Sackmann, E.,** Radical accumulation in liver microsomal membranes during biotransformation of aromatic amines and nitro compounds, *Naunyn Schmiedebergs Arch. Exp. Pathol. Pharmakol.,* 274, 189, 1972.
86. **Floyd, R. A., Soong, L. M., and Calver, P. L.,** Horse radish peroxidase/hydrogen peroxide-catalyzed oxidation of the carcinogen *N*-hydroxy-*N*-acetyl-2-aminofluorene as effected by cyanide and ascorbate, *Cancer Res.,* 36, 1510, 1976.
87. **Floyd, R. A., Soong, L. M., Walker, R. N., and Stuart, M.,** Lipid hydroperoxide activation of *N*-hydroxy-*N*-acetylaminofluorene via a free radical route, *Cancer Res.,* 36, 2761, 1976.
88. **Yang, S. P.,** Dietary fat affects tumor growth in rats, quoted in *Chem. Eng. News,* Sept. 5, 1977, 22.
89. **Floyd, R. A. and Soong, L. M.,** Obligatory free radical intermediate in the oxidative activation of the carcinogen *N*-hydroxy-2-acetylaminofluorene, *Biochim. Biophys. Acta,* 498, 244, 1977.
90. **Irving, C. C.,** Interaction of chemical carcinogens with DNA, in *Methods in Cancer Research,* Vol. 7, Busch, H., Ed., Academic Press, New York, 1973, chap. 5.
91. **Kriek, E.,** On the mechanism of action of carcinogenic aromatic amines. I. Binding of 2-acetylaminofluorene and *N*-hydroxy-2-acetylaminofluorene to rat-liver nucleic acids in vivo. *Chem. Biol. Interact.,* 1, 3, 1969.
92. **Kriek, E.,** Persistent binding of a new reaction product of the carcinogen *N*-hydroxy-*N*-2-acetylaminofluorene with guanine in rat liver DNA *in vivo, Cancer Res.,* 32, 2042, 1972.
93. **Westra, J. G., Kriek, E., and Hittenhausen, H.,** Identification of the persistently bound form of the carcinogen *N*-acetyl-2-aminofluorene to rat liver DNA *in vivo, Chem. Biol. Interact.,* 15 149, 1976.
94. **Weinstein, I. B. and Grunberger, D.,** Structural and functional changes in nucleic acids modified by chemical carcinogens, in *Chemical Carcinogenesis,* Ts'o, P. and DiPaolo, J., Eds., Marcel Dekker, New York, 1974, 217.
95. **Miller, J. A. and Miller, E. C.,** The metabolic activation of carcinogenic aromatic amides and amines, in *Prog. in Exp. Tumor Res.,* 11, 273, 1969.
96. **Fuchs, R. and Daune, M.,** Physical studies on deoxyribonucleic acid after covalent binding of a carcinogen, *Biochemistry,* 11, 2659, 1972.
97. **Kapuler, A. M. and Michelson, A. M.,** The reaction of the carcinogen *N*-acetoxy-2-acetylaminofluorene with DNA and other polynucleotides and its stereochemical implications, *Biochim. Biophys. Acta,* 232, 436, 1971.
98. **Kriek, E. and Reitsema, J.,** Interaction of the carcinogen *N*-acetoxy-2-acetylaminofluorene with polyadenylic acid: dependence of reactivity on conformation, *Chem. Biol. Interact.,* 3, 397, 1971.
99. **Swenson, D. H., Farmer, P. B., and Lawley, P. D.,** Identification of the methylphosphotriester of thymidylyl 3′-5′ thymidine as a product from reaction of DNA with the carcinogen MNU, *Chem. Biol. Interact.,* 15, 91, 1976.
100. **King, C. M., Shayman, M. A., and Thissen, M. R.,** Reaction of arylhydroxylamines and phosphate of RNA; cleavage of the nucleic acid chain, *Proc. Am. Assoc. Cancer Res.,* 16, 475, 1975.
101. **Janss, D. H. and Irving, C. C.,** Radioactivity in rat mammary gland after the administration of 2-acetylaminofluorene-9-¹⁴C and its *N*-hydroxy metabolite, *J. Natl. Cancer Inst.,* 49, 765, 1972.
102. **King, C. M. and Shayman, M. A.,** Reaction *in vivo* of *N*-hydroxy-2-fluorenylacetamide with RNA and DNA of gastrointestinal tract and liver of the rat, *Proc. Am. Assoc. Cancer Res.,* 15, 166, 1974.
103. **Kriek, E.,** On the mechanism of action of carcinogenic aromatic amines. II. Binding of *N*-hydroxy-*N*-acetyl-4-aminobiphenyl to rat liver nucleic acids *in vivo, Chem. Biol. Interact.,* 3, 19, 1971.
104. **Westra, J. G.,** Mechanism of action of aromatic amines, in Abstracts 11th Int. Cancer Congress, Vol. 2, Casa Editrice Ambrosiana, Milano, 1974, 38.
105. **Kriek, E.,** Binding of aromatic amines to DNA and RNA, in *Proc. 11th Int. Cancer Congress, Vol. 2, Chemical and Viral Oncogenesis,* Bucalossi, P., Veronesi, U., and Cascinelli, N., Eds., Excerpta Medica, Amsterdam, 1975, 36.

106. King, C. M., Traub, N. R., Cardona, R. A., and Howard, R. B., Comparative adduct formation of 4-aminobiphenyl and 2-aminofluorene derivatives with macromolecules in isolated liver parenchymal cells, *Cancer Res.*, 36, 2374, 1976.

107. Stromberg, K. and Reuber, M. D., Influence of age and sex on hepatic lesions induced by chemical carcinogens: ingestion of N-4-(4'-fluorobiphenyl) acetamide by Buffalo strain rats, *J. Natl. Cancer Inst.*, 44, 1047, 1970.

108. Reuber, M. D., Hyperplastic and neoplastic lesions of the kidney in Buffalo rats of varying ages ingesting N-4-(4'-fluorobiphenyl)acetamide, *J. Natl. Cancer Inst.*, 54, 427, 1975.

109. Stromberg, K. and Reuber, M. D., Histopathology of breast lesions induced in BUF rats of varying ages by ingestion of N-4-(4'-fluorobiphenyl)acetamide, *J. Natl. Cancer Inst.*, 54, 1223, 1975.

110. Scribner, J. D. and Naimy, N. K., Adducts between the carcinogen 2-acetamidophenanthrene and adenine and guanine of DNA, *Cancer Res.*, 35, 1416, 1975.

111. Lin, J. K., Schmall, B., Sharpe, I. D., Miura, I., and Miller, J. A., N-substitution of the carbon-8 in guanosine and deoxyguanosine by the carbinogen N-benzoyloxy-N-methyl-4-aminoazobenzene *in vitro*, *Cancer Res.*, 35, 832, 1975.

112. Lin, J. K., Miller, J. A., and Miller, E. C., Structures of hepatic nucleic acid-bound dyes in rats given the carcinogen N-methyl-4-aminoazobenzene, *Cancer Res.*, 35, 844, 1975.

113. Lin, J. K. and Fok, K. F., Chemically induced binding of the hepatocarcinogen N-monomethyl-4-aminoazobenzene to nucleic acids *in vitro*, *Cancer Res.*, 33, 529, 1973.

114. Warwick, G. P. and Roberts, J. J., Persistent binding of butter yellow metabolites to rat liver DNA, *Nature*, 213, 1206, 1967.

115. Shubik, P., Pietra, G., and Della Porta, G., Studies of skin carcinogenesis in the Syrian golden hamster, *Cancer Res.*, 20, 100, 1960.

116. Scribner, J. D. and Miller, J. A., Synthesis of 2-nitroanthracene and N-hydroxy-2-anthrylamine, *J. Chem. Soc.*, p. 5377, 1965.

117. Scribner, J. D., Miller, J. A., and Miller, E. C., Nucleophilic substitution on carcinogenic N-acetoxy-N-arylacetamides, *Cancer Res.*, 30, 1570, 1970.

118. Scribner, J. D. and Naimy, N. K., Reactions of the carcinogens N-acetoxy-4-acetamidostilbene and N-hydroxy-4-aminostilbene, *Proc. Am. Assoc. Cancer Res.*, 18, 521, 1977.

119. Watabe, T. and Akamatsu, K., Accumulation of an epoxy intermediate during the hepatic microsomal metabolism of *cis*-stilbene to *threo*-stilbene glycol due to the inhibition of epoxide hydrase by *trans*-stilbenimine, *Biochem. Pharmacol.*, 23, 1845, 1974.

120. Yost, Y., Gutmann, H. R., and Rydell, R. E., The carcinogenicity of fluorenylhydroxamic acids and N-acetoxy-N-fluorenylacetamides for the rat as related to the reactivity of the esters toward nucleophiles, *Cancer Res.*, 35, 447, 1975.

121. Gutmann, H. R., Leaf, D. S., Yost, Y., Rydell, R. E., and Chen, S. C., Structure-activity relationships of N-acylarylhydroxylamines in the rat, *Cancer Res.*, 30, 1485, 1970.

122. Irving, C. C., Influence of the aryl group on the reaction of glucuronides of N-arylacethydroxamic acids with polynucleotides, *Cancer Res.*, 37, 524, 1977.

123. Fuchs, R. R. P., Levèvre, J. F., Pouyet, J., and Daune, M. P., Comparative orientation of the fluorene residue in native DNA modified by N-acetoxy-N-2-acetylaminofluorene and two 7-halogeno derivatives, *Biochemistry*, 15, 3347, 1976.

124. Harvan, D. J., Has, J. R., and Lieberman, M. W., Adduct formation between the carcinogen N-acetoxy-2-acetylaminofluorene and synthetic polydeoxyribonucleotides, *Chem. Biol. Interact.*, 17, 203, 1977.

125. Metzger, G., Wilhelm, F. X., and Wilhelm, M. L., Distribution along DNA of the bound carcinogen N-acetoxy-N-2-acetylaminofluorene in chromatime modified *in vitro*, *Chem. Biol. Interact.*, 15, 257, 1976.

126. Ramanathan, R., Rajalakshmi, S., and Sarma, D. S. R., Non random nature of ³H-N-hydroxy-2-acetylaminofluorene and its subsequent removal from rat liver chromatin DNA, *Chem. Biol. Interact.*, 14, 375, 1976.

127. Kriek, E., Difference in binding of 2-acetylaminofluorene to rat liver deoxyribonucleic acid and ribosomal ribonucleic acid in vivo, *Biochim. Biophys. Acta*, 161, 273, 1968.

128. Scribner, J. D. and Naimy, N. K., Inhibition of DNA degradation by bound 2-acetamidofluorene, *Proc. Am. Assoc. Cancer Res.*, 16, 258, 1975.

129. Ames, B. N., Gurney, E. G., Miller, J. A., and Bartsch, H., Carcinogens as frameshift mutagens: metabolites and derivatives of 2-acetylaminofluorene and other aromatic amine carcinogens, *Proc. Natl. Acad. Sci. U.S.A.*, 19, 3128, 1972.

130. Fukuda, S. and Yamamoto, N., Detection of activating enzymes for 4-nitroquinoline-1-oxide activation with a microbial assay system, *Cancer Res.*, 32, 435, 1972.

131. Durston, W. and Ames, B., A simple method for the detection of mutagens in urine: studies with the carcinogen 2-acetylaminofluorene, *Proc. Natl. Acad. Sci. U.S.A.*, 71, 737, 1974.

132. **Stout, D. L., Baptist, J. N., Matney, Th. S., and Shaw, C. R.,** N-hydroxy-2-aminofluorene: the principal mutagen produced from N-hydroxy-2-acetylaminofluorene by a mammalian supernatant enzyme preparation, *Cancer Lett.,* 1, 269, 1976.

133. **Hong, S. J. and Piette, L. H.,** Electron spin resonance spin-label studies of intercalation of ethidium bromide and aromatic amine carcinogens in DNA, *Cancer Res.,* 36, 1159, 1976.

134. **Barry, E. J. and Gutmann, H. R.,** Protein modification by activated carcinogens. I. The acetylation of ribonuclease by N-acetoxy-2-fluorenylacetamide, *J. Biol. Chem.,* 248, 2730, 1973.

135. **Moyer, G. H., Gumbiner, B., and Austin, G. E.,** Binding of N-hydroxy acetylaminofluorene to eu- and heterochromatic fractions of rat liver in vivo, *Cancer Lett.,* 2, 259, 1977.

136. **Kriek, E.,** unpublished data, 1977.

137. **Kriek, E.,** unpublished data, 1969.

138. **Scribner, J. D.,** personal communication.

Chapter 2

POLYCYCLIC AROMATIC HYDROCARBON METABOLITES: THEIR REACTIONS WITH NUCLEIC ACIDS

David H. Phillips and Peter Sims

TABLE OF CONTENTS

I. INTRODUCTION

The first pure chemicals that were shown to cause cancer in experimental animals were the polycyclic aromatic hydrocarbons, dibenz[a,h]anthracene and benzo[a]pyrene. A number of polycyclic hydrocarbons, including benzo[a]pyrene, are formed during the incomplete combustion of organic materials and thus are widespread atmospheric pollutants. Over the years, much work has been carried out on investigations into how compounds of this class cause cancer, and two of the main areas of investigation have concerned the metabolism of the hydrocarbons and their reactions with the macromolecules present in the cells of tissues treated with the compounds. In recent years, the two areas of investigation have become linked together, since it was realized that the hydrocarbons undergo metabolic activation within cells to intermediates that react covalently with cellular macromolecules and in particular with nucleic acids.

The covalent binding of a polycyclic hydrocarbon to the DNA of mouse skin was first noted by Heidelberger and Davenport.[1] The hydrocarbon used in these experiments was [³H]-labeled dibenz[*a,h*]anthracene, but in later work Brookes and Lawley[2] used a series of six hydrocarbons, each labeled with tritium, and showed that the amount of hydrocarbon bound to the DNA, but not to the RNA or protein of mouse skin treated with any one of these hydrocarbons, was related to the carcinogenic activity of the compound, as measured by Iball's index. A more detailed study by Goshman and Heidelberger[3] confirmed the earlier observations and showed that the binding that is measured represents the true extent of metabolic reaction between the hydrocarbons and the DNA of mouse skin.

Diamond et al.[4] showed that the multiplication of transformed rodent cells or normal or transformed human cells was not inhibited by treatment with 7,12-dimethylbenz[*a*]anthracene, whereas the multiplication of normal embryonic rodent cells was. They also showed that the amount of hydrocarbon bound to the DNA of the normal rodent cells was 10 to 15 times greater than that bound to the DNA of transformed rodent or normal or embryonic human cells. These results suggested that there were differences in metabolizing abilites between the two types of cells. Brookes and Heidelberger[5] found that when rodent embryo cells were treated with 7,12-dimethylbenz[*a*]anthracene, binding of the hydrocarbon to DNA occurred, and they were able to carry out preliminary enzymic degradation and fractionation procedures on the isolated DNA that suggested that the hydrocarbon was covalently bound to one or more of the bases of DNA.

These early observations gave rise to the concept that since the hydrocarbons do not possess reactive groups, their metabolic activation was necessary before they could react with nucleic acids. Attempts were therefore made to link the metabolism of hydrocarbons in cells to the levels of their reactions with cellular DNA. The enzymes thought most likely to be involved in this metabolic activation were the mono-oxygenases present in the endoplasmic reticulum of most cells, and this idea was supported by the results of experiments in which [³H]-labeled hydrocarbons were incubated with rat liver microsomal systems (which contain the mono-oxygenase) in the presence of DNA.[6,7] Thus, studes on the metabolism of the hydrocarbons seemed essential if an understanding of the way in which the compounds react, both with DNA and with other cellular macromolecules, was to be gained. It is the purpose of this chapter to review those pathways of polycyclic hydrocarbon metabolism that give rise to reactive intermediates and to consider the nature of the products that are formed as a consequence of the reactions of those intermediates with nucleic acids, together with the biological events induced by the hydrocarbons and their derivatives that probably occur because of these reactions. So far the activation of only one polycyclic hydrocarbon, benzo[*a*]pyrene, has been studied in depth, but some information on the activation of others is available. The structural formulas of the hydrocarbons considered in this review are shown in Figure 1.

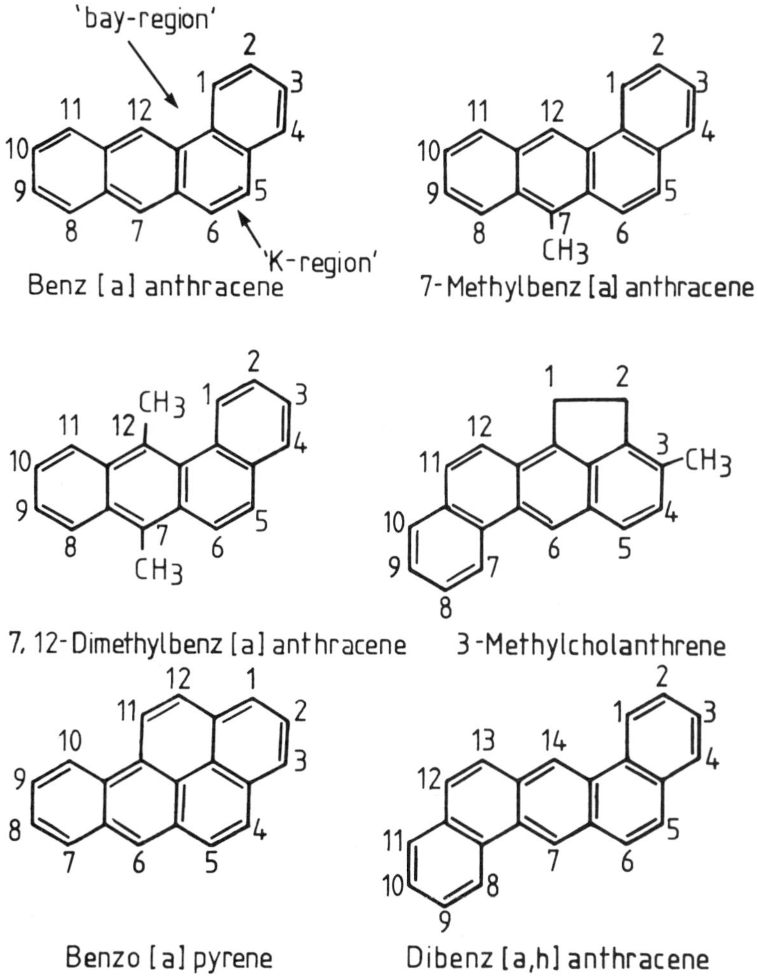

FIGURE 1. Structural formulae of the polycyclic hydrocarbons referred to in the text. The K-region and the bay-region of one of them, benz[a]anthracene, are indicated.

II. METABOLIC PATHWAYS INVOLVED IN THE ACTIVATION OF POLYCYCLIC AROMATIC HYDROCARBONS

A. Overall Metabolic Pathways

There now seems little doubt that all polycyclic hydrocarbons are metabolized by essentially similar pathways that lead to similar types of products, irrespective of whether or not the particular hydrocarbon will induce tumors in experimental animals. Moreover, the patterns of products that are formed from any one hydrocarbon do not appear to depend to any great extent on the source of the tissue under examination, although there are quantitative differences.

It is not intended to review in detail the metabolism of the hydrocarbons since the earlier aspects of this work have been discussed previously.[8] Some of the more important metabolic routes of the hydrocarbon, benzo[a]pyrene, are shown in Figure 2. Much of the more recent work has been carried out with this hydrocarbon, and much use has been made of sensitive, high-pressure liquid chromatographic techniques. The investigations have been concerned mainly with the identification and measurement of metabolites of benzo[a]pyrene, first identified in rat liver preparations, in a number

of tissues derived from animals of various strains and species. Differences in the proportions of the various metabolites of benzo[*a*]pyrene, shown in Figure 2, have also
been reported. Thus, for example, the metabolism of benzo[*a*]pyrene has been studied
in liver microsomal fractions from rats pretreated with 3-methylcholanthrene,[9-11] from
normal and 3-methylcholanthrene-treated rats and mice,[12] Rhesus monkeys,[13] and
from humans.[14] The ability of rat liver nuclei to metabolize the hydrocarbon has also
been reported.[15] The metabolism of benzo[*a*]pyrene by microsomal fractions from the
lungs of genetically-responsive and nonresponsive mice[16] and from Rhesus monkeys[13]
has also been examined. Other investigators have studied the metabolism of benzo[*a*]-
pyrene in rodent embryo cells,[17] in human lymphocytes[14] and epithelial cells,[19] in rat
intestinal epithelial cells,[19] in homogenates of mouse epidermis,[20] and in rat colon in
culture.[21] Use has also been made of human bronchial[22,23] and rat and hamster tracheal
and lung tissues[23] in organ culture and isolated perfused rat and hamster lungs.[24] Other
hydrocarbons appear to have been studied in less detail in recent years, but investigations on the metabolism of 7,12-dimethylbenz[*a*]anthracene by rat or hamster liver
microsomal fractions,[25,26] of 7-methylbenz[*a*]anthracene by rat liver homogenates and
microsomal fractions,[27] and by mouse skin in organ culture[27] have been reported. The
relationship of the observations made in some of these experiments to the in vivo reactions of benzo[*a*]pyrene with nucleic acids is not yet clear.

With benzo[*a*]pyrene, the metabolites most usually detected in experiments of the
type described above are the phenols and dihydrodiols shown in Figure 2, although
other, often unidentified, metabolites have been reported. Quinones are also formed,
but these appear to arise from the nonenzymic oxidation of phenols. The phenols
themselves appear to be metabolized further, but little is known of the products that
are formed. The dihydrodiols are thought to arise from the hydrocarbons via the intermediate formation of simple epoxides as first suggested in 1950 by Boyland,[28] and
there is now evidence that the phenol, 3-hydroxybenzo[*a*]pyrene, also arises from an
epoxide intermediate, the unstable benzo[*a*]pyrene 2,3-oxide.[29] The simple epoxides
can conveniently be divided into two groups, the K-region and the non-K-region epoxides, according to the type of aromatic double bond on which they are formed, the K-

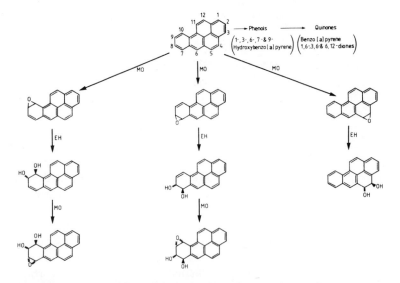

FIGURE 2.   The major pathways involved in the metabolism of benzo[*a*]pyrene.
The *anti*-isomers of the diol-epoxides are shown. MO — Mono-oxygenase; EH —
Epoxide hydratase.

region being the phenanthrene type of aromatic double bond present in the polycyclic hydrocarbons shown in Figure 1. There is now abundant evidence[8] that epoxides are formed from the parent hydrocarbons in microsomal systems. Because of their ease of synthesis,[30-32] much work over recent years has been concerned both with the biochemical and biological properties of the K-region epoxides and with their reactions with nucleic cids. This latter work is reviewed in Section V.

Both types of epoxides are further metabolized to dihydrodiols by the epoxide hydratases present on the endoplasmic reticulum of the cells of most tissues. The properties of these enzymes have been reviewed by Oesch.[33] Until quite recently, both the K-region and the non-K-region dihydrodiols were considered to be detoxification products, but it now appears that some of the non-K-region dihydrodiols are further metabolized to products that are intimately concerned in the reactions of hydrocarbons with cellular nucleic acids that are described in Sections III and VI.

The non-K-region dihydrodiols all possess isolated olefinic double bonds adjacent to the hydroxyl groups so that it might be expected that metabolism of the dihydrodiols would lead to epoxidation of those double bonds to give vicinal diol-epoxides. The formation of a diol-epoxide from the 8,9-dihydrodiol of benz[a]anthracene by a rat liver microsomal fraction was first demonstrated by Booth and Sims,[34] and, although the stereochemistry of this diol-epoxide was not established at that time, the problem of the stereochemistry of the diol-epoxides in general and that of the dihydrodiols from which they are derived has become of increasing importance. Thus, the (−)-enantiomer of the 7,8-dihydrodiol of benzo[a]pyrene is more active than the (+)-enantiomer in initiating skin tumors in mice,[35] and the diol-epoxides derived from the (−)-7,8-dihydrodiol are more active as mutagens in *Salmonella typhimurium* strains and in Chinese hamster V79 cells than the diol-epoxides derived from the (+)-7,8-dihydrodiol.[36]

Work on the non-K-region dihydrodiols and the diol-epoxides derived from them has been greatly facilitated by the development of methods of synthesis. Thus, synthetic routes leading to the preparation of the *trans*-7,8- and 9,10-dihydrodiols of benzo [a] pyrene,[37] the *trans* -1,2-, 3, 4-, 8,9-, and 10, 11- dihydrodiols of benz[a]anthracene,[38] and the *trans*-10,11-dihydrodiol of 7-methylbenz[a]anthracene[39] have been described. An oxidative procedure that leads to the formation of the *trans*-1,2-,3,4-, and 8,9-dihydrodiols of 7-methylbenz[a]anthracene directly from the hydrocarbon has also been described.[40] Methods have also been developed for the conversion of the non-K-region dihydrodiols into the isomeric diol-epoxides of both benzo[a]pyrene[39,41-44] and benz[a]anthracene[39,45] and for the synthesis of non-K-region epoxides,[46,47] the metabolic precursors of the non-K-region dihydrodiols.

B. Formation and Metabolism of Dihydrodiols

Since the dihydrodiols that are formed from the hydrocarbons arise by the further metabolism of simple epoxides, they would be expected to have the *trans*-configuration. This has been confirmed in the relatively few instances where the configurations of the non-K-region dihydrodiols have been investigated in detail, either by NMR spectroscopy or by chromatographic comparisons with the synthetic *trans*-compounds. With the K-region dihydrodiols, where both *cis*- and *trans*-isomers of a particular dihydrodiol are often available, the metabolic dihydrodiols have the mobilities of the *trans*- and not of the *cis*-compounds on chromatograms.[8] The dihydrodiols are formed from the epoxides by enzymic reactions and should therefore be optically active, but, except for the dihydrodiols derived from benzo[a]pyrene, little is known of the optical activities of these metabolites. With benzo[a]pyrene, all three known metabolic dihydrodiols, the *trans*-4,5-dihydrodiol, the *trans*-7,8-dihydrodiol, and the *trans*-9,10-dihydrodiol are formed mainly as the (−)-enantiomers when the hydrocarbon is incubated with rat liver microsomal fractions.[48,49] In the case of the 7,8-dihydrodiol of benzo-

[a]pyrene, the synthetic racemic compound has been resolved into its optically active enantiomers by the separation, by high-pressure liquid chromatography, of the di(-)-menthoxyacetates,[50,51] or the di(-)-α-methoxy-α-trifluoromethylphenylacetates.[49] Comparisons by Yang et al.[52] of the optical rotation of the resolved synthetic (-)-enantiomer of the *trans*-7,8-dihydrodiol of benzo[a]pyrene with that of the metabolically formed dihydrodiol showed that the latter contained 97% of the (-)-enantiomer. Thakker et al.,[49] using both chemical and optical methods, showed that the dihydrodiol formed by metabolism contained more than 90% of the (-)-enantiomer. Yang et al.,[52,53] consider that the dihydrodiol arises by two steps, a stereospecific oxygenation of the 7,8-double bond of benzo[a]pyrene to give essentially a single enantiomer of the 7,8-epoxide, followed by a stereospecific hydration of the 7,8-epoxide by epoxide hydratase to give an optically pure (-)-*trans*-7,8-dihydrodiol. They also claim that the synthetic racemic 7,8-epoxide of benzo[a]pyrene is converted by rat liver microsomal preparations into a 7,8-dihydrodiol containing 86% of the (-)-enantiomer. However, in similar experiments, Thakker et al.[49] found only an 8% excess of the (-) over the (+)-enantiomer when a chemical method to determine the proportions of each isomer present was used. Although there is no direct evidence, it seems likely that dihydrodiols derived from other hydrocarbons also arise by stereospecific pathways when their parent hydrocarbons are metabolized in microsomal systems.

Metabolism of dihydrodiols leading to products other than diol-epoxides has also been reported. Thakker et al.[49] showed that the 7,8-dihydrodiol of benzo[a]pyrene is converted by microsomal systems into a phenolic metabolite that is possibly the 6-hydroxy derivative of the 7,8-dihydrodiol. It has also been reported by Booth and Sims[54] that the 9,10-dihydrodiol of benzo[a]pyrene, but not the 7,8-dihydrodiol, is dehydrogenated to the related catechol by rat liver microsomal or soluble fractions. Investigations of these alternative pathways may be of importance, since such pathways may lead to a detoxification rather than an activation of the dihydrodiols.

C. Formation and Reactions of Diol-Epoxides

Vicinal diol-epoxides are formed by the action of microsomal mono-oxygenases on non-K-region dihydrodiols by the addition of oxygen to the olefinic double bond adjacent to the hydroxyl groups. In these diol-epoxides, the hydroxyl groups necessarily have the *trans*-configuration, but two stereoisomers are possible for a diol-epoxide derived from a particular *trans*-dihydrodiol, in which the epoxide oxygen is either *cis* or *trans* to the benzylic hydroxyl group.* It has been pointed out by Hulbert[55] and by Yagi et al.[41] that, in the isomers in which the epoxide oxygen is *cis* to the benzylic hydroxyl group (the *syn*-isomers), anchimeric assistance to attack by nucleophiles is possible because, when these isomers are in the quasi-diaxial configuration, the interatomic distances between the epoxide oxygen and the hydrogen of the benzylic hydroxyl group are short enough for strong interactions (hydrogen bonding) to take place between them, as shown in Figure 3. With the second type of isomers, where the epoxide oxygen is *trans* to the benzylic hydroxyl group (the *anti*-isomers), no such interac-

---

* Various forms of nomenclature have been used in describing the stereochemistry of the diol-epoxides. The two isomers were originally called *cis* or *trans* according to whether the oxygen function was on the same or the opposite side of the tetrahydrobenzene ring to the benzylic hydroxyl group. Harvey and co-workers favor the term *syn* and *anti*, and for simplicity this form is used throughout this chapter. The systematic names for the *syn*-7,8-diol-9,10-epoxide of benzo[a]pyrene are either, 7β, 8α-dihydroxy-9β, 10β-epoxy-7,8,9,10-tetrahydrobenzo[a]pyrene or r-7, t-8-dihydroxy-c-9,10-oxy-7,8,9,10-tetrahydrobenzo[a]pyrene, where r indicates the reference substituent and c and t substituents *cis* or *trans* to the reference constituent. Other diol-epoxides are similarly named.

With the isomers of the 7,8-diol-9,10-epoxide of benzo[a]pyrene in particular, Gelboin and co-workers[52] call the *anti*-isomer, diol-epoxide I and the *syn*-isomer, diol-epoxide II, whereas Jerina and co-workers[44] call the *syn*-isomer, diol-epoxide 1 and the *anti*-isomer, diol-epoxide I and the *anti*-isomer, diol-epoxide 2.

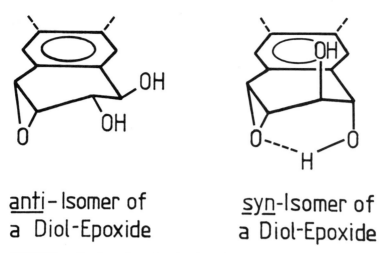

anti-Isomer of
a Diol-Epoxide

syn-Isomer of
a Diol-Epoxide

FIGURE 3.   Configurations of *anti-*and *syn-*isomers of a vicinal diol-epoxide.

tion is possible. At first sight, therefore, it would seem that the former isomer might
be more reactive both chemically and biologically than the latter, and it thus becomes
important to know which isomers are produced when the parent dihydrodiols are metabolized by microsomal mono-oygenases. Jerina and colleagues have measured the
second-order rate constants for the reactions between pairs of *syn* and *anti-*isomers of
diol-epoxides derived from benz[*a*]anthracene[45] and benzo[*a*]pyrene[41] with 4-nitrothio-
phenolate in dry *tert-*butanol and find that the *anti-*isomers are 60 to 130 times less
reactive than the corresponding *syn-*isomers. However, tests in biological systems have
shown that in general, although the *syn-*isomers are more active in bacterial systems,
the *anti-*isomers are more active in mammalian systems (see Section VI).

Most of the investigations into the configurations of the diol-epoxides that are
formed from dihydrodiols by metabolism have employed the 7,8-dihydrodiol of
benzo[*a*]pyrene as substrate. Because both isomers of the expected diol-epoxide, the
7,8-diol-9,10-epoxide, react rapidly with water, it has not proved possible to isolate
the diol-epoxides as such. However, the composition of the mixtures of stereoisomeric
tetrols that is formed when a particular diol-epoxide reacts with water depends on the
stereochemistry of the diol-epoxide. Thus, each of the isomeric forms of the 7,8-diol-
9,10-epoxides of benzo[*a*]pyrene can, in theory, yield one or more of the three isomers
shown in Figure 4. Several groups of workers[49,56-58] have shown that, in practice, each
isomeric diol-epoxide gives rise to only two isomers of the tetrol; the *syn-*isomer yielding the 7,9/8,10- and the 7,9,10/8-tetrol and the *anti-*isomer, the 7,10/8,9- and the 7/
8,9,10-tetrol.* The ratios of the isomeric tetrols formed when a 7,8-diol-9,10-epoxide
of benzo[*a*]pyrene reacts with water appear to depend on pH, the reaction being acid-
catalyzed at low pH and spontaneous at higher pH.[59] Since the various isomeric tetrols
can be separated by high-pressure liquid chromatography, it is possible to determine
the relative proportions of the isomers of the diol-epoxides formed from the 7,8-dihy-
drodiol in microsomal systems from an examination of the composition of the mixture
of tetrols present at the end of the incubation. The first report on experiments of this
type by Huberman et al.[60] indicated that the major metabolite formed by rat liver
microsomal fractions from a *trans-*7,8-dihydrodiol (presumably the (−)-isomer), prepared by the microsomal metabolism of the hydrocarbon, was mainly the *anti-*form

*   The nomenclature used here for the tetrols is that used by Gelboin's group[56] where, for example, a 7,10/
      8,9-tetrol indicates that the 10-hydroxy group is *cis* and the 8- and 9-hydroxy groups are *trans* to the 7-
      hydroxy group.

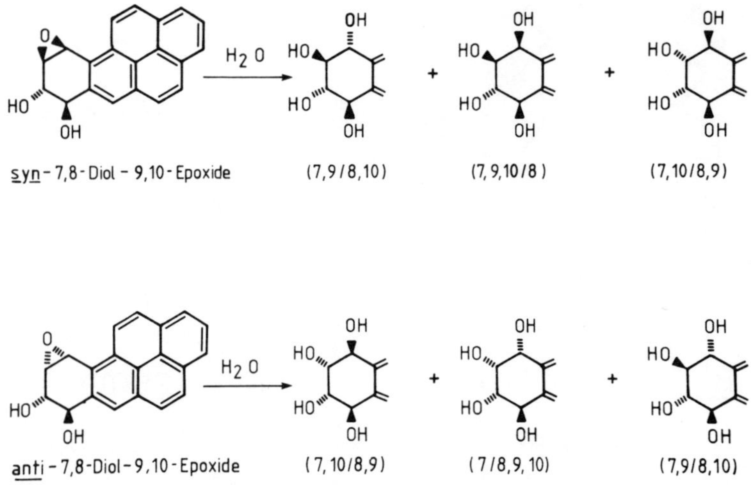

FIGURE 4.   Structures of isomeric tetrols that could arise from the hydration of the isomeric 7,8-diol-9,10-epoxides of benzo[a]pyrene.

of the diol-epoxide. Later Thakker et al.[61] showed that the (±)-*trans*-dihydrodiol was converted into both isomeric forms of the diol-epoxide by microsomal fractions from both normal and phenobarbitone- and 3-methylcholanthrene-treated rats and by purifed cytochrome P-448 and P-450 systems. Thakker et al.[49] have also shown that the metabolism of the 7,8-dihydrodiol in some of these systems was dependent on its stereochemistry, the (−) enantiomer of the dihydrodiol yielding 70 to 86% of the *anti*-isomer of the diol-epoxide and the (+)-enantiomer yielding 82 to 92% of the *syn*-isomer. Similar stereoselectivity in the conversion of the (−)-dihydrodiol into the *anti*-diol-epoxide has been observed by Yang et al. for a rat liver microsomal fraction[52] and for cultured human bronchus.[62]

Thus, it seems clear that with benzo[a]pyrene, the 7,8-diol-9,10-oxide is formed from the hydrocarbon by three stereospecific steps involving oxygenation of the 7,8-bond by the microsomal mono-oxygenase, the hydration of the 7,8-epoxide to form the (−)-7,8-dihydrodiol by the microsomal epoxide hydratase, and the oxygenation of the vicinal 9,10-double bond of the (−)-7,8-dihydrodiol by the microsomal mono-oxygenase to form mainly the *anti*-isomer of the 7,8-diol-9,10-epoxide. The hydration of the diol-epoxides to form tetrols appears to be a nonenzymic process, since the presence or absence of epoxide hydratase does not affect the ratio of products formed from either of the isomers of the diol-epoxides.[61]

It has also been reported by Yang and Gelboin[63] that the isomeric benzo[a]pyrene diol-epoxides are each reduced nonenzymically by NADPH to trihydroxy compounds, the *anti*-isomer yielding 7/8,9-trihydroxy- and the *syn*-isomer, 7,9/8-trihydroxy-7,8,9,10,10-pentahydrobenzo[a]pyrene. The presence of one or the other of these products among the metabolites formed when the 7,8-dihydrodiol is metabolized by microsomal fractions povides additional evidence for the stereochemical structures of the diol-epoxide intermediates. Whether or not these triols are formed during the in vivo metabolism of the hydrocarbon is not known.

III. THE IN VITRO ACTIVATION OF POLYCYCLIC HYDROCARBON DERIVATIVES

A. The Role of Metabolism

Conclusive evidence that metabolism is a prerequisite of polycyclic hydrocarbon covalent interaction with DNA and other cellular macromolecules was first obtained by

Grover and Sims[6] and by Gelboin,[7] who showed that hydrocarbon binding to DNA was mediated by the metabolizing enzymes present in rat liver microsomal fractions; the DNA that was isolated contained covalently bound hydrocarbon residues as determined by the radioactivity present in the DNA samples even after they had been put through a number of purification procedures. In the absence of the cofactors necessary for the function of the mono-oxygenase system, the levels of radioactivity were greatly reduced, showing that the mono-oxygenase was involved in the activation processes. These observations have been amply confirmed for both liver and lung microsomal fractions by other workers,[64-67] and it has also been established that nuclear preparations from rodent livers and lungs possess the necessary enzyme activity to bind polycyclic hydrocarbons to nuclear macromolecules.[68-73] However, it should be noted that such nuclear preparations commonly contain nuclei that have outer nuclear membranes with residual tags of endoplasmic reticulum attached to them.[74] It is thus not clear whether the enzyme activity associated with nuclear preparations is due principally to a distinct nuclear mono-oxygenase system, or to the microsomal enzymes in the residual endoplasmic reticulum present in these preparations. Certainly comparison between both the carbon monoxide difference spectra of cytochrome P-450 and the catalytic properties of the mixed-function mono-oxygenase systems of nuclear and microsomal preparations indicates that both preparations are similar.[75]

B. Activation of Epoxides and Dihydrodiols

Once the conditions for binding of polycyclic hydrocarbons to DNA had been established, attention turned to the types of metabolites that, when added to in vivo and in vitro metabolizing systems, resulted in covalent binding. Kuroki et al.[76] studied the binding of benz[a]anthracene and dibenz[a,h]anthracene and their K-region epoxides, cis-dihydrodiols and phenols to the DNA, RNA, and proteins of exponentially growing hamster embryo cells in culture found that the derivatives, particularly the epoxides, bound to a greater extent than the parent hydrocarbons. It should be emphasized, however, that reaction of a metabolite directly with cellular macromolecules or the further metabolism to such a reactive species does not mean that the particular metabolite is necessarily an intermediate in the binding of the parent hydrocarbon, since the latter could bind as a result of an entirely different metabolic process. Thus, the K-region epoxides were shown subsequently not to be reactive intermediates formed from polycyclic hydrocarbons in vivo (reviewed in Section V), although this did not preclude the involvement of epoxides of some sort in the metabolic activation of polycyclic hydrocarbons.

Attention was drawn to the further metabolism of non-K-region dihydrodiols by the report of Borgen et al.[77] that when the [³H]-labeled dihydrodiols derived from the metabolism of benzo[a]pyrene were further metabolized by hamster liver microsomal preparations in the presence of DNA, the level of reaction of one metabolite, the 7,8-dihydrodiol, with DNA greatly exceeded that of benzo[a]pyrene itself. This observation was confirmed in studies using rat liver preparations by Sims et al.[78] and by Thompson et al.[79] The further metabolism of the 7,8-dihydrodiol of benzo[a]pyrene and the concomitant binding to DNA was also demonstrated in hamster embryo cells in culture,[78] in cultured human bronchial mucosa,[80] and in mouse skin in vivo.[80] Harris and co-workers showed that a series of polycyclic hydrocarbons bind to macromolecules in cultured human bronchi[81,82] and that the 7,8-dihydrodiol of benzo[a]pyrene was more active than either benzo[a]pyrene or several other metabolites including phenols, the K-region 4,5-dihydrodiol, and the non-K-region 9,10-dihydrodiol, in binding to DNA.[62] This inability of the 4,5- and 9,10-dihydrodiol to bind to DNA has been noted by other workers[77-80] and is discussed further in Section VI. Booth and Sims[34] had earlier shown that a non-K-region dihydrodiol of benz[a]anthracene could be further metabolized at the olefinic double bond adjacent to the dihydrodiol grouping to yield a vicinal diol-epoxide (see Section II), and it was proposed by Sims et al.[78] that this new type of metabolite might be responsible for binding of polycyclic hydrocarbons to nucleic acids in vivo. There is now extensive evidence supporting this hypothesis which is reviewed in detail in Section VI. The remainder of this section reviews the status of metabolites other than simple epoxides or diol-epoxides in the metabolic activation of polycyclic hydrocarbons. The majority of studies have investigated metabolites of benzo[a]pyrene, and data on other hydrocarbons are sparse.

C. Activation of Phenols

6-Hydroxybenzo[a]pyrene is a major transient metabolite of benzo[a]pyrene that undergoes autooxidation to produce the three stable 1,6-, 3,6-, and 6,12-benzo[a]pyrene diones.[83] In ethanol-phosphate buffer solution, 6-hydroxybenzo-[a]pyrene spontaneously reacts with DNA forming covalent bonds and causing strand breakages,[84] probably via some reactive species formed in the autooxidation of this metabolite. To account for these reactions, Nagata et al.[85] proposed the formation of a 6-phenoxy-free radical intermediate derived from 6-hydroxybenzo[a]pyrene, while Flesher and Sydnor[86] proposed an alternative mechanism of metabolic activation involving the formation of 6-hydroxymethylbenzo[a]pyrene. However, Blackburn et al.[87] showed that the 6 position of benzo[a]pyrene was not significantly involved in the liver microsome-mediated binding of benzo[a]pyrene to DNA: photochemical binding of [6-³H]-benzo[a]pyrene to DNA resulted in the loss of 92% of its tritium content, while binding using rat liver microsomal preparations showed a loss of only 20% of tritium. Similar tritium retention studies on the metabolic activation of benzo[a]pyrene in cells also discounted the involvement of the 6 position.[88]

3-Hydroxybenzo[a]pyrene is also a metabolite of of benzo[a]pyrene[89,90] and has been shown to bind covalently to DNA in the presence of rat lung microsomal fractions.[91] However, the reaction does not appear to occur in vivo, as no binding to DNA was detected in the skin of mice to which 3-hydroxybenzo[a]pyrene had been administered topically in solution.[80]

Osborne et al.[92] showed that metabolism of double-labeled [³H], [¹⁴C]-benzo[a]pyrene by rat liver microsomal fractions yielded 3-hydroxybenzo[a]pyrene with 30% loss of tritium, a mixture of quinones with 50% loss of tritium, and three dihydrodiol metabolites that had retained all the tritium of the parent hydrocarbon. DNA that was isolated from mouse embryo cells that had been exposed to the double-labeled benzo[a]pyrene and DNA to which this hydrocarbon bound following in vitro rat liver microsomal incubation were each degraded enzymically and the hydrocarbon-deoxyribonucleoside products separated by chromatography on Sephadex LH20® columns using a technique developed by Baird and Brookes.[93] The tritium contents of the products obtained from both DNA samples were very close to those of the original double-labeled benzo[a]pyrene. These results are inconsistent with the 3-phenol or a quinone intermediate being responsible for the reaction with DNA, but consistent with a diol-epoxide intermediate as proposed by Sims et al.[78]

Meehan et al.[94] showed, using benzo[a]pyrene specifically labeled with tritium at the 1, 3, and 6 positions, that none of these positions was involved in the microsome-mediated binding of benzo[a]pyrene to poly(G), and they subsequently provided fluorescence evidence (see chapter 4) which confirmed the involvement in this binding of the 7,8,9,10-ring of the hydrocarbon.[95]

Wislocki et al.[96] have demonstrated the high carcinogenicity of 2-hydroxybenzo[a]-pyrene on mouse skin, but there is no evidence for the formation of this phenol as a metabolite of benzo[a]pyrene and, although nothing is known of the metabolism of this phenol, it seems unlikely that a derivative of 2-hydroxybenzo[a]pyrene is involved in the metabolic activation of benzo[a]pyrene in vivo.

Brookes et al.[97] showed that purine moieties in DNA react with the metabolically activated hydrocarbon derivative in vivo; the DNA of mouse embryo cells was specifically labeled with either tritiated deoxyadenosine or deoxycytidine, and the cells were then treated with either 7-methylbenz[a]anthracene or benzo[a]pyrene. When the DNA was isolated and degraded to nucleosides and the products fractionated by Sephadex LH20® column chromatography, radioactive hydrocarbon-nucleosides were obtained from the DNA prelabeled with deoxyadenosine, but no such radioactive products were obtained from the DNA prelabeled with deoxycytidine.

Comparisons of the Sephadex LH20® elution profiles of enzyme digests of DNA modified by microsomal incubations with hydrocarbon have revealed additional artifactual product peaks arising from these incubations that are not related to the metabolic activation of the hydrocarbon in vivo. Thus, while a single hydrocarbon-nucleoside peak is obtained when benzo[a]pyrene is metabolized by cells,[78] King et al.[98] obtained five peaks from the rat liver microsome-induced binding of benzo[a]pyrene to DNA, and Nebert et al.[99] reproducibly found nine peaks when using mouse liver microsomal fractions to effect metabolism and binding. Grover[74] has pointed out that the appearance of extra products is not surprising in view of the artificially high levels of mono-oxygenase activity of the microsomal preparations (the experimental animals are frequently pretreated with an inducer of the mono-oxygenase enzymes, and epoxide hydratase activity is not comparably augmented), the high levels of cofactors, especially NADPH, that are used for the optimum function of the mono-oxygenase system, and the absence from purified microsomal preparations of deactivating enzymes such as the soluble glutathione transferases.

Thompson et al.[79] showed that a mixture of phenols derived from benzo[a]pyrene became bound to DNA in the presence of microsomal fractions, although to a lesser extent than did the 7,8-dihydrodiol of benzo[a]pyrene. It was further shown by King et al.[100] that a major peak eluting from Sephadex LH20® columns that is not observed in in vivo studies[78,80] was derived from 9-hydroxybenzo[a]pyrene, and these workers suggested that 9-hydroxybenzo[a]pyrene 4,5-oxide was the derivative whose reaction with DNA yielded this microsome-mediated benzo[a]pyrene-DNA product.

IV. THE DISTRIBUTION OF BINDING OF POLYCYCLIC HYDROCARBONS IN DNA

Relatively little information is available on the actual distribution of hydrocarbon binding in DNA. Mouse skin DNA is separable into two species, satellite and main band DNA; the satellite DNA is thought to be composed of about a million copies of a repeated sequence of approximately 100 to 400 base pairs while main band DNA contains unique, nonrepeating sequences.[101] Zeiger et al.[102] isolated the mouse satellite and main band epidermal DNA after the topical application of [³H]-labeled 7,12-dimethylbenz[a]anthracene to mouse skin and found that the amount of hydrocarbon bound per milligram of DNA was the same for both satellite and mainband DNA. Meunier and Chauveau[66] examined the microsome-mediated binding of benzo[a]pyrene to calf thymus DNA and found that, although the benzo[a]pyrene metabolites(s) does not exhibit a preferential binding to one satellite DNA, the levels of binding to all satellite DNAs were higher than those to main band DNA. Metabolites of polycyclic hydrocarbons are known to react preferentially with the guanine bases in DNA (see Section V), and it may be that these results reflect the G$_+$C content in the different DNA species.[103,104] Zytkovicz et al.[105] found that the binding of benzo[a]pyrene in mouse embryo cells was largely localized in a particular subnuclear fraction isolated by sucrose gradient centrifugation of sheared nuclei from cells exposed to the hydrocarbon. This fraction has been shown to be more transcriptionally active than other fractions and to have greater nonhistone protein and RNA contents.[106]

Bowden et al.[107] demonstrated that the binding of 7,12-dimethylbenz[a]anthracene was reproducibly greater to nonreplicating DNA than to replicating DNA and that the skin epidermal DNA to which the hydrocarbon was bound was able to serve as a template for further DNA synthesis.[108]

The accessibility of DNA in chromatin can determine the distribution of binding of a carcinogen. The structure of chromatin can be visualized as a string of beads, or nucleosomes, of complexed DNA and histones, with connecting interbead, or spacer, regions of DNA.[109] Jahn and Litman[110] have demonstrated that the incubation of benzo[a]pyrene with calf thymus nuclei in the presence of NADPH and rat liver microsomal fractions results in the hydrocarbon binding preferentially to nuclease-accessible regions of DNA in chromatin; this implies that benzo[a]pyrene binds primarily to the spacer regions of DNA.[111]

V. THE REACTIONS OF K-REGION EPOXIDES WITH NUCLEIC ACIDS

More than 20 years after the idea that epoxides are primary metabolites of polycyclic hydrocarbons was first postulated,[28] the formation of epoxides of phenanthrene, benz[a]anthracene, 7-methylbenz[a]anthracene, 7,12-dimethylbenz[a]anthracene, pyrene, benzo[a]pyrene, and dibenz[a,h]anthracene was directly demonstrated in rat and hamster liver microsomal systems.[112-117] As these first-discovered epoxides were all K-region epoxides, attention was naturally focused on the properties of the epoxides formed at this reactive region. The K-region epoxides were relatively easy to synthesize and could be readily obtained labeled with tritium. Grover and Sims[118] showed that the K-region epoxides of phenanthrene and dibenz[a,h]anthracene reacted with DNA, RNA, and histone in the absence of any metabolizing systems, conditions in which the parent hydrocarbons and their respective K-region dihydrodiols did not react. They further showed that these epoxides and also the K-region epoxides of benz[a]anthracene and 7-methylbenz[a]anthracene reacted mainly with the purine moieties of nucleic acids: they reacted to a greater extent with DNA and RNA, in aqueous ethanol solution, than with apurinic acid, and in similar experiments with polyribonucleotides, they were reactive towards poly(G), less reactive towards poly(A), poly(X), and poly(I), but did not react appreciably with poly(U) or poly(C).[119]

Swaisland et al.[120] separated hydrolysates of RNA, poly(G), and poly(A) that had been allowed to react with either benz[a]anthracene 5,6-oxide or 7,12-dimethylbenz[a]anthracene 5,6-oxide by Sephadex LH20® column chromatography and showed that, of the two RNA products resulting from reactions with benz[a]anthracene 5,6-oxide, one resulted from reaction with guanine and the other from reaction with adenine. With 7,12-dimethylbenz[a]anthracene 5,6-oxide, six RNA products were separated, two of which resulted from reaction with guanine and three from reaction with adenine; the sixth product was not identified.

Weinstein and co-workers[121] investigated the reaction of 7,12-dimethylbenz[a]anthracene 5,6-oxide with synthetic homopolymers and nucleic acids and obtained the highest level of reaction with poly(G), and they also obtained some reaction with GMP and dGMP. Separation by high-pressure liquid chromatography of the hydrolysates of poly(G) and poly(A) that had been allowed to react with the epoxide yielded four major products in the case of poly(G) and two in the case of poly(A).[122] Analysis of the UV, circular dichroic, mass, and proton magnetic resonance spectra of the poly(G) reaction products revealed that all four products resulted from the reaction of the epoxide with the 2-amino group of guanine; in two of the products, the amino group was conjugated with the 6 position of 7,12-dimethyl-benz[a]anthracene, and in the other two, with the 5 position of the hydrocarbon[123] as shown in Figure 5.

K-Region epoxides were found to cause the malignant transformation of rodent cells in culture,[124] to be mutagenic in a variety of systems including mammalian cells,[125] bacteria,[126] and bacteriophage T_2h^+ [127] and appeared to have the requisite chemical reactivity to qualify them for the role of ultimate carcinogenic forms of the polycyclic hydrocarbons. However, they are generally weaker carcinogens than their parent hydrocarbons[128-132] and, although such a lack of carcinogenic activity may be due to the failure of an ultimate carcinogen to penetrate cell membranes and interact with its critical target, this is unlikely with the K-region epoxides since it was eventually shown that they were not the major metabolites involved in the binding of hydrocarbons to nucleic acids in vivo. Baird et al. compared the Sephadex LH20® elution profiles of hydrolysates of DNA[133] and RNA[134] isolated from mouse embryo cells that had been treated with 7-methylbenz[a]anthracene with the profiles of hydrolysates of DNA and RNA that had been reacted with 7-methylbenz[a]anthracene 5,6-oxide in aqueous ethanol: it was found that the profiles were dissimilar. This finding suggests that the binding of 7-methylbenz[a]anthracene to nucleic acids in cells does not involve metabolic activation at the K-region to form an epoxide. However, Thompson et al.[135] in studies in which 7-methylbenz[a]anthracene was incubated in the presence of DNA with liver microsomal fractions prepared from rats treated with 3-methylcholanthrene, obtained Sephadex LH20® elution profiles of DNA-hydrolysates that differed from those obtained from the DNA of mouse embryo cells treated with 7-methylbenz[a]anthracene, and they suggested that the K-region epoxide made a significant contribution to the binding of the hydrocarbon to DNA mediated by rat liver microsomal fractions. It thus appears that, at least with 7-methylbenz[a]anthracene, the rat liver microsomal system is not a good model for the in vivo activation of the hydrocarbon.

The situation with benzo[a]pyrene is different for it was found, using methods similar to those described above, that the DNA-bound products of this hydrocarbon did not arise via the K-region epoxide, either in mouse embryo cell cultures that had been treated with [³H]-labeled benzo[a]pyrene[136] or when benzo[a]pyrene was metabolized by rat liver microsomal fractions in the presence of DNA.[98] Blackburn et al.[137] arrived at the same conclusion from studies of the extent of loss of tritium from labeled benzo[a]pyrene that became bound to the DNA of mouse kidney cells.

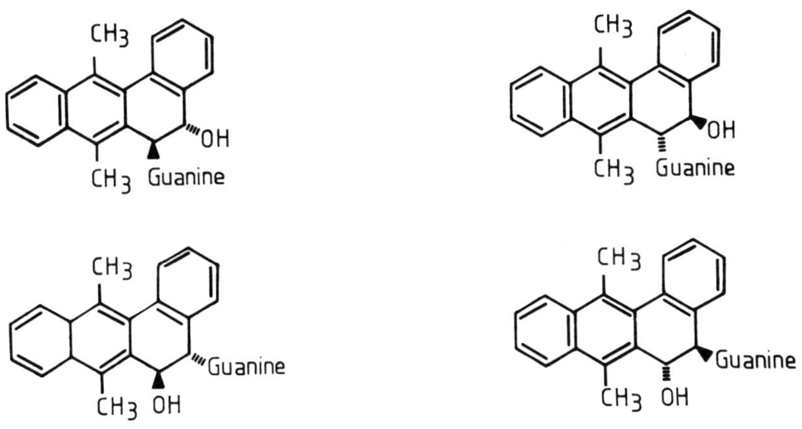

FIGURE 5.   Structures of the products arising from the reaction of 7,12-dimethylbenz[a]anthracene 5,6-oxide with the guanine residues in poly(G).

Thus, despite the formation of the K-region epoxide from benzo[a]pyrene in liver-metabolizing systems[113] and the covalent reactions that occur between the epoxide and nucleic acid in neutral solution,[136] no hydrocarbon-nucleoside products derived from the K-region epoxide have been isolated when benzo[a]pyrene is metabolized in the presence of DNA.[98,136] The observation of Murray et al.[138] may be relevant to this paradox; they observed the production of 4-hydroxybenzo[a]pyrene when benzo[a]pyrene 4,5-oxide was incubated in the presence of poly(G) or DNA. Phenol formation was not detected when the epoxide was incubated in the absence of nucleic acid, and these workers proposed that in addition to the formation of stable epoxide-polynucleotide products, there was a second type of reaction that involved the formation of an unstable, transient epoxide-polynucleotide complex that decomposed spontaneously to yield the K-region phenol and an unchanged polynucleotide. This latter reaction offers one explanation for the failure to detect K-region epoxide-nucleoside products when benzo[a]pyrene is metabolized in the presence of DNA.

VI. THE REACTIONS OF DIOL-EPOXIDES WITH NUCLEIC ACIDS

A. Diol-Epoxides as Reactive Metabolites of Polycyclic Hydrocarbons

Although the K-region epoxides did not appear to be involved in the metabolic activation of polycyclic hydrocarbons, the possibility of the involvement of epoxides of some other sort was not ruled out. Simple non-K-region epoxides did not seem likely candidates, however, because the hydrocarbon-nucleoside products formed in cells that had been treated with the parent hydrocarbon were more polar and therefore eluted earlier with a water-methanol gradient from Sephadex LH20® columns than those that were derived from the reaction of a simple epoxide with DNA.[133,136] It was known that non-K-region dihydrodiols, which are indeed more polar than simple epoxides, were formed by rat liver preparations and underwent further metabolism to even more polar products,[139] possibly via epoxide intermediates. Then, as mentioned in Section III, the non-K-region 7,8-dihydrodiol of benzo[a]pyrene was shown to be further metabolized to a product or products that reacted extensively with DNA.[77] Booth and Sims[34] demonstrated the formation of a vicinal diol-epoxide, the 8,9-diol-10,11-epoxide of benz[a]anthracene, by the action on microsomal mono-oxygenases on the olefinic double bond of the *trans*-8,9-dihydrodiol (see Section II), and Swaisland et al.[140] showed that when this diol-epoxide was allowed to react with DNA in solution, among the hydrolysis products were hydrocarbon-nucleosides possessing chromatographic properties on Sephadex LH20® similar to those of the hydrocarbon-DNA adducts obtained from hamster embryo cells that had been treated in culture with benz[a]anthracene. Other vicinal diol-epoxides of benz[a]anthracene, for example, those formed on the 1,2,3,4-ring, were not then available for comparison in this study. Sims et al.[78] then showed that the hydrolysis products of DNA that were allowed to react with the 7,8-diol-9,10-epoxide of benzo[a]pyrene coeluted from Sephadex LH20® columns with the hydrolysis products of the DNA isolated from cells treated with the parent hydrocarbon. The synthetic diol-epoxide was obtained by treating the *trans*-7,8-dihydrodiol, a metabolite isolated from the microsomal incubation of benzo[a]pyrene, with *m*-chloroperoxybenzoic acid; although the stereochemistry of this diol-epoxide was not then known, it was subsequently shown to be the *anti*-isomer.[43]

B. Metabolic Activation of Benzo[a]pyrene

The low levels of reactions between nucleic acids and polycyclic hydrocarbons in vivo (one hydrocarbon molecule per 10^4 to 10^5 nucleotides) necessitate the use of very sensitive detection methods. One such technique (already discussed in detail in Volume

I, Chapter 4) employs an extremely sensitive phonton-counting spectrophotofluorimeter to compare the fluorescence spectra of DNA isolated from cells or tissues treated with polycyclic hydrocarbons with those of DNA modified by chemical reactions with hydrocarbon derivatives in solution. Using this technique, Daudel et al.[141] have shown that benzo[a]pyrene retains an intact pyrene nucleus when bound to DNA in mouse skin, a finding that is consistent with the formation of a diol-epoxide in the 7,8,9,10-ring lvanovic et al.[142] confirmed this by low temperature fluorescence spectroscopy using a conventional spectrophotofluorimeter: at low temperatures the quenching processes were considerably reduced and allowed the detection of the fluorescence emission of DNA-bound benzo[a]pyrene isolated from hamster embryo cells.

Although fluorescence studies give useful information about which ring of a polycyclic hydrocarbon is involved in metabolic activation, they do not distinguish the actual sites of reaction. For example, in the case of the diol-epoxides derived from benzo[a]pyrene, the reaction products formed both from DNA and a 7,8-diol-9,10-epoxide and from DNA and a 9,10-diol-7,8-epoxide retain the same pyrene aromatic nucleus, and therefore have identical fluorescence spectra.

Grover et al.[80] obtained [³H]-labeled *trans*-dihydrodiol metabolites from large scale incubations of [³H]-labeled benzo[a]pyrene with rat liver preparations and applied them to mouse skin, a tissue in which benzo[a]pyrene is carcinogenic. After 24 hr, the mice were killed and the epidermal DNA isolated, hydrolyzed, and the nucleosides chromatographed on Sephadex LH20® columns. The 7,8-dihydrodiol gave rise to hydrocarbon-nucleosides indistinguishable in their chromatographic properties from those arising from the reaction of the 7,8-diol-9,10-epoxide with DNA in solution; the 4,5- and 9,10-dihydrodiols failed to yield hydrocarbon-nucleosides. The 4,5-dihydrodiol, being a K-region derivative, cannot give rise to a simple vicinal diol-epoxide because it lacks an olefinic bond adjacent to the diol grouping. Although K-region dihydrodiols can be further metabolized by microsomal oxidation on other double bonds to give nonvicinal diol-epoxides that can give rise to glutathione conjugates,[143] there is no evidence to suggest that these types of nonvicinal diol-epoxides are involved in the metabolic activation of the parent hydrocarbons. The 9,10-dihydrodiol is probably largely metabolized by a pathway that does not involve the formation of a diol-epoxide (see Section II), and this may account, at least in part, for its failure to yield hydrocarbon-nucleoside products in vivo.

King et al.[144] investigated the reaction between the *syn*- and *anti*-isomers of the 7,8-diol-9,10-epoxide of benzo[a]pyrene and DNA and showed that the use of borate buffer in place of water in the solvent gradient used to elute Sephadex LH20® columns enabled the hydrolyzed hydrocarbon-DNA products obtained from the two isomers to be separated. They reported that the microsome-mediated binding to DNA of the *trans*-7,8-dihydrodiol involved exclusively the *anti*-diol-epoxide and that benzo[a]-pyrene binding to DNA in baby hamster kidney cells involved predominantly the *anti*-diol-epoxide. Baird and Diamond[145] also used borate buffer in column eluants, but they found that the nature of the benzo[a]pyrene-DNA adducts isolated from hamster embryo cells depended on the length of time that the cells were exposed to the hydrocarbon; after 4 hr the adducts resulted from the reaction of the *syn*-isomer, but after 24 hr or longer most of the adducts resulted from the reaction of the *anti*-isomer with cellular DNA. Remsen et al.[146] have also demonstrated the formation of benzo-[a]pyrene-DNA adducts derived from both isomers in mouse embryo fibroblasts after their treatment with benzo[a]pyrene, and both isomers are reported to be involved in the binding of the hydrocarbon to the DNA of mouse skin.[147]

Several research groups have investigated the structures of the nucleic acid adducts formed when benzo[a]pyrene is incubated with mammalian tissues in culture. Thus, Weinstein et al.[148] found that when benzo[a]pyrene was incubated with cultured bovine bronchial mucosa, one of the major adducts formed with RNA was identical to the product formed in the chemical reaction of the *anti*-7,8-diol-9,10-epoxide with poly(G) as shown by an examination of the ribonucleoside derivatives obtained by hydrolysis of the polymers. Thus, diol-epoxides, in common with simple epoxides,[119] show a greater reactivity towards poly(G) than towards other polyribonucleotides.[149,150] Jeffrey et al.[151] deduced from circular dichroism and from NMR spectra that the adduct is formed by covalent bonding between the 10 position of the diol-epoxide and the 2-amino group of guanine. The absolute configuration of this adduct was established by Weinstein and colleagues,[152] and the adduct was shown to be derived initially from the (−)-enantiomer of the *trans*-7,8-dihydrodiol and to have the structure shown in Figure 6. Both Yagi et al.[153] and Yang et al.[48,52] have also assigned absolute configurations to the dihydrodiol and to the diol-epoxide intermediates.

Koreeda et al.[154] reported that the alkylation of poly(G) by the *syn*-7,8-diol-9,10-epoxide also involved the 2-amino group of guanine and the 10 position of the hydrocarbon derivative. The diol-epoxide was sufficiently reactive to alkyate inorganic phosphate, and minor products of the reaction of the diol-epoxide with poly(G) had properties that suggested that the alkylation of the phosphodiester linkages of poly(G) first produced labile phosphotriesters. A later report[147] indicated that the *anti*-isomer could also alkylate phosphate groups. Both the *syn*- and *anti*-diol-epoxide isomers caused strand scission in superhelical DNA in vitro;[155] kinetic analysis of this minor reaction, which accounts for less than 1% of the DNA modification by diol-epoxide, implicates the formation of phosphotriesters, hydrolysis of which would cause the DNA strand to be cleaved.

The reactions of the diol-epoxides with DNA have not been characterized fully, although Osborne et al.[256] have proposed a structure for the reaction of the *anti*-isomer with DNA analogous to that described for the RNA adduct.[152] Meehan et al.[157] found that 92% of the reaction of the *anti*-diol-epoxide with DNA involved covalent interaction of the diol-epoxide with deoxyguanosine, with minor reaction occurring with deoxyadenosine and deoxycytidine, and they also provided evidence that the optical enantiomers present in the racemic mixture of the diol-epoxide used did not react with DNA to the same extent. The mass spectrum of the main deoxyguanosine adduct was consistent with a structure in which the 2-amino group of the base is attached to the 10 position of the hydrocarbon. Jeffrey et al.[158] have compared the RNA and DNA adducts formed in the treatment of human bronchial explants with benzo[a]pyrene. Metabolic activation of benzo[a]pyrene in this tissue is particularly relevant as polycyclic hydrocarbons are suspected of being carcinogenic in the human respiratory tract, and Grover et al.[80] have shown that benzo[a]pyrene becomes bound to DNA in human bronchial mucosa by a similar mechanism to that in mouse skin where the hydrocarbon is known to be active. High-pressure liquid chromatographic analysis of the RNA adducts obtained from human bronchial epithelium revealed profiles consisting of four

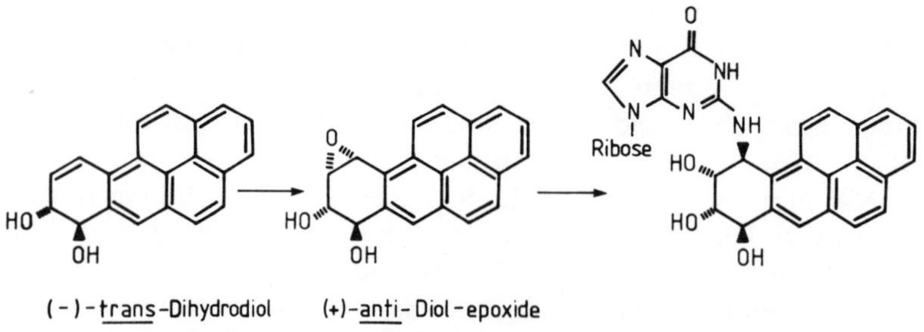

(−)-*trans*-Dihydrodiol   (+)-*anti*-Diol-epoxide

FIGURE 6.   The formation of the benzo[a]pyrene-guanine adduct in vivo, deriving from a single enantiomer of the 7,8-dihydrodiol.

distinct product peaks similar to the profile obtained in the analysis of samples derived from bovine bronchial tissue.[148] The chromatographic profiles of the DNA adducts obtained both from bovine and human tissues were simpler: in both cases, most of the products formed a single peak that cochromatographed with one of the adducts derived from the reaction of poly(dG) with the *anti*-7,8-diol-9,10-epoxide. The authors suggest several reasons for the greater heterogeneity of RNA adducts: either that the double-stranded nature of DNA may make its modification more selective, that the greater reactivity of the *syn*-diol-epoxide compared to the *anti*-isomers[41] may prevent them reaching the nuclear-DNA from the cytoplasm, or that a more stereospecific nuclear mono-oxygenase system may be responsible for the biosynthesis of the reactive metabolites in the nucleus. The failure to obtain DNA adducts derived from the *syn*-diol-epoxide may also be related to the length of time of exposure of the tissue to the hydrocarbon, since experiments with hamster embryo cells indicated that there may be adducts formed from the *syn*-isomer shortly after exposure that are rapidly excised and therefore not found at later times.[145]

There are considerable biological data supporting the involvement of a 7,8-diol-9,10-epoxide of benzo[a]pyrene in the metabolic activation of this hydrocarbon. Carcinogenicity studies have shown that the 7,8-epoxide[159] and the 7,8-dihydrodiol[160-163] of benzo[a]pyrene, both of which are intermediates in the formation of the 7,8-diol-9,10-epoxides, are active when applied to mouse skin. The *trans*-7,8-dihydrodiol and the *anti*-isomer of the diol-epoxide are highly active as carcinogens in newborn mice when administered i.p.,[164] however, the *anti*- and *syn*-isomers are inactive and weakly active, respectively, as carcinogens when applied topically to the skin of adult mice.[163] The high chemical reactivity of the diol-epoxides may account for their lack of significant carcinogenic activity on mouse skin.

Transformation studies in M2 mouse fibroblasts[165] and hamster embryo cells[166] have indicated that the *trans*-7,8-dihydrodiol is more active in inducing malignant transformations than benzo[a]pyrene itself. The dihydrodiol is also more mutagenic than benzo[a]pyrene in *S. typhimurium* TA 98 in the presence of rat liver microsomal fractions.[167]

Mutagenicity studies on the diol-epoxides themselves indicate that the *anti*-7,8-diol-9,10-epoxide is a more potent mutagen than the *syn*-isomer in V79 Chinese hamster cells,[60,168-170] while the reverse is the case in strains of *S. typhimurium*.[169,171]

In all of these biological studies, racemic mixtures of compounds were tested. It has since been demonstrated by Levin et al.[35] that the (−)-*trans*-7,8-dihydrodiol is much more potent as a tumor initiator on mouse skin than the corresponding (+)-enantiomer, and Wood et al.[36] have shown that there are differences in mutagenic activity among the optical enantiomers of the 7,8-diol-9,10-epoxides; the (+)-enantiomer of the *anti*-diol-epoxide and the (−)-enantiomer of the *syn*-diol-epoxide, both of which are derived from the (−)-*trans*-7,8-dihydrodiol, are more mutagenic in V79 cells and *S. typhimurium* TA 98 and TA 100 than their respective optical enantiomers.

C. Extension of the Diol-Epoxide Hypothesis to Other Polycyclic Hydrocarbons

The results of the investigations of the role of a diol-epoxide in the metabolic activation of benzo[a]pyrene have led to generalizations that can be applied to other polycyclic aromatic hydrocarbons. A feature of the 7,8-diol-9,10-epoxide of benzo[a]pyrene is the presence of an epoxide on a saturated, angular benzo-ring which forms part of the bay-region of the hydrocarbon (see Figure 1). It has been proposed[172] that such an entity is of structural importance in the mutagenicity and carcinogenicity of polycyclic hydrocarbons, and quantum mechanical calculations have predicted that, for a given hydrocarbon, bay-region carbonium ions on saturated angular benzo-rings should be more easily formed than non-bay-region carbonium ions.[173] Furthermore, the effect of substituents such as fluorine atoms that might be expected to hinder the formation of bay-region carbonium ions is to reduce the carcinogenicity of a given aromatic polycyclic ring system.[172] Metabolic formation of a dihydrodiol at the two carbon atoms most distant from the bay-region of an angular benzo-ring, e.g., at positions 7 and 8 of benzo[a]pyrene, would provide a nonaromatic (olefinic) double bond, the vicinal 9,10-bond in the case of the 7,8-dihydrodiol of benzo[a]pyrene, at the bay-region where epoxide formation can then take place.[78]

Both the importance of saturation of the benzo-ring and of the formation of an epoxide at the bay-region have been demonstrated by several studies. Benzo[a]pyrene 9,10-oxide (a bay-region epoxide in which the benzo-ring is unsaturated) is only weakly mutagenic in strains of *S. typhimurium*,[174] while the 7,8,9,10-tetrahydro-9,10-epoxide has a mutagenic activity comparable with that of the *syn*-7,8-diol-9,10-epoxide;[169] the *anti*-7,8-diol-9,10-epoxide is more reactive towards DNA in aqueous solution than is the isomeric non-bay-region diol-epoxide, *anti*-9,10-diol-7,8-epoxide,[150] and the former was also more active in inducing mutations[170,171] and malignant transformations[170] in mammalian cells.

Whether or not the diol-epoxide[78] and bay-region[172] hypotheses have a general application to other polycyclic hydrocarbons remains to be established, but the state of knowledge of the metabolic activation of benz[a]anthracene, 7-methyl-benz[a]anthracene, 7,12-dimethylbenz[a]anthracene, and 3-methylcholanthrene will be described with reference to these working hypotheses.

D. Metabolic Activation of Benz[a]anthracene

Studies on the five possible *trans*-dihydrodiols of of benz[a]anthracene have shown that the 3,4-dihydrodiol is metabolized by a highly purified mono-oxygenase system to products that are ten times more mutagenic in *S. typhimurium* TA 100 than are the metabolites of benz[a]anthracene or the other four dihydrodiols.[175] Also, the 3,4-dihydrodiol is 10 to 20-fold more active in initiating tumors in mouse skin than is benz[a]anthracene, while the other dihydrodiols are less active than the hydrocarbon.[176] The *syn*- and *anti*-isomers of the 3,4-diol-1,2-epoxide, which possess epoxide groups adjacent to the bay-region, are several times more mutagenic in *S. typhimurium* TA 100 and V79 Chinese hamster cells than the correponding isomers of the non-bay-region 8,9-diol-10,11-epoxides or 10,11-diol-8,9-epoxides.[177] These studies suggest that one or both of the 3,4-diol-1,2-epoxides of benz[a]anthracene are the ultimately reactive forms of this hydrocarbon. In contrast, an earlier report by Swaisland et al.[140] showed that the hydrocarbon-nucleoside adducts from DNA that had been reacted with the *anti*-8,9-diol-10,11-epoxide of benz[a]anthracene eluted from Sephadex LH20® columns in the same fractions as the [³H]-labeled nucleoside adducts from the DNA of cells treated with [³H])-labeled benz[a]anthracene. Also the 8,9-dihydrodiol was more mutagenic than the parent hydrocarbon in *S. typhimurium* TA 100 in the presence of microsomal fractions of rat liver, and the *anti*- 8,9-diol-10,11-epoxide was mutagenic without further metabolism.[167] However, the hydrocarbon-nucleoside adducts formed when the other diol-epoxides are allowed to react with DNA may also elute in the same fractions as those derived from the *anti*-8,9-diol-10,11-epoxide; the study of Tierney et al.[27] on 7-methylbenz[a]anthracene (see Section VI. E) has indicated that Sephadex LH20® chromatography does not appear to give good resolution of hydrocarbon-nucleoside adducts formed from diol-epoxides derived from positionally isomeric dihydrodiols.

E. Metabolic Activation of 7-Methylbenz[a]anthracene

Fluorescence spectral studies, of the type described in Volume I, Chapter 4, on the mechanism of the activation of 7-methylbenz[a]anthracene in mouse skin and hamster embryo cells show that the hydrocarbon moiety bound to DNA retains an anthracene-rather than a phenanthrene-type aromatic nucleus, indicating that the 1,2,3,4-ring is involved in metabolic activation.[178] Tierney et al.[27] detected all five possible *trans*-dihydrodiols, the 1,2-, 3,4-, 5,6-, 8,9-, and 10,11-compounds, as metabolites of 7-methylbenz[a]anthracene in mouse skin, and investigated their roles, together with those of the related vicinal diol-epoxides, in the metabolic activation of the parent hydrocarbon in mouse skin. The application to mouse skin of [³H]-labeled samples of either the 1,2- or the 3,4-dihydrodiol resulted in their reaction with DNA and, after hydrolysis of the DNA, in the detection of [³H]-labeled nucleoside products; the chromatographic properties of these products were similar to those of the products resulting from application of the parent hydrocarbon; no [³H]-labeled nucleoside products were isolated following the application of the [³H]-labeled 8,9-dihydrodiol. These results are consistent with the 1,2,3,4-ring being involved in the metabolic activation of 7-methylbenz-[a]anthracene, but unequivocable data as to which of the related vicinal diol-epoxides, the 1,2-diol-3,4-epoxide or the 3,4-diol-1,2-epoxide, is the reactive intermediate in vivo, were not obtained; products believed to be the *anti*-isomers of both synthetic diol-epoxides, when allowed to react with DNA in solution, gave rise to UV-absorbing nucleoside adducts that were inseparable by Sephadex LH20® chromatography from the [³H]-labeled nucleoside adducts that were obtained from the hydrolysates of the DNA from mouse skin treated with [³H]-7-methylbenz[a]anthracene in vivo.

In studies on microsome-mediated mutagenesis in *S. typhimurium* TA 98, the 3,4-dihydrodiol of 7-methylbenz[a]anthracene was more active than either the parent hydrocarbon or the 1,2-, 5,6-, and 8,9-dihydrodiols.[179] The 3,4-dihydrodiol was also more active than the hydrocarbon and these other dihydrodiols in inducing mutations in V79 Chinese hamster cells and in inducing malignant transformation in M2 mouse fibroblasts.[180] Also, the 3,4-dihydrodiol has a higher tumor-initiating activity on mouse skin than 7-methylbenz[a]anthracene, while of the other dihydrodiols tested, the 8,9- is only weakly active and the 1,2- and 5,6-dihydrodiols are almost inactive.[181] These results, taken in conjunction with the studies on DNA binding in mouse skin,[27,178] suggest that metabolic activation of 7-methylbenz[a]anthracene most likely involves the formation of a 3,4-diol-1,2-epoxide, a conclusion consistent with both the diol-epoxide and the bay-region hypotheses.

F. Metabolic Activation of 7,12-Dimethylbenz[a]anthracene

The metabolic activation of 7,12-dimethylbenz[a]anthracene, the most potent carcinogen in the benz[a]anthracene series, has, by comparison, been little studied. Baird and Dipple[182] compared the photosensitivity of the products that are bound to DNA when the hydrocarbon is incubated with hamster embryo cell cultures with the photosensitivity of various model compounds. The DNA-bound products, 9,10-dimethylanthracene and 7,12-dimethylbenz[a]anthracene itself, were all photosensitive under conditions in which the 5,6-dihydro and 8,9,10,11-tetrahydro derivatives of the carcinogen were not; this suggests that when 7,12-dimethylbenz[a]anthracene becomes bound to DNA in cells, it either retains the aromatic benz[a]anthracene nucleus or is metabolically activated in the 1,2,3,4-ring, thus retaining an aromatic anthracene nucleus. Vigny et al.[183] have studied the fluorescence emission spectrum of the hydrocarbon bound to the DNA of mouse skin and found it to be characteristic of a substituted anthracene nucleus, implying that activation of the 1,2,3,4-ring had occurred. Moschel et al.[184] reached the same conclusion from an examination of the fluorescence excitation and emission spectra of the hydrocarbon-nucleoside adducts, separated by Sephadex LH20® chromatography from hydrolysates of the DNA isolated from 7,12-dimethylbenz[a]anthracene-treated mouse embryo cells. Furthermore, these adducts displayed similar susceptibilities to acid hydrolysis as those found for the products of reaction of poly(G) with a vicinal diol-epoxide of benzo[a]pyrene.[154] The 1,2,3,4-ring of 7,12-dimethylbenz[a]anthracene is an angular benzo-ring of the type required to support the bay-region hypothesis, but these studies do not of themselves show whether, if indeed a vicinal diol-epoxide is involved, it is a bay region 3,4-diol-1,2-epoxide or an isomeric non-bay-region 1,2-diol-3,4-epoxide that is the metabolically generated reactive intermediate. Blackburn et al.[185] found that when 7,12-dimethylbenz[a]anthracene, specifically labeled with tritium in the 7-methyl group, becomes bound to DNA in an in vivo system, some of this radioactive labeling was displaced. Ivanovic et al.[186] have therefore proposed that metabolism of the 7-methyl group to a hydroxymethyl group may precede metabolic activation in the 1,2,3,4-ring. The metabolism of methyl groups to hydroxymethyl groups in 7,12-dimethylbenz[a]anthracene is well established.[187]

G. Metabolic Activation of 3-Methylcholanthrene

Two studies on the metabolic activation of 3-methylcholanthrene have been reported. In one, Vigny et al.[183] painted the skin of mice with the hydrocarbon, the DNA was isolated and purified, and its fluorescence spectrum examined (as described in Volume I, Chapter 4). The spectrum resembled that of anthracene rather than that of phenanthrene, thus indicating the involvement of the 7,8,9,10-ring of 3-methylcholanthrene in the interactions with the nucleic acid. This ring is the angular benzo-ring equivalent to the 1,2,3,4-ring of benz[a]anthracene and its methyl derivatives (see Figure 1).

The second study by King et al.[188] was carried out in mouse embryo cells in culture. The DNA obtained from these cells after they had been treated with 3-methylcholanthrene was hydrolyzed enzymically to deoxyribonucleosides and the hydrolysate fractionated by Sephadex LH20® and high-pressure liquid chromatography to give five hydrocarbon-nucleoside products. Metabolites tentatively identified as the 9,10-dihydrodiol and one of its hydroxylated derivatives were obtained from microsomal incubations of the hydrocarbon, and these were further metabolized in the presence of DNA. Hydrolysis of this DNA yielded modified nucleosides that were identified in their chromatographic properties with some of the products obtained from the embryo cells. The fluorescence spectra of the products from both sources were similar and showed that they were all probably derived either from the 9,10-diol-7,8-epoxide or from its hydroxylated derivatives. It was also shown that the K-region epoxide, 3-methylcholanthrene 11,12-oxide was not involved in the reactions of the hydrocarbon with the DNA of mouse embryo cells. The results thus indicate that in common with the other hydrocarbons so far investigated, it is the bay-region diol-epoxide that reacts with the DNA of cells treated with the parent hydrocarbon.

VII. CONCLUSIONS

With benzo[a]pyrene, the evidence now seems quite clear that:

1. The reactive intermediates that are involved in the reactions with nucleic acids when tissues are treated with the hydrocarbon are diol-epoxides.
2. The diol-epoxides involved are the 7,8-diol-9,10-epoxides rather than the isomeric 9,10-diol-7,8-epoxides.
3. The *anti*-isomer of the 7,8-diol-9,10-epoxide is the isomer most concerned in these reactions, although some involvement of the *syn*-isomer seems likely.
4. The diol-epoxides involved in the reactions with nucleic acids are bay-region epoxides, and these are more reactive chemically than non-bay-region epoxides.
5. The biological activities of the bay-region diol-epoxides or of the dihydrodiol that can give rise to the bay-region diol-epoxides by metabolism are greater than non-bay-region diol-epoxides or their parent dihydrodiol.

With the isomeric 7,8-diol-9,10-epoxides of benzo[a]pyrene, the *syn*-isomer is the most active as a mutagen in bacterial systems and the *anti*-isomer the most active in mammalian systems, but the reason for these differences in biological activities is not clear.

Other hydrocarbons have not been studied in such detail, but with benz-[a]anthracene, 7-methylbenz[a]anthracene, 7,12-dimethylbenz[a]anthracene, and 3-methylcholanthrene the available evidence suggests that it is the bay-region epoxides that are involved in the reactions with nucleic acids that occur in treated tissues. With benz[a]anthracene and 7-methylbenz[a]anthracene, the dihydrodiols that can give rise to bay-region epoxides are the most active in biological systems.

It is clear that, at least with benzo[a]pyrene derivatives, the (−)-enantiomer of the 7,8-dihydrodiol, the enantiomer that is formed by metabolism, is more active biologically than the (+)-enantiomer. If the biological effects are initiated by the reactions with nucleic acids of one or the other of the optically active diol-epoxides derived from the (−)-dihydrodiol, then the differential effects are not unexpected since they would arise from reactions in which both electrophile and nucleophile have chiral centers. It should also be pointed out that the in vivo reaction of hydrocarbons with nucleic acids so far described involves the whole of the RNA or DNA present in a particular tissue. It is therefore not possible to directly link these observed interactions with the induction of the biological events, since these events occur in only a small proportion of the cells being treated.

REFERENCES

1. Heidelberger, C. and Davenport, G. R., Local functional components of carcinogenesis, *Acta Unio Int. Contra Cancrum.*, 17, 55, 1961.
2. Brookes, P. and Lawley, P. D., Evidence for the binding of polynuclear aromatic hydrocarbons to the nucleic acids of mouse skin: relation between carcinogenic power of hydrocarbons and their binding to deoxyribonucleic acid, *Nature (London)*, 202, 781, 1964.
3. Goshman, L. M. and Heidelberger, C., Binding of tritium-labeled polycyclic hydrocarbons to DNA of mouse skin, *Cancer Res.*, 27, 1678, 1967.
4. Diamond, L., Defendi, V., and Brookes, P., The interaction of 7,12-dimethylbenz[a]anthracene with cells sensitive and resistant to toxicity induced by this carcinogen, *Cancer Res.*, 27, 890, 1967.
5. Brookes, P. and Heidelberger, C., Isolation and degradation of DNA from cells treated with tritium-labeled 7,12-dimethylbenz[a]anthracene: studies on the nature of the binding of this carcinogen to DNA, *Cancer Res.*, 29, 157, 1969.
6. Grover, P. L. and Sims, P., Enzyme-catalyzed reactions of polycyclic hydrocarbons with deoxyribonucleic acid and protein in vitro, *Biochem. J.*, 110, 159, 1968.
7. Gelboin, H. V., A microsome-dependent binding of benzo[a]pyrene to DNA, *Cancer Res.* 29, 1272, 1969.
8. Sims, P. and Grover, P. L., Epoxides in polycyclic aromatic hydrocarbon metabolism and carcinogenesis, *Adv. Cancer Res.*, 20, 165, 1974.
9. Holder, G., Yagi, H., Dansette, P., Jerina, D. M., Levin, W., Lu, A. Y. H., and Conney, A. H., Effects of inducers and epoxide hydrase on the metabolism of benzo[a]pyrene by liver microsomes and a reconstituted system: analysis by high pressure liquid chromatography, *Proc. Natl. Acad. Sci. U.S.A.*, 71, 4356, 1974.
10. Selkirk, J. K., Croy, R. G., Roller, P. P., and Gelboin, H. V., High-pressure liquid chromatographic analysis of benzo[a]pyrene metabolism and covalent binding and the mechanism of action of 7,8-benzoflavone and 1,2-epoxy-3,3,3-trichloropropane, *Cancer Res.*, 34, 3474, 1974.
11. Yang, S. K., Selkirk, J. K., Plotkin, E. V., and Gelboin, H. V., Kinetic analysis of the metabolism of benzo[a]pyrene to phenols, dihydrodiols, and quinones by high-pressure chromatography compared to analysis by aryl hydrocarbon hydroxylase assay, and the effect of enzyme induction, *Cancer Res.*, 35, 3642, 1975.

12. Holder, G. M., Yagi, H., Jerina, D. M., Levin,W., Lu, A. Y. H., and Conney, A. H., Metabolism of benzo[a]pyrene. Effect of substrate concentration and 3-methylcholanthrene pretreatment on hepatic metabolism by microsomes from rats and mice, *Arch. Biochem. Biophys.,* 170, 557, 1975.

13. Hundley, S. G. and Freudenthal, R. I., High-pressure liquid chromatography analysis of benzo[a]pyrene metabolism by microsomal enzymes from Rhesus liver and lung, *Cancer Res.,* 37, 244, 1977.

14. Selkirk, J. K., Croy, R. G., Whitlock, J. P. Jr., and Gelboin, H. V., *In vitro* metabolism of benzo-[a]pyrene by human liver microsomes and lymphocytes, *Cancer Res.,* 35, 3651, 1975.

15. Bresnick, E., Stoming, T. A., Vaught, J. B., Thakker, D. R., and Jerina, D.M., Nuclear metabolism of benzo[a]pyrene and of (±)-trans-7,8-dihydroxy-7,8-dihydrobenzo[a]pyrene. Comparative chromatographic analysis of alkylated DNA, *Arch. Biochem. Biophys.,* 183, 31, 1977.

16. Seifried, H. E., Birkett, D. J., Levin, W., Lu, A. Y. H., Conney, A. H., and Jerina, D. M., Metabolism of benzo[a]pyrene. Effect of 3-methylcholanthrene pretreatment on metabolism by microsomes from lungs of genetically "responsive" and "nonresponsive" mice, *Arch. Biochem. Biophys.,* 178, 256, 1977.

17. Selkirk, J. K., Croy, R. G., Wiebel, F. J., and Gelboin, H. V., Differences in benzo[a]pyrene metabolism between rodent liver microsomes and embyronic cells, *Cancer Res.,* 36, 4476, 1976.

18. Fox, C. H., Selkirk, J. K., Price, F. M., Croy, R. G., Sanford, K. K., and Cottler-Fox, M., Metabolism of benzo[a]pyrene by human epithelial cells *in vitro, Cancer Res.,* 35, 3551, 1975.

19. Stohs, S. J., Grafström, R. C., Burke, M. D., and Orrenius, S., Benzo[a]pyrene metabolism by isolated rat intestinal epithelial cells, *Arch. Biochem. Biophys.,* 179, 71, 1977.

20. Berry, D. L., Bracken, W. R., Slaga, T. J., Wilson, N. M., Butty, S. G., and Juchau, M. R., Benzo[a]pyrene metabolism in mouse epidermis. Analysis by high pressure liquid chromatography and DNA binding, *Chem. Biol. Interact.,* 18, 129, 1977.

21. Autrup, H., Harris, C. C., Fugaro, S., and Selkirk, J. K., Effect of various chemicals on the metabolism of benzo[a]pyrene by cultured rat colon, *Chem. Biol. Interact.,* 18, 337, 1977.

22. Harris, C. C., Autrup, H., Stoner, G., Yang, S. K., Leutz, J. C., Gelboin, H. V., Selkirk, J. K., Connor, R. J., Barrett, L. A., Jones, R. T., McDowell, E., and Trump, B. F., Metabolism of benzo[a]pyrene and 7,12-dimethylbenz[a] anthracene in cultured human bronchus and pancreatic duct, *Cancer Res.,* 37, 3349, 1977.

23. Cohen, G. M., Haws, S. M., Moore, B. P., and Bridges, J. W., Benzo[a]pyren-3-yl hydrogen sulphate, a major ethyl acetate-extractable metabolite of benzo[a]pyrene in human, hamster and rat lung cultures, *Biochem. Pharmacol.,* 25, 2561, 1976.

24. Cohen, G. M. and Moore, B. P., Metabolism of [³H]benzo[a]pyrene by different portions of the respiratory tract, *Biochem. Pharmacol.,* 25, 1623, 1976.

25. Gentil, A., Lasne, C., and Chouroulinkov, I., Metabolism of 7,12-dimethylbenz[a]anthracene by hamster liver homogenates, *Xenobiotica,* 4, 537, 1974.

26. Yang, S. K. and Dower, W. V., Metabolic pathways of 7,12-dimethylbenz[a]anthracene in hepatic microsomes, *Proc. Natl. Acad. Sci. U.S.A.,* 72, 2601, 1975.

27. Tierney, B., Hewer, A., Walsh, C., Grover, P. L., and Sims, P., The metabolic activation of 7-methylbenz[a]anthracene in mouse skin, *Chem. Biol. Interact.,* 18, 179, 1977.

28. Boyland, E., The biological significance of metabolism of polycyclic compounds, *Biochem. Soc. Symp.,* 5, 40, 1950.

29. Yang, S. K., Roller, P. P., Fu, P. P., Harvey, R. G., and Gelboin, H. V., Evidence for a 2,3-epoxide as an intermediate in the microsomal metabolism of benzo[a]pyrene to 3-hydroxybenzo[a]pyrene, *Biochem. Biophys. Res. Commun.,* 77, 1176, 1977.

30. Newman, M. S. and Blum, S., A new cyclization reaction leading to epoxides of aromatic hydrocarbons, *J. Am. Chem. Soc.,* 86, 5598, 1964.

31. Goh, S. H. and Harvey, R. G., K-Region arene oxides of carcinogenic aromatic hydrocarbons, *J. Am. Chem. Soc.,* 95, 242, 1973.

32. Dansette, P. and Jerina, D. M., A facile synthesis of arene oxides at the K regions of polycyclic hydrocarbons, *J. Am. Chem. Soc.,* 96, 1224, 1974.

33. Oesch, F., Mammalian epoxide hydrases: inducible enzymes catalysing the inactivation of carcinogenic and cytotoxic metabolites derived from aromatic and olefinic compounds, *Xenobiotica,* 3, 305, 1973.

34. Booth, J. and Sims, P., 8,9-Dihydro-8,9-dihydroxybenz[a]anthracene-10,11-oxide: a new type of polycyclic aromatic hydrocarbon metabolite, *FEBS Lett.,* 47, 30, 1974.

35. Levin, W., Wood, A. W., Chang, R. L., Slaga, T. J., Yagi, H., Jerina, D. M., and Conney, A. H., Marked differences in the tumor-initiating activity of optically pure (+)- and (−)-*trans*-7,8-dihydroxy-7,8-dihydrobenzo[a]-pyrene on mouse skin, *Cancer Res.,* 37, 2721, 1977.

36. Wood, A. W., Chang, R. L., Levin, W., Yagi, H., Thakker, D. R., Jerina, D. M., and Conney, A. H., Differences in mutagenicity of the optical enantiomers of the diastereomeric benzo[a]pyrene 7,8-diol-9,10-epoxides, *Biochem. Biophys. Res. Commun.,* 77, 1389, 1977.

37. McCaustland, D. J., Fischer, D. L., Kolwyck, K. C., Duncan, W. P., Wiley, J. C., Menon, C. S., Engel, J. F., Selkirk, J. K., and Roller, P. P., Polycyclic aromatic hydrocarbon derivatives: synthesis and physiochemical characterization, in *Carcinogenesis*, Vol. 1, Freudenthal, R. I. and Jones, P. W., Eds., Raven Press, New York, 1976, 349.

38. Lehr, R. E., Schaefer-Ridder, M., and Jerina, D. M., Synthesis and properties of the vicinal trans dihydrodiols of anthracene, phenanthrene, and benzo[a]anthracene, *J. Org. Chem.*, 42, 736, 1977.

39. Fu, P. P. and Harvey, R. G., Synthesis of the diols and diolepoxides of carcinogenic hydrocarbons, *Tetrahedron Lett.*, 2059, 1977.

40. Tierney, B., Abercrombie, B., Walsh, C., Hewer, A., Grover, P. L., and Sims, P., The preparation of dihydrodiols from 7-methylbenz[a]anthracene, *Chem. Biol. Interact.*, 21, 289, 1978.

41. Yagi, H, Hernandez, O., and Jerina, D. M., Synthesis of (±)-7β,8α-dihydroxy-9β,10β-epoxy-7,8,9,10-tetrahydrobenzo[a]pyrene, a potential metabolite of the carcinogen benzo[a]pyrene with stereochemistry related to the antileukemic triptolides, *J. Am. Chem. Soc.*, 97, 6881, 1975.

42. McCaustland, D. J., Duncan, W. P., and Engel, J. F., Labeled metabolites of polycyclic aromatic hydrocarbons. V. *trans*-7,8-Dihydrobenzo[a]-pyrene-7,8-diol-^{14}C and (±)-7α,8β-dihydroxy-9β,10β-epoxy-7,8,9,10-tetrahydrobenzo[-a-]pyrene-7-^{14}C, *J. Labelled Compd.*, 12, 442, 1976.

43. Beland, F. A. and Harvey, R. G., The isomeric 9,10-oxides of *trans*-7,8-dihydroxy-7,8-dihydrobenzo[a]pyrene, *J. Chem. Soc. Chem. Commun.*, 84, 1976.

44. Yagi, H., Thakker, D. R., Hernandez, O., Koreeda, M., and Jerina, D. M., Synthesis and reactions of the highly mutagenic 7,8-diol 9,10-epoxides of the carcinogen benzo[a]pyrene, *J. Am. Chem. Soc.*, 99, 1604, 1977.

45. Lehr, R. E., Schaefer-Ridder, M., and Jerina, D. M., Synthesis and reactivity of diol epoxides derived from non-K-region *trans*-dihydrodiols of benzo[a]anthracene, *Tetrahedron Lett.*, 539, 1977.

46. McCaustland, D. J. and Engel, J. F., Metabolites of polycyclic aromatic hydrocarbons. II. Synthesis of 7,8-dihydrobenzo[a]pyrene-7,8-diol and 7,8-dihydrobenzo[a]pyrene-7,8-epoxide, *Tetrahedron Lett.*, 2549, 1975.

47. Yagi, H. and Jerina, D. M., A general synthetic method for non-K-region arene oxides, *J. Am. Chem. Soc.*, 97, 3185, 1975.

48. Yang, S. K. and Gelboin, H. V., Microsomal mixed-function oxidases and opoxide hydratase convert benzo[a]pyrene stereospecifically to optically active dihydroxydihydrobenzo[a]pyrenes, *Biochem. Pharmacol.*, 25, 2221, 1976.

49. Thakker, D. R., Yagi, H., Akagi, H., Koreeda, M., Lu, A. Y. H., Levin, W., Wood, A. W., Conney, A. H., and Jerina, D. M., Metabolism of benzo[a]pyrene. VI. Stereoselective metabolism of benzo[a]pyrene and benzo[a]pyrene 7,8-dihydrodiol to diol epoxides, *Chem. Biol. Interact.*, 16, 281, 1977.

50. Yang, S. K., Gelboin, H. V., Weber, J. D., Sankaran, V., Fischer, D. L., and Engel, J. F., Resolution of optical isomers by high pressure liquid chromatography. The separation of benzo[a]pyrene *trans*-diol derivatives, *Anal. Biochem.*, 78, 520, 1977.

51. Harvey, R. G. and Cho, H., Efficient resolution of the dihydrodiol derivatives of benzo[a]pyrene by high-pressure liquid chromatography of the related (−)-dimenthoxyacetates, *Anal. Biochem.*, 80, 540, 1977.

52. Yang, S. K., McCourt, D. W., Leutz, J. C., and Gelboin, H. V., Benzo[a]pyrene diol epoxides: mechanism of enzymatic formation and optically active intermediates, *Science*, 196, 1199, 1977.

53. Yang, S. K., Roller, P. P., and Gelboin, H. V., Enzymatic mechanism of benzo[a]pyrene conversion to phenols and diols and an improved high-pressure liquid chromatographic separation of benzo[a]pyrene derivatives, *Biochemistry*, 16, 3680, 1977.

54. Booth, J. and Sims, P., Different pathways involved in the metabolism of the 7,8- and 9,10-dihydrodiols of benzo[a]pyrene, *Biochem. Pharmacol.*, 25, 979, 1976.

55. Hulbert, P. B., Carbonium ion as ultimate carcinogen of polycyclic aromatic hydrocarbons, *Nature* (London), 256, 146, 1975.

56. Yang, S. K., McCourt, D. W., Gelboin, H. V., Miller, J. R., and Roller, P. P., Stereochemistry of the hydrolysis products and their acetonides of two stereoisomeric benzo[a]pyrene 7,8-diol 9,10-epoxides, *J. Am. Chem. Soc.*, 99, 5124, 1977.

57. Yang, S. K., McCourt, D. W., Roller, P. P., and Gelboin, H. V., Enzymatic conversion of benzo[a]pyrene leading predominantly to the diol-epoxide r-7,t-8-dihydroxy-t-9,10-oxy-7,8,9,10-tetrahydrobenzo[a]pyrene through a single enantiomer of r-7,t-8-dihydroxy-7,8-dihydrobenzo[a]pyrene *Proc. Natl. Acad. Sci. U.S.A.*, 73, 2594, 1976.

58. Keller, J. W., Heidelberger, C., Beland, F. A., and Harvey, R. G., Hydrolysis of *syn*- and *anti*-benzo[a]pyrene diol epoxides: stereochemistry, kinetics, and the effect of an intramolecular hydrogen bond on the rate of *syn*-diol epoxide solvolysis, *J. Am. Chem. Soc.*, 98, 8276, 1976.

59. Whalen, D. L., Montemarano, J. A., Thakker, D. R., Yagi, H., and Jerina, D. M., Changes of mechanisms and product distributions in the hydrolysis of benzo[a]pyrene-7,8-diol 9,10-epoxide metabolites induced by changes in pH, *J. Am. Chem. Soc.*, 99, 5522, 1977.

60. Huberman, E., Sachs, L., Yang, S. K., and Gelboin, H. V., Identification of mutagenic metabolites of benzo[a]pyrene in mammalian cells, *Proc. Natl. Acad. Sci. U.S.A.*, 73, 607, 1976.

61. Thakker, D. R., Yagi, H., Lu, A.Y.H., Levin, W., Conney, A. H., and Jerina, D. M., Metabolism of benzo[a]pyrene: conversion of (±)-*trans*-7,8-dihydroxy-7,8-dihydrobenzo[a]pyrene to highly mutagenic 7,8-diol-9,10-epoxides, *Proc. Natl. Acad. Sci. U.S.A.*, 73, 3381, 1976.

62. Yang, S. K., Gelboin, H. V., Trump, B. F., Autrup, H., and Harris, C. C., Metabolic activation of benzo[a]pyrene and binding to DNA in cultured human bronchus, *Cancer Res.*, 37, 1210, 1977.

63. Yang, S. K., Gelboin, H. V., Nonenzymatic reduction of benzo[a]pyrene diol-epoxides to trihydroxypentahydrobenzo[a]pyrenes by reduced nicotinamide adenine dinucleotide phosphate, *Cancer Res.*, 36, 4185, 1976.

64. Wang, I. Y., Marver, H. S., Rasmussen, R. E., and Crocker, T. T., Enzymatic conversion of benzo[a]pyrene, *Arch. Intern. Med.*, 128, 125, 1971.

65. Hey-Ferguson, A. and Bresnick, E., The binding of 3-methylcholanthrene to macromolecular components of rat liver preparations, *Mol. Pharmacol.*, 7, 183, 1971.

66. Meunier, M. and Chauveau, J., Binding of benzo[a]pyrene metabolite(s) to main and satellite calf thymus DNA's *in vitro*, *FEBS Lett.*, 31, 327, 1973.

67. Bogdan, D. P. and Chmielewicz, Z. F., Studies on interactions between polynucleotides and benzo[a]pyrene (BaP) in the presence of aryl hydrocarbon hydroxylase (AHH), *Proc. Am. Assoc. Cancer Res.*, 14, 49, 1973.

68. Rogan, E. G. and Cavalieri, E., 3-Methylcholanthrene-inducible binding of aromatic hydrocarbons to DNA in purified rat liver nuclei, *Biochem. Biophys. Res. Commun.*, 58, 1119, 1974.

69. Rogan, E. G., Mailander, P., and Cavalieri, E., Metabolic activation of aromatic hydrocarbons in purified rat liver nuclei: induction of enzyme activities and binding to DNA with and without monooxygenase-catalyzed formation of active oxygen, *Proc. Natl. Acad. Sci. U.S.A.*, 73, 457, 1976.

70. Jerström, B., Vadi, H., and Orrenius, S., Formation in isolated rat liver microsomes and nuclei of benzo[a]pyrene metabolites that bind to DNA, *Cancer Res.*, 36, 4107, 1976.

71. Pezzuto, J. M., Lea, M. A., and Yang, C. S., Binding of metabolically activated benzo[a]pyrene to nuclear macromolecules, *Cancer Res.*, 36, 3647, 1976.

72. Alexandrov, K., Brookes, P., King, H. W. S., Osborne, M. R., and Thompson, M. H., Comparison of the metabolism of benzo[a]pyrene and binding to DNA caused by rat liver nuclei and microsomes, *Chem. Biol. Interact.* 12, 269, 1976.

73. Vaught, J. and Bresnick, E., Binding of polycyclic hydrocarbons to nuclear components *in vitro*, *Biochem. Biophys. Res. Commun.*, 69, 587, 1976.

74. Grover, P. L., Reactions of polycyclic hydrocarbon metabolites with DNA, in *In Vitro Metabolic Activation in Mutagenesis Testing*, de Serres, F. J., Fouts, J. R., Bend, J. R., and Philpot, R. M. Eds., Elsevier/North Holland Biomedical Press, Amsterdam, 1977, 295.

75. Pezzuto, J. M., Lea, M. A., and Yang, C. S., The role of microsomes and nuclear envelope in the metabolic activation of benzo[a]pyrene leading to binding with nuclear macromolecules, *Cancer Res.*, 37, 3427, 1977.

76. Kuroki, T., Huberman, E., Marquardt, H., Selkirk, J. K., Heidelberger, C., Grover, P. L., and Sims, P., Binding of K-region epoxides and other derivatives of benz[a]anthracene and dibenz[a,h]anthracene to DNA, RNA and proteins of transformable cells, *Chem. Biol. Interact.*, 4, 389, 1971/2.

77. Borgen, A., Darvey, H., Castagnoli, N., Crocker, T. T., Rasmussen, R. E., and Wang, I. Y., Metabolic conversion of benzo[a]pyrene by Syrian hamster liver microsomes and binding of metabolites to deoxyribonucleic acid, *J. Med. Chem.*, 16, 502, 1973.

78. Sims, P., Grover, P. L., Swaisland, A., Pal, K., and Hewer, A., Metabolic activation of benzo[a]pyrene proceeds by a diol-epoxide, *Nature (London)*, 252, 326, 1974.

79. Thompson, M. H., King, H. W. S., Osborne, M. R., and Brookes, P., Rat liver microsome-mediated binding of benzo[a]pyrene metabolites to DNA, *Int. J. Cancer*, 17, 270, 1976.

80. Grover, P. L., Hewer, A., Pal, K., and Sims, P., The involvement of a diol-epoxide in the metabolic activation of benzo[a]pyrene in human bronchial mucosa and in mouse skin, *Int. J. Cancer*, 18, 1, 1976.

81. Harris, C. C., Genta, V. M., Frank, A. L., Kaufman, D. G., Barrett, L. A., McDowall, E. M., and Trump, B. F., Carcinogenic polynuclear hydrocarbons bind to macromolecules in cultured human bronchi, *Nature* (London), 252, 68, 1974.

82. Harris, C. C., Frank, A. L., van Haaften, C., Kaufman, D. G., Connor, R., Jackson, F., Barrett, L. A., McDowall, E. M., and Trump, B. F., Binding of [³H] benzo[a]pyrene to DNA in cultured human bronchus, *Cancer Res.*, 36, 1011, 1976.

83. Lorentzen, R. J., Caspary, W. J., Lesko, S. A., and Ts'o, P. O. P., The autoxidation of 6-hydroxybenzo[a]pyrene and 6-oxobenzo[a]pyrene radical, reactive metabolites of benzo[a]pyrene, *Biochemistry*, 14, 3970, 1975.

84. Ts'o, P. O. P., Caspary, W. J., Cohen, B. I., Leavitt, J. C., Lesko, S. A., Lorentzen, R. J., and Schechtman, L. M., Basic mechanisms in polycyclic hydrocarbon carcinogenesis, in *Chemical Carcinogenesis*, Part A, Ts'o, P. O. P. and DiPaolo, J. A. Eds.,Marcel Dekker, New York, 1974, 113.

85. Nagata, C., Tagashira, Y., and Kodama, M., Metabolic activation of benzo[a]pyrene: significance of the free radical, in *Chemical Carcinogenesis*, Part A, Ts'o, P. O. P. and DiPaolo, J. A. Eds., Marcel Dekker, New York, 1974, 87.

86. Flesher, J. W. and Sydnor, K. L. Possible role of 6-hydroxymethylbenzo[a]pyrene as a proximate carcinogen of benzo[a]pyrene and 6-methylbenzo[a]pyrene, *Int. J. Cancer*, 11, 433, 1973.

87. Blackburn, G. M., Milne, G. M., and Orgee, L., Displacement of tritium from 6-tritiobenzo[a]pyrene on covalent binding to DNA, *J. Chem. Soc. Chem. Commun.*, 359, 1976.

88. King, H. W. S., Thompson, M. H., Osborne, M. R., Harvey, R. G., and Brookes, P., The binding of benzo[a]pyrene to DNA does not involve substitution at the 6 position, *Chem. Biol. Interact.*, 12, 425, 1976.

89. Wiebel, F. J., Selkirk, J. K., Gelboin, H. V., Haugen, D. A., van der Hoeven, T. A., and Coon, M. J., Position-specific oxygenation of benzo[a]pyrene by different forms of purified cytochrome P-450 from rabbit liver, *Proc. Natl. Acad. Sci. U.S.A.*, 72, 3917, 1975.

90. Selkirk, J. K., Croy, R. G., and Gelboin, H. V., High-pressure liquid chromatographic separation of 10 benzo[a]pyrene phenols and the identification of 1-phenol and 7-phenol as new metabolites, *Cancer Res.*, 36, 922, 1976.

91. Capdevila, J., Jerström, B., Vadi, H., and Orrenius, S., Cytochrome P-450-linked activation of 3-hydroxyenzo[a]pyrene, *Biochem. Biophys. Res. Commun.*, 65, 894, 1975.

92. Osborne, M. R., Thompson, M. H., King, H. W. S., and Brookes, P., Retention of tritium during the binding of tritiated benzo[a]pyrene to DNA, *Int. J. Cancer*, 16, 659, 1975.

93. Baird, W. M. and Brookes, P., Isolation of the hydrocarbon-deoxyribonucleoside products from the DNA of mouse embryo cells treated in culture with 7-methylbenz[a]anthracene-³H, *Cancer Res.*, 33, 2378, 1973.

94. Meehan, T., Warshawsky, D., and Calvin, M., Specific positions involved in enzyme catalyzed covalent binding of benzo[a]pyrene to poly(G), *Proc. Natl. Acad. Sci. U.S.A.*, 73, 1117, 1976.

95. Meehan, T., Straub, K., and Calvin, M., Elucidation of hydrocarbon structure in an enzyme-catalyzed benzo[a]pyrene-poly(G) covalent complex, *Proc. Natl. Acad. Sci. U.S.A.*, 73, 1437, 1976.

96. Wislocki, P. G., Chang, R. L., Wood, A. W., Levin, W., Yagi, H., Hernandez, O., Mah, H. D., Dansette, P. M., Jerina, D. M., and Conney, A. H., High carcinogenicity of 2-hydroxybenzol[a]pyrene on mouse skin, *Cancer Res.*, 37, 2608, 1977.

97. Brookes, P., Jones, P., and Amos, J., The nature of the deoxyribonucleosides involved in the binding of carcinogenic hydrocarbons to the DNA of mouse embryo cells, *Int. J. Cancr*, 15, 912, 1975.

98. King, H. W. S., Thompson, M. H., and Brookes, P., The benzo[a]pyrene deoxyribonucleoside products isolated from DNA after metabolism of benzo[a]pyrene by rat liver microsomes in the presence of DNA, *Cancer Res.*, 35, 1263, 1975.

99. Nebert, D. W., Boobis, A. R., Yagi, H., Jerina, D. M., and Kouri, R., Genetic differences in benzo[a]pyrene carcinogenic index *in vivo* and in mouse cytochrome $P_2$450-mediated benzo[a]pyrene metabolite binding to DNA *in vitro*, in *Biological Reactive Intermediates*, Jallow, D. J., Kocsis, J. J., Snyder, R., and Vainio, H. Eds., Plenum Press, New York, 1977, 125.

100. King, H. W. S., Thompson, M. H., and Brookes, P., The role of 9-hydroxybenzo[a]pyrene in the microsome mediated binding of benzo[a]pyrene to DNA, *Int. J. Cancer*, 18, 339, 1976.

101. Waring, M. and Britten, R. J., Nucleotide sequence repetitions: a rapidly reassociating fraction of mouse DNA, *Science*, 154, 791, 1966.

102. Zeiger, R. S., Salomon, R., Kinoshita, N., and Peacock, A., The binding of 9,10-dimethyl-1,2-benzanthracene to mouse epidermal satellite DNA *in vivo*, *Cancer Res.*, 32, 643, 1972.

103. Schildkraut, C. L., Marmur, J., and Doty, P., Determination of the base composition of deoxyribonucleic acid from its buoyant density in CsC1, *J. Mol. Biol.*, 4, 430, 1962.

104. Corneo, G., Ginelli, E., Soave, C., and Bernardi, G., Isolation and characterization of mouse and Guinea pig satellite deoxyribonucleic acids, *Biochemistry*, 7, 4373, 1968.

105. Zytkovicz, T., Moses, H. L., and Spelsberg, T. C., The binding of benzo[a]pyrene and N-methyl-N'-nitro-N-nitrosoguanidine to subnuclear fractions of AKR mouse embryo cells in culture, *Int. J. Cancer*, 20, 408, 1977.

106. Webster, R. A., Moses, H. L., and Spelsberg, T. C., Separation and characterization of transcriptionally active and inactive nuclear subfractions of AKR mouse embryo cells, *Cancer Res.*, 36, 2896, 1976.

107. Bowden, G. T., Shapas, B. G., and Boutwell, R. K., The binding of 7,12-dimethylbenz[a]anthracene to replicating and non-replicating DNA in mouse skin, *Chem. Biol. Interact.*, 8, 379, 1974.

108. Bowden, G. T. and Boutwell, R. K., The replication of mouse skin epidermal DNA to which is bound 7,12-dimethylbenz[a]anthracene, *Chem. Biol. Interact.*, 9, 15, 1974.

109. Oudet, P., Gross-Bellard, M., and Chambon, P., Electron microscopic and biochemical evidence that chromatin structure is a repeating unit, *Cell*, 4, 281, 1975.

110. **Jahn, C. L. and Litman, G. W.,** Distribution of covalently bound benzo[a]pyrene in chromatin, *Biochem. Biophys. Res. Commun.,* 76, 534, 1977.

111. **Noll, M.,** Internal structure of the chromatin subunit, *Nucleic Acids Res.,* 1, 1573, 1974.

112. **Grover, P. L., Hewer, A., and Sims, P.,** Epoxides as microsomal metabolites of polycyclic hydrocarbons, *FEBS Lett.,* 18, 76, 1971.

113. **Keysell, G. R., Booth, J., Grover, P. L., Hewer, A., and Sims, P.,** The formation of K-region epoxides as hepatic microsomal metabolites of 7-methylbenz[a]anthracene and 7,12-dimethylbenz[a]anthracene and their 7-hydroxymethyl derivatives, *Biochem. Pharmacol.,* 22, 2853, 1973.

114. **Grover, P. L., Hewer, A., and Sims, P.,** Formation of K-region epoxides as microsomal metabolites of pyrene and benzo[a]pyrene, *Biochem. Pharmacol.,* 21, 2713, 1972.

115. **Wang, I. Y., Rasmussen, R. E., and Crocker, T. T.,** Isolation and characterization of an active DNA-binding metabolite of benzo[a]pyrene from hamster liver microsomal incubation systems, *Biochem. Biophys. Res. Commun.,* 49, 1142, 1972.

116. **Selkirk, J. K., Croy, R. G., and Gelboin, H. V.,** Isolation by high pressure liquid chromatography and characterization of benzo[a]pyrene-4,5-epoxide as a metabolite of benzo[a]pyrene, *Arch. Biochem. Biophys.,* 168, 322, 1975.

117. **Selkirk, J. K., Huberman, E., and Heidelberger, C.,** An epoxide is an intermediate in the microsomal metabolism of the chemical carcinogen dibenz[a,h]anthracene, *Biochem. Biophys. Res. Commun.,* 43, 1010, 1971.

118. **Grover, P. L. and Sims, P.,** Interactions of the K-region epoxides of phenanthrene and dibenz[a,h]anthracene with nucleic acids and histone, *Biochem. Pharmacol.,* 19, 2251, 1970.

119. **Grover, P. L. and Sims, P.,** K-Region epoxides of poycyclic hydrocarbons: reactions with nucleic acids and polyribonucleotides, *Biochem. Pharmacol.,* 22, 661, 973.

120. **Swaisland, A. J., Grover, P. L., and Sims, P.,** Reactions of polycyclic hydrocarbon epoxides with RNA and polyribonucleotides, *Chem. Biol. Interact.,* 9, 317, 1974.

121. **Blobstein, S. H., Weinstein, I. B., Grunberger, D., Weisgras, J., and Harvey, R. G.,** Products obtained after *in vitro* reaction of 7,12-dimethylbenz[a]anthracene 5,6-oxide with nucleic acis, *Biochemistry,* 14, 3451, 1975.

122. **Jeffrey, A. M., Blobstein, S. H., Weinstein, I. B., and Harvey, R. G.,** High-presure liquid chromatography of carcinogen-nucleoside conjugates: separation of 7,12-dimethylbenzanthracene derivatives, *Anal. Biochem.,* 73, 378, 1976.

123. **Jeffrey, A. M., Blobstein, S. H., Weinstein, I. B., Beland, F. A., Harvey, R. G., Kasai, H., and Nakanishi, K.,** Structure of 7,12-dimethylbenz[a]anthracene-guanosine adducts, *Proc. Natl. Acad. Sci. U. S. A.,* 73, 2311, 1976.

124. **Grover, P. L., Sims, P., Huberman, E., Marquardt, H., Kuroki, T. and Heidelberger, C.,** *In vitro* transformation of rodent cells by K-region derivatives of polycyclic hydrocarbons, *Prc. Natl. Acd. Sci. U.S.A.,* 68, 1098, 1971.

125. **Huberman, E., Aspiras, L., Heidelberger, C., Grover, P. L., and Sims, P.,** Mutagenicity to mammalian cells of epoxides and other derivatives of polycyclic hydrocarbons, *Proc. Natl. Acad. Sci. U.S.A.,* 68, 3195, 1971.

126. **Ames, B. N., Sims, P., and Grover, P. L.,** Epoxides of carcinogenic polycyclic hydrocarbons are frameshift mutagens, *Science,* 176, 47, 1972.

127. **Cookson, M. J., Sims, P., and Grover, P. L.,** Mutagenicity of epoxides of polycyclic hydrocarbons correlates with carcinogenicity of parent hydrocarbons, *Nature* (London) *New Biol.,* 234, 186, 1971.

128. **Miller, E. C. and Miller, J. A.,** Low carcinogeniciy of the K-region epoxides of 7-methylbenz[a]anthracene and benz[a]anthracene in the mouse and rat, *Proc. Soc. Exp. Biol. Med.,* 124, 915, 1967.

129. **Boyland, E. and Sims, P.,** The carcinogenic activities in mice of compounds related to benz[a]anthracene, *Int. J. Cancer,* 2, 500, 1967.

130. **Sims, P.,** The carcinogenic activities in mice of compounds related to 3-methylcholanthrene, *Int. J. Cancer,* 2, 505, 1967.

131. **Van Duuren, B. L., Langseth, L., Goldschmidt, B. M., and Orris, L.,** Carcinogenicity of epoxides, lactones and peroxy compounds. VI. Structure and carcinogenic activity, *J. Natl. Cancer Inst.,* 39, 1217, 1967.

132. **Flesher, J. ., Harvey, R. G., and Sydnor, K. L.,** Oncogenicity of K-region epoxides of benzo[a]pyrene and 7,12-dimethylbenz[a]anthracene, *Int. J. Cancer,* 1, 351, 1976.

133. **Baird, W. M., Dipple, A., Grover, P. L., Sims, P., and Brookes, P.,** Studies on the formation of hydrocarbon-deoxyribonucleoside products by the binding of derivatives of 7-methylbenz[a]anthracene to DNA in aqueous solution and in mouse embryo cells in culture, *Cancer Res.,* 33, 2386, 1973.

134. **Baird, W. M., Grover, P. L., Sims., P., and Brookes, P.,** Comparison of the products of the reaction of 7-methylbenz[a]anthracene 5,6-oxide and RNA, with those formed in 7-methylbenz[a]anthracene-treated cells, *Cancer Res.,* 36, 2306, 1976.

135. Thompson, M. H., Osborne, M. R., King, H. W. S., and Brookes, P., The 7-mthylbenz[a] anthracene deoxyribonucleoside products isolated from DNA after metabolism of the carcinogen by rat liver microsomes in the presence of DNA, *Chem. Biol. Interact.*, 14, 13, 1976.

136. Baird, W. M., Harvey, R. G., and Brookes, P., Comparison of the cellular DNA-bound products of benzo[a]pyrene with the products formed by the reaction of benzo[a]pyrene-4,5-oxide with DNA, *Cancer Res.*, 35, 54, 1975.

137. Blackburn, G. M., Taussig, P. E., and Will, J. P., Binding of benzo[a]pyrene to DNA investigated by tritium displacement, *J. Chem. Soc. Chem. Commun.*, 907, 1974.

138. Murray, A. W., Grover, P. L., and Sims, P., The conversion of benzo[a]pyrene 4,5-oxide into 4-hydroxybenzo[a]pyrene in the presence of polyriboguanylic acid, *Chem. Biol Interact.* 13, 57, 1976.

139. Booth, J., Keysell, G. R., and Sims, P., Formation of glutathione conjugates as metabolites of 7,12-dimethylbenz[a]anthracene by rat liver homogenates, *Biochem. Pharmacol.*, 22, 1781, 1973.

140. Swaisland, A. J., Hewer, A., Pal, K., Keysell, G. R., Booth, J., Grover, P. L., and Sims, P., Polycyclic hydrocarbon epoxides: the involvement of 8,9-dihydro-8,9-dihydroxybenz[a]anthracene 10,11-oxide in reactions with the DNA of benz[a]anthracene-treated hamster embryo cells, *FEBS Lett.*, 47, 34, 1974.

141. Daudel, P., Duquesne, M., Vigny, P., Grover, P. L., and Sims, P., Fluorescence spectral evidence that benzo[a]pyrene-DNA products in mouse skin arise from diol-epoxides, *FEBS Lett.*, 57, 250, 1975.

142. Ivanovic, V., Geacintov, N. E., and Weinstein, I. B., Cellular binding of benzo[a]pyrene to DNA characterized by low temperature fluorescence, *Biochem. Biophys. Res. Commun.*, 70, 1172, 1976.

143. Keysell, G. R., Booth, J., and Sims, P., Glutathione conjugates as metabolites of benz[a]anthracene, *Xenobiotica*, 5, 349, 1975.

144. King, H. W. S., Osborne, M. R., Beland, F. A., Harvey, R. G., and Brookes, P., (±)-7α,8β-Dihydroxy-9β,10β-epoxy-7,8,9,10-tetrahydrobenzo[a]pyrene is an intermediate in the metabolism and binding to DNA of benzo[a]pyrene, *Proc. Natl. Acad. Sci. U.S.A.*, 73, 2679, 1976.

145. Baird, W. M. and Diamond, L., The nature of benzo[a]pyrene-DNA adducts formed in hamster embryo cells depends on the length of time of exposure to benzo[a]pyrene, *Biochem. Biophys. Res. Commun.*, 77, 162, 1977.

146. Remsen, J., Jerina, D., Yagi, H. and Cerutti, P., *In vitro* reaction of radioactive 7β,8α-dihydroxy-9α,10α-epoxy-7,8,9,10-tetrahydrobenzo[a]pyrene and 7β,8α-dihydroxy-9β,10β-epoxy-7,8,9,10-tetrahydrobenzo[a]pyrene with DNA, *Biochem. Biophys. Res. Commun.*, 74, 934, 1977.

147. Moore, P. D., Koreeda, M., Wislocki, P. G., Levin, W., Conney, A. H., Yagi, H. and Jerina, D. M., In vitro reactions of the diastereomeric 9,10-epoxides of (+) and (−)-trans-7,8-dihydroxy-7,8-dihydrobenzo[a]pyrene with polyguanylic acid and evidence for formation of an enantiomer of each diastereomeric 9,10-epoxide from benzo[a]pyrene in mouse skin, in ACS Symp. Series, No. 44, *Drug Metabolism Concepts*, Jerina, D. M., Ed., American Chemical Society, Washington, D.C., 1977, 127.

148. Weinstein, I. B., Jeffrey, A. M., Jennette, K. W., Blobstein, S. H., Harvey, R. G., Harris, C., Autrup, H., Kasai, H., and Nakanishi, K., Benzo[a]pyrene diol epoxides as intermediates in nucleic acid binding in vitro and in vivo, *Science*, 193, 592, 1976.

149. Jennette, K. W., Jeffrey, A. M., Blobstein, S. H., Beland, F. A., Harvey, R. G., and Weinstein, I. B., Nucleoside adducts from the in vitro reation of benzo[a]pyrene-7,8-dihydrodiol 9,10-oxide or benzo[a]pyrene 4,5-oxide with nucleic acids, *Biochemistry*, 16, 932, 1977.

150. Phillips, D. H., Grover, P. L., and Sims, P., Some properties of vicinal diol-epoxides derived from benz[a]anthracene and benzo[a]pyrene, *Chem. Biol. Interact.*, 20, 63, 1978.

151. Jeffrey, A. M., Jennette, K. W., Blobstein, S. H., Weinstein, I. B., Beland, F. A., Harvey, R. G., Kasai, H., Miura, I., and Nakanishi, K., Benzo[a]pyrene-nucleic acid derivative found in vivo: structure of a benzo[a]pyrentetrahydrodiol epoxide-guanosine adduct, *J. Am. Chem. Soc*, 98, 5714, 1976.

152. Nakanishi, K., Kasai, H., Cho, H., Harvey, R. G., Jeffrey, A. M., Jennette, K. W., and Weinstein, I. B., Absolute configuration of a ribonucleic acid adduct formed in vivo by metabolism of benzo-[a]pyrene, *J. Am. Chem. Soc.*, 99, 258, 1977.

153. Yagi, H., Akagi, H., Thakker, D. R., Mah, H. D., Koreeda, M., and Jerina, D. M., Absolute stereochemistry of the highly mutagenic 7,8-diol 9,10-epoxides derived from the potent carcinogen trans-7,8-dihydroxy-7,8-dihydrobenzo[a]pyrene, *J. Am. Chem. Soc.*, 99, 2358, 1977.

154. Koreeda, M., Moore, P. D., Yagi, H., Yeh, H. J. C., AND Jerina, D. M., Alkylation of polyguanylic acid at the 2-amino group and phosphate by the potent mutaen (±)-7β,8α-dihydroxy-9β,10β-epoxy-7,8,9,10-tetrahydrobenzo[a]pyrene, *J. Am. Chem. Soc.*, 8, 6720, 1976.

155. Gamper, H. B., Tung, A. S.-C., Straub, K., Bartholomew, J. C., and Calvin, M., DNA strand scission by benzo[a]pyrene diol epoxides, *Science*, 197, 671, 1977.

156. Osborne, M. R. Beland, F. A., Harvey, R. G., and Brookes, P., The reaction of (±)7α,8β-dihydroxy-9β,10β-epoxy-7,8,9,10-tetrahydrobenzo[a]pyrene with DNA, *Int. J. Cancer*, 18, 362, 1976.

157. Meehan, T., Straub, K., and Calvin, M., Benzo[*a*]pyrene diol epoxide covalently binds to deoxyguanosine and deoxyadenosine in DNA, *Nature*London), 269, 725, 1977.

158. Jeffrey, A. M., Weinstein, I. B., Jennette, K. W., Grzeskowiak, K., Nakanishi, K., Harvey, R. G., Autrup, H., nd Harris, C., Structures of benzo[*a*]pyrene-nucleic acid adducts formed in human and bovine bronchial explants, *Nature*(London), 269, 348, 1977.

159. Levin, W., Wood, A. W., Yagi, H., Dansette, P. M., Jerina, D. M., and Conney, A. H., Carcinogenicity of benzo[*a*]pyrene 4,5-, 7,8- and 9,10-oxides on mouse skin, *Proc. Natl. Acad. Sci. U.S.A.*, 73, 243, 1976.

160. Chouroulinkov, I., Gentil, A., Grover, P. L., and Sims, P., Tumour-initiating activities on mouse skin of dihydrodiols derived from benzo[*a*]pyrene, *Br. J. Cancer*, 34, 523, 1976.

161. Slaga, T. J., Viaje, A., Berry, D. L., Bracken, W., Buty, S. G., and Scribner, J. D., Skin tumor initiating ability of benzo[*a*]pyrene 4,5- 7,8- and 7,8-diol-9,10-epoxides and 7,8-diol, *Cancer Lett.*, 2, 115, 1976.

162. Levin, W., Wood, A. W., Yagi, H., Jerina, D. M., and Conney, A. H., (±)-*trans*-7,8-Dihydroxy-7,8-dihydrobenzo[*a*]pyrene: a potent skin carcinogen when applied topically to mice, *Proc. Natl. Acad. Sci. U.S.A.*, 73, 3867, 1976.

163. Levin, W., Wood, A. W., Wislocki, P. G., Kapitulnik, J., Yagi, H., Jerina, D. M., and Conney, A. H., Carcinogenicity of benzo-ring derivatives of benzo[*a*]pyrene on mouse skin, *Cancer Res.*, 37, 3356, 1977.

164. Kapitulnik, J., Levin, W., Conney, A. H., Yagi, H., and Jerina, D. M., Benzo[*a*]pyrene 7,8-dihydrodiol is more carcinogenic than benzo[*a*]pyrene in newborn mice, *Nature*, 266, 378, 1977.

165. Marquardt, H., Grover, P. L., and Sims, P., *In vitro* malignant transformation of mouse fibroblasts by non-K-region dihydrodiols derived from 7-methylbenz[*a*]anthrcene, 7,12-dimethylbenz[*a*]anthracene and benzo[*a*]pyrene, *Cancer Res.*, 36, 2059, 1976.

166. Mager, R., Huberman, E., Yang, S. K., Gelboin, H. V., and Sachs, L., Transformation of normal hamster cells by benzo[*a*]pyrene diol-epoxide, *Int. J. Cancer*, 19, 814, 1977.

167. Malaveille, C., Bartsch, H., Grover, P. L., and Sims, P., Mutagenicity of non-K-region diols and diol-epoxides of benz[*a*]anthracene and benzo[*a*]pyrene in *S. typhimurium* TA100, *Biochem. Biophys. Res. Commun.*, 66, 693, 1975.

168. Newbold, R. F. and Brookes, P., Exceptional mutagenicity of a benzo[*a*]pyrene diol epoxide in cultured mammalian cells, *Nature*(London), 261, 52, 1976.

169. Wood, A. W., Wislocki, P. G., Chang, R. L., Levin, W., Lu, A. Y. H., Yagi, H., Hernandez, O., Jerina, D. M., and Conney, A. H., Mutagenicity and cytotoxicity of benzo[*a*]pyrene benzo-ring epoxides, *Cancer Res.*, 36, 3358, 1976.

170. Marquardt, H., Baker, S., Grover, P. L., and Sims, P., Malignant transformation and mutagenesis in mammalian cells induced by vicinal diol-epoxides derived from benzo[*a*]pyrene, *Cancer Lett.*, 3, 31, 1977.

171. Malaveille, C., Kuroki, T., Sims, P., Grover, P. L., and Bartsch, H., Mutagenicity of isomeric diol-epoxides of benzo[*a*]pyrene and benz[*a*]anthracene in *S. typhimurium* TA98 and TA100 and in V79 Chinese hamster cells, *Mutat. Res.*, 44, 313, 1977.

172. Jerina, D. M. and Daly, J. W., Oxidation at carbon, in *Drug Metabolism—from Microbe to Man*, Parke, D. V. and Smith, R. L., Eds., Taylor and Francis, London,

173. Jerina, D. M., Lehr, R. E., Yagi, H., Hernandez, O., Dansette, P. M., Wislocki, P. G., Wood, A. W., Chang, R. L., Levin, W., and Conney, A. H., Mutagenicity of benzo[*a*]pyrene derivatives and the description of a quantum mechanical model which predicts the ease of carbonium ion formation from diol epoxides, in *In Vitro Metabolic Activation in Mutagenesis Testing*, de Serres, F. J., Fouts, J. R., Bend, J. R., and Philpot, R. M.,Eds., Elsevier/North Holland Biomedical Press, Amsterdam, 1976, 159.

174. Wislocki, P. G., Wood, A. W., Chang, R. L., Levin, W., Yagi, H., Hernandez, O., Dansette, P. M., Jerina, D. M., and Conney, A. H., Mutagenicity and cytotoxicity of benzo[*a*]pyrene arene oxides, phenols, quinones and dihydrodiols in bacterial and mammalian cells, *Cancer Res.*, 36, 3350, 1976.

175. Wood, A. W., Levin, W., Lu, A. Y. H., Ryan, D., West, S. B., Lehr, R. E., Schaefer-Ridder, M., Jerina, D. M., and Conney, A. H., Mutagenicity of metabolically activated benzo[*a*]anthracene 3,4-dihydrodiol: evidence for bay region activation of carcinogenic polycyclic hydrocarbons, *Biochem. Biophys. Res. Commun.*, 72, 680, 1976.

176. Wood, A. W., Levin, W., Chang, R. L., Lehr, R. E., Schaefer-Ridder, M., Karle, J. M., Jerina, D. M., and Conney,A. H., Tumorigenicity of five dihydrodiols of benz[*a*]anthracene on mouse skin: exceptional activity of benz[*a*]anthracene 3,4-dihydrodiol, *Proc. Natl. Acad. Sci. U.S.A.*, 74, 3176, 1977.

177. Wood, A. W., Chang, R. L., Levin, W., Lehr, R. E., Schaefer-Ridder, M., Karle, J. M., Jerina, D. M., and Conney, A. H., Mutagenicity and cytotoxicity of benz[*a*]anthracene diol epoxides and tetrahydro-epoxides: exceptional activity of the bay region 1,2-epoxides, *Proc. Natl. Acad. Sci. U.S.A.*, 74, 2746, 1977.

178. **Vigny, P., Duquesne, M., Coulomb, H., Lacombe, C., Tierney, B., Grover, P. L., and Sims, P.,** Metabolic activation of polycyclic hydrocarbons. Fluorescence spectral evidence is consistent with metabolism at the 1,2- and 3,4-double bonds of 7-methylbenz[a]anthracene, *FEBS Lett.,* 75, 9, 1977.

179. **Malaveille, C., Tierney, B., Grover, P. L., Sims, P., and Bartsch, H.,** High microsome-mediated mutagenicity of the 3,4-dihydrodiol of 7-methylbenz[a]anthracene in *S. typhimurium* TA 98, *Biochem. Biophys. Res. Commun.,* 75, 427, 1977.

180. **Marquardt, H., Baker, S., Tierney, B., Grover, P. L. and Sims, P.,** The metabolic activation of 7-methylbenz[a]anthracene: the induction of malignant transformation and mutation in mammalian cells by non-K-region dihydrodiols, *Int. J. Cancer,* 19, 828, 1977.

181. **Chouroulinkov, I., Gentil,A., Tierney, B., Grover, P. L., and Sims, P.,** The metabolic activation of 7-methylbenz[a]anthracene in mouse skin: high tumour-initiating activity of the 3,4-dihydrodiol, *Cancer Lett.* 3, 247, 1977.

182. **Baird, W. M. and Dipple, A.,** Photosensitivity of DNA-bound 7,12-dimethylbenz[a]anthracene, *Int. J. Cancer,* 20, 427, 1977.

183. **Vigny, P., Duquesne, M., Coulomb, H., Tierney, B., Grover, P. L., and Sims, P.,** Flourescence spectral studies on the metabolic activation of 3-methylcholanthrene and 7,12-dimethylbenz[a]anthracene in mouse skin, *FEBS Lett.,* 28, 278, 1977.

184. **Moschel, R. C., Baird, W. M., and Dipple, A.,** Metabolic activation of the carcinogen 7,12-dimethylbenz[a]anthracene for DNA binding, *Biochem. Biophys. Res. Commun.,* 76, 1092, 1977.

185. **Blackburn, G. M., Flavell, A. J., Paussio, P. E., and Will, J. P.,** Binding of 7,12-dimethylbenz[a]anthracene to DNA investigated by tritium displacement, *J. Chem. Soc. Chem. Commun.,* 358, 1975.

186. **Ivanovic, V., Geacintov, N. E., Jeffrey, A. M., Fu, P. P., Harvey, R. G., and Weinstein, I. B.,** Cell and microsome mediated binding of 7,12-dimethylbenz[a]anthracene to DNA studied by fluorescence spectroscopy, *Cancer Lett.,* 4, 131, 1978.

187. **Boyland, E. and Sims, P.,** Metabolism of polycyclic compounds. The metabolism of 7,12-dimethylbenz[a]anthracene by rat-liver homogenates, *Biochem. J.,* 95, 780, 1965.

188. **King, H. W. S., Osborne, M. R., and Brookes, P.,** The metabolism and DNA binding of 3-methylcholanthrene, *Int. J. Cancer,* 20, 564, 1977.

Chapter 3

CONFORMATIONAL CHANGES IN NUCLEIC ACIDS MODIFIED BY CHEMICAL CARCINOGENS

D. Grunberger and I. B. Weinstein

TABLE OF CONTENTS

I. INTRODUCTION*

A. General Considerations

It has become an axiom in carcinogenesis that many, and perhaps all, carcinogens become covalently bound to nucleic acids in the tissue. It also appears that this interaction is critical to the carcinogenic process (for reviews, see References 1 and 2). This covalent modification can introduce important changes, not only in the primary structure of nucleic acids, but also in the conformation (three-dimensional structure) of the nucleic acids at the sites of modification. Since distortions in nucleic acid structure are likely to have functional consequences, a detailed description of these conformational changes seems essential if we are to ultimately understand the carcinogenic process at the molecular level.

B. Basic Principles of Nucleic Acid Conformation

X-Ray diffraction and a variety of spectral techniques have provided extensive information on the conformations of nucleosides, oligonucleotides, and single- and double-strand nucleic acids. (For details, see reviews by Ward and Reich[3] and by Sundaralingam.[4]) These studies indicate that two major structural aspects influence the conformation of nucleosides and polynucleotides. These are the relative orientation of the base and sugar residues at the glycosyl bond (Figure 1) and the type of pucker in the sugar ring (Figure 2). In polynucleotides, the series of single bonds which form the phosphodiester linkages between adjacent nucleotides can also provide sites of rotation during conformational distortions of the polymer (Figure 2). Rotational "flexibility" of the backbone is possible at the $C^{3'}$-$C^{4'}$ bond and the internucleotide P - O bonds.

The major conformational parameter is the relative orientation of the base to the sugar, which is defined in terms of a torsion angle ϕ CN. The latter refers to the angle formed between the plane of the base and the $C^{1'}$-O bond of the sugar, viewed along the glycosyl bond (Figure 1).[5] There are two ranges of torsional angles within which stable conformations of nucleosides are assumed, the *anti* and the *syn,* and each of these ranges cover more than 90°. X-Ray crystallographic data of normal nucleosides have revealed that the vast majority of these compounds correspond to the *anti* conformation.[6,7] The nuclear magnetic resonance (NMR) and circular dichroism (CD) data are in agreement with the X-ray data. On the other hand, bulky substituents in position 6 in pyrimidines or in position 8 in purines force the nucleosides to change their conformation from the usually preferred *anti* to the *syn* position. Well-known examples are the 8-bromo substituted purine nucleosides or 6-methyl pyrimidine nucleosides.[8,9,10] The nucleoside conformation in double-stranded DNA or RNA helices is usually restricted to *anti,* since this conformation is indispensable for ordinary base pairing in structures of the Watson-Crick type.

In nucleosides, the five-membered furanose ring of the sugar residue is puckered so that all of the carbon atoms are displaced by about 0.5 Å from the plane formed by the remaining four atoms (Figure 2). In most nucleosides, the sugar residues have either the $C^{2'}$ *endo* or the $C^{3'}$ *endo* form, i.e., the respective carbons are located on the same side of the sugar plane as $C^{5'}$. Variations in the sugar pucker could alter nucleic acid conformation, although these have not, to our knowledge, been identified with carcinogen modification.

In a DNA helix with Watson-Crick geometry (DNA-B), all of the nucleoside residues

---

* Abbreviations: BP, benzo[a]pyrene; BPDE, benzo[a]pyrene 7,8-diol 9,10-oxide; AAF, *N*-2-acetylaminofluorene; AAFF, *N*-2-acetylamino-7-fluorofluorene; AAIF, *N*-2-acetylamino-7-iodofluorene; HPLC, high-pressure liquid chromatography; CD, circular dichroism; NMR and PMR, nuclear and proton magnetic resonance; A, adenosine; G, guanosine; U, uridine; C, cytidine. In DNA studies A, G, U, and C refer to the corresponding deoxynucleosides.

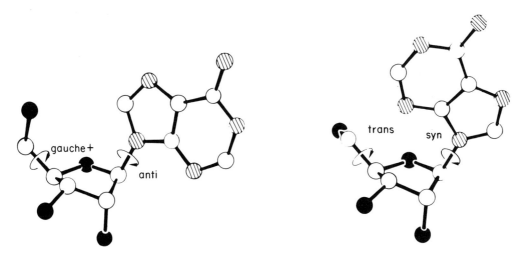

FIGURE 1.   Illustrations of the *anti* and *syn* conformations around the glycosyl bond. (From Sundaralingam, M., *Structure and Conformation of Nucleic Acid and Protein-Nucleic Acid Interactions,* (Part 5), University Park Press, Baltimore, 1975, 487. With permission.)

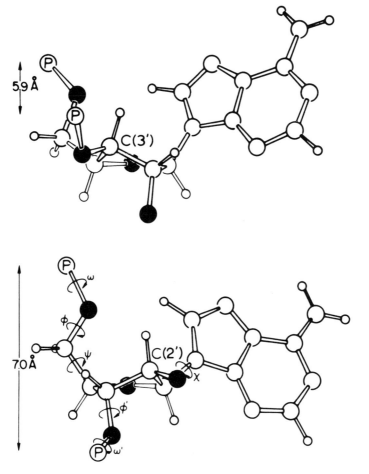

FIGURE 2.   The two preferred or rigid nucleotide units. $C^{3'}$-*endo* (top), $C^{2'}$-*endo* (bottom). The torsion angle Ψ' is *gauche* in $C(3')$-*endo* and *trans* in $C(2')$-*endo*. (From Sundaralingam, M., *Structure and Conformation of Nucleic Acid and Protein-Nucleic Acid Interactions,* (Part 5), University Park Press, Baltimore, 1975, 487. With permission.)

are in the *anti* conformation and the deoxyribose residues have the $C^{2'}endo$ structure. The *anti* conformation is essential for base pairing between the complementary strands in the helix and it also appears to be essential for Watson-Crick-type base pairing during nucleic acid replication, transcription, and codon-anticodon recognition. Stabilization of the helix structure involves base-pairing and base-stacking energies, as well as the short-range intramolecular interactions associated with the polynucleotide backbone.[4]

The conformation of the sugar residues plays a major role in determining the overall conformation of the nucleic acid. In the DNA-B helix, the sugar residues are $C^{2'}endo$, whereas, in double helical RNA and in the DNA-A helix (an alternative structure for double-stranded DNA), they are apparently $C^{3'}endo$. In both types of helices, however, there is the *anti* orientation of the bases and the *gauche* conformation of the backbone $C^{4'}$-$C^{5'}$ bond. The differences in sugar pucker are associated with marked differences in the dimensions of the major and minor grooves of the helix. In $C^{2'}endo$ double helices, the vertical dimensions of the major and minor grooves differ much more from each other than in $C^{3'}endo$ helices. On the other hand, in $C^{3'}endo$ helices, differences in the depths of the two grooves are more striking than in $C^{2'}endo$ helices.[4] In terms of possible conformational distortions, it is of interest that the $C^{2'}endo$ sugars of DNA provide more flexibility of the helix than do the $C^{3'}endo$ sugars of RNA.

Although there has been a tendency to think of the DNA helix as a rigid rod-like structure, it is apparent that in the packaging of DNA that occurs in viruses and in cellular chromatin, the double helix must be folded into a higher order structure and that this folding must be associated with either a continuous or discontinuous deformation of the backbone structure of a Watson-Crick helix. The latter distortions have been termed "Kinks" by Crick and Klug,[11] and their possible existence and structure is an active area of current research. Sobel et al.[12] have postulated that kinks produced by bending a linear helix laterally, so as to open up a wedge-like space in the minor groove, may provide the initial sites for insertion of intercalating drugs, for the binding of certain DNA-associated proteins, and for the unwinding of the helix during denaturation and strand separation.

What are the general implications of the above described conformational aspects of nucleic acids in terms of covalent attachment of various carcinogens? Carcinogens are known to bind to various bases and positions in DNA and RNA as has been described in some detail in Volume II, Chapter 2. A *priori*, we might predict that depending on the size of the carcinogen and its site of substitution, there might be no appreciable change in nucleic acid conformation, alterations in conformation at the glycoside bond, rotations of the backbone residues, and possbile changes in sugar puckering. In addition, the accessibility to carcinogen attack of residues in the nucleic acid structure would depend upon such factors as base pairing and stacking, the dimensions of the major and minor grooves, and the overall stability of the helix.

The methylation or ethylation of bases by the simple alkylating agents does not appear to present major steric problems,[13] nor would we expect major conformational distortions of the helix. Such modifications can, however, impair Watson-Crick base pairing and, in the case of N^7 substitution on purines, results in depurination due to labilization of the glycoside bond (see Volume I, Chapters 1 and 5). In addition, the formation of phosphotriesters can result in chain scissions.[13]

The covalent attachment of bulky carcinogens like AAF, BP, aflatoxin, and safrole does, however, present steric problems and, depending on the sites of substitution, may be associated with major distortions in the native conformation of nucleic acids. In this chapter, we will largely confine our discussion to results obtained with AAF- and BP-modified nucleic acids, since no detailed information is yet available on the conformations of nucleic acids modified with other bulky carcinogens.

The conformational changes in nucleic acids associated with noncovalent binding and intercalation with certain drugs and carcinogens have been reviewed in detail elsewhere.[14-16]Since the available evidence indicates that, with most carcinogens, covalent rather than physical binding to nucleic acids is critical to the carcinogenic process, physical binding and intercalation will not be reviewed in this chapter.

C. Methods of Analysis

Conformational changes associated with covalent modification by chemical carcinogens can be studied either with low-molecular-weight oligonucleotides, which mimic relatively well the situation in macromolecules, or with polymeric nucleic acids as model compounds.[17,18]The smallest unit that can be studied, which has many of the local interactions also present in a polymer, is a dinucleoside monophosphate (dimer). As in naturally occurring nucleic acids, it has a phosphate linkage between the $O^{3'}$and the $O^{5'}$of the two sugar residues. Further, neighboring bases interact strongly in dimers, as in polymers. CD and NMR spectroscopy are the two most powerful methods used for studying the conformation of dimers in solution.[19-21]and the results are more readily interpreted than those obtained with higher-molecular-weight polymers. Dynamic changes in the conformation of the dimers can be induced by altering the solvent conditions in terms of polarity, pH, etc., or in the extreme case, the properties of dimers can be reversibly altered so that they may approach that of the constituent monomers.[22-25]CD can be used to monitor changes which are characteristic of the loss, or presence, of base-stacking interactions.[23,24]Similarly, NMR spectra can be used to monitor stacking interactions between the bases in dimers and the effects of modified residues,[26,27]Utilizing the latter methods and computer-generated molecular models, we were able to propose a new model for AAF-modified dimers which we named "the base displacement model".[28,29]This model also proved to be valid for AAF-modified DNA molecules.[30,31]

Analysis of the conformation of carcinogen-modified, high-molecular-weight nucleic acids is, of course, much more difficult. Techniques that have proved to be useful include thermal denaturation, formaldehyde denaturation, intrinsic viscosity, nucleic acid hybridization, electric dichroism, susceptibility to single-strand specific nucleases, and fluorescence spectroscopy. The application of these techniques is illustrated in various sections of this chapter.

The most precise description of nucleic acid conformation comes from X-ray diffraction studies. Thus far, this technique has not been extensively applied to nucleosides or nucleic acids modified by chemical carcinogens largely because of the difficulties of preparing samples for X-ray diffraction studies.

II. CONFORMATION OF NUCLEIC ACIDS CONTAINING CONVALENTLY BOUND N-2-ACETYLAMINOFLUORENE

A common feature of most chemical carcinogens is that they are metabolically converted to electrophilic forms that react with nucleophilic centers in nucleic acids and proteins.[1,32]This has been demonstrated with alkylnitrosamines, N-2-acetylaminofluorene (AAF), polycyclic aromatic hydrocarbons, aflatoxin, and other carcinogens.[1,13,32,33]Miller et al.[34] first demonstrated that both RNA and DNA can react nonenzymatically in vitro with the N-acetoxy derivative of AAF. The major product obtained from hydrolysates of the modified DNA is N-(deoxyguanosine-8-yl)AAF.[35] There is also a minor component, 3-(deoxyguanosin-N^2-yl)AAF.[36,69]The same two nucleic acid derivatives were found in rat-liver DNA when AAF was administered in vivo.[1] Since modification of the C^8 or N^2 positions of G could be associated with different conformational changes, we have studied the conformations of both

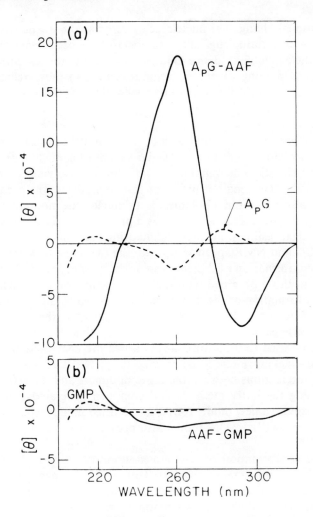

FIGURE 3.   Circular dichroism spectra comparing (a) ApG
to ApG*AAF* and (b) GMP to AAF-GMP. (With permission from
Grunberger, D., Nelson, J. H., Cantor, C. R., and Weinstein,
I. B., *J. Mol. Biol.*, 62, 331, 1971. Copyright by Academic
Press, Inc. (London) Ltd.)

types of adducts. We have termed the conformational changes associated with the C^8
modification the "base displacement model".[28,29] Evidence for this model is described
below.

A. The Base Displacement Model

The first feature of this model is that the attachment of the AAF residue to the 8
position of G is associated with a change in glycosidic N^9-$C^{-1'}$conformation from the
anti conformation of nucleosides in nucleic acids with Watson-Crick geometry to the
syn conformation. Evidence for this is restricted to a study of molecular models of
AAF-G which indicates severe steric hindrance between AAF and the ribose, or deoxyribose, of the nucleoside, unless the guanine base is rotated on the glycoside bond
from the *anti* conformation. This change to the *syn* conformation is similar to the
change that occurs with the substitution of bromine at the 8 position of GMP.[9,10]

The second major feature of this model is that there is a stacking interaction between
AAF and a base adjacent to the substituted G residue. Direct evidence for this in
oligonucleotides has been obtained from both CD and PMR spectra.[37-39]The CD results obtained with ApG are illustrated in Figure 3. At wavelengths greater than 290

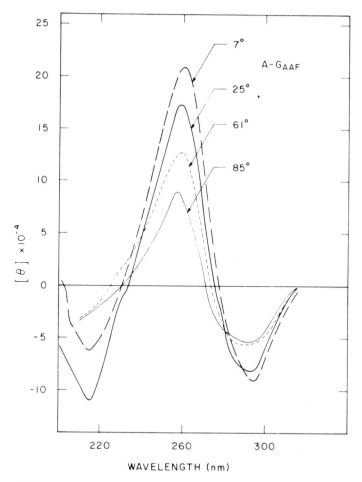

FIGURE 4.   Temperature dependence of the circular dichroism spectrum of A-G$_{AAF}$ in 0.005 M phosphate buffer (pH 7). (With permission from Grunberger, D., Nelson, J. H., Cantor, C. R., and Weinstein, I. B., *J. Mol. Biol.*, 62, 331, 1971. Copyright by Academic Press Inc. (London) Ltd.)

nm, where most of the light absorption is due to AAF, the dichroism of AAF-modified ApG (A-G$_{AAF}$) is much greater than that of the modified monomer GMP (AAF-GMP). The optical activity in the 240 to 280 nm spectral region is also very pronounced. The intense bands in the spectra of this and other AAF-modified oligomers are probably the result of intramolecular interaction between the transition dipoles of fluorene and the adjacent base residue. It is unlikely that they reflect intermolecular interactions because the concentrations of the dimers are relatively low ($10^{-5}M$), there is no salt other than buffer in the solutions, and the spectra are concentration independent over the 10^{-4} to $10^{-5}M$ range. A reversible temperature dependence of the CD spectrum of ApG$_{AAF}$, and of several other AAF-modified oligomers, is observed when the solvent is changed from H$_2$O to MeOH (Figures 4 and 5).[38] These properties are also characteristic of stacking interactions.

Additional evidence of a stacking interaction between AAF and the adjacent base is obtained from PMR spectra;[38] this is illustrated in Figure 6. Since both adenine and fluorene have significant aromaticity, we have been able to monitor possible fluorene-adenine interactions in ApG$_{AAF}$ and G$_{AAF}$pA by comparing their PMR spectra with those of ApG, GpA, pG$_{AAF}$, and $_{AAF}$Gp. The H^2 and H^8 adenine signals of both ApG$_{AAF}$ and G$_{AAF}$pA are shifted considerably upfield relative to the corresponding signals in

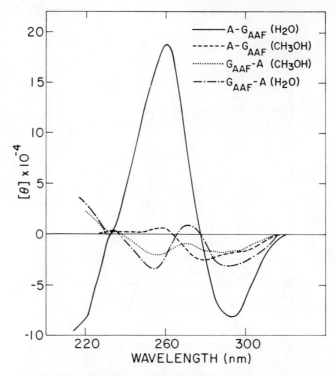

FIGURE 5.   Comparison of the circular dichroism spectra of Ap-G_{AAF} and $_{AAF}$GpA in water (0.005 M phosphate buffer, pH 7) and in methanol. — , ApG$_{AAF}$ (H$_2$O); ---, ApG$_{AAF}$ (CH$_3$OH); $\cdots\cdots$, $_{AAF}$GpA(CH$_3$OH); — · — · —, $_{AAF}$GpA (H$_2$O). (With permission from Grunberger, D., Nelson, J. H., Cantor, C. R., and Weinstein, I. B., *J. Mol. Biol.*, 62, 331, 1971. Copyright by Academic Press, Inc. (London) Ltd.)

the unmodified molecules. Analogous higher field shifts are observed for the fluorene ring protons of ApG$_{AAF}$ and G$_{AAF}$pA when referenced to the corresponding protons of pG$_{AAF}$ and $_{AAF}$Gp, respectively. These upfield shifts are characteristic of stacking[21,26]and provide convincing evidence that the adenine and fluorene planes are intramolecularly stacked in the AAF-modified dinucleotides. These changes are best illustrated in a computer-generated display of molecular models. The computer display allows one to readily perform rotation around appropriate bond angles while obtaining a three-dimensional image of the molecular structures on a video-screen (Figure 7).[38]

Figure 7A displays the conformation of a single dinucleoside monophosphate, ApG, in which the ribose-phosphate-ribose backbone has a right-handed helical conformation analogous to that found in double helical DNA, with each of the bases in the *anti* conformation and stacked coplanar to each other. In the display of ApG-AAF (Figure 7B), the guanine base has been rotated around the glycosidic bond to the *syn* conformation to avoid the problem of steric hindrance discussed above. In addition, the guanine base has been displaced from its normal coplanar relation with the adjacent adenine residue by the planar AAF molecule, and the latter is now stacked with the neighboring adenine residue.

A similar model called the "insertion-denaturation model" for AAF-modified DNA has been proposed by Fuchs and Daune.[31,40]They modified native calf thymus DNA with *N*-acetoxy-AAF, or with the 7-fluoro (AAFF) and 7-iodo (AAIF) derivatives of *N*-acetoxy-AAF. The technique of electric dichroism was then used to determine the orientation of the covalently bound fluorene ring to the long axis of the DNA. The

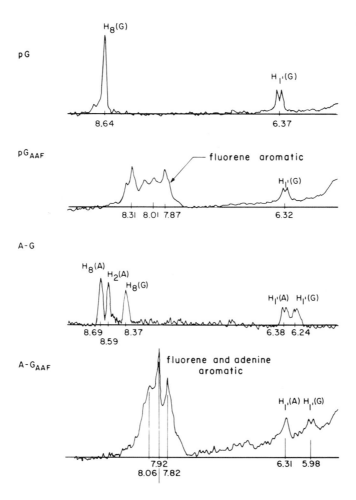

FIGURE 6. Proton magnetic resonance spectra of the aromatic and H₁ protons of pG, Pg$_{AAF}$, ApG, and ApG$_{AAF}$. Chemical shifts are ppm downfield from external tetramethylsilane. Spectral assignments are shown above the resonance signals with the appropriate nucleoside indicated in parentheses. The solvent is 0.005 M deuterated phosphate buffer in D₂O at pD ≏ 7. (With permission from Grunberger, D., Nelson, J. H., Cantor, C. R., and Weinstein, I. B., *J. Mol. Biol.*, 62, 331, 1971. Copyright by Academic Press, Inc. (London) Ltd.)

results clearly indicated that in the case of DNA-AAF and DNA-AAFF, the fluorene ring lies almost perpendicular to the helix axis, the angle being 80°. On the other hand, with the iodo derivative, DNA-AAIF, they found the angle between the transition moment of the fluorene molecule and the helix axis to be only 60°. The results obtained with DNA-AAF and DNA-AAFF are consistent with those observed with AAF-modified dimers, as well as other physical studies on AAF-modified DNA described by Fuchs and Daune[31,40]and Levine et al.,[30] since the base displacement or "base insertion" model would predict an angle of orientation approaching 90°. On the other hand, the 60° angle obtained with DNA-AAIF is not compatible with the latter model. The different conformation of DNA-AAIF can be explained by the fact that the bulky iodine atom (which has a van der Waals' diameter of 4.3, compared to 2.4 and 2.7 for H and F, respectively) would be expected to prevent insertion of the iodofluorene between base plates in native DNA, which are separated by a distance of 3.4Å.[31,41]It seems likely, therefore, that in the case of DNA-AAF and DNA-AAFF, the fluorene

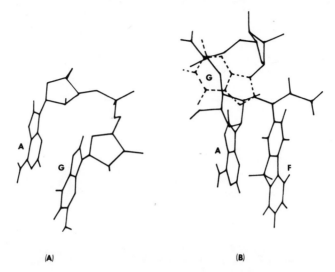

(A)   (B)

FIGURE 7.   Computer display of three-dimensional structures of ApG and ApG$_{AAF}$. (A) The conformation of ApG with Watson-Crick type geometry. (B) The base displacement model of ApG$_{AAF}$. The fluorene and adenine rings are stacked, and the displaced guanosine in *syn* conformation is represented by dashed lines. (With permission from Grunberger, D., Nelson, J. H., Cantor, C. R., and Weinstein, I. B., *J. Mol. Biol.*, 62, 331, 1971. Copyright by Academic Press, Inc. (London) Ltd.)

ring is inserted into the helix almost perpendicular to the helix axis, whereas with DNA-AAIF, the iodine substituted fluorene residue lies along the phosphate-sugar backbone outside the DNA helix. It is interesting from this point of view that AAF and AAFF are strong carcinogens, but AAIF apparently lacks carcinogenic activity.[42]

In separate electric dichroism studies on DNA-AAF, Chang et al.[43] also measured the angle of orientation of the fluorene ring with respect to the DNA helix axis and obtained an angle of 60°, which is in apparent contradiction with the 80° angle obtained by Fuchs et al.[40] Chang et al.,[43] however, measured the orientation of the fluorene ring after renaturation of a DNA sample which had been reacted with the carcinogen in a denatured state. It is possible that during the renaturation step, the arrangement between base plates and the fluorene rings is not the same as in a DNA sample modified in the native state. Moreover, Chang et al.[43] studied a DNA-AAF sample in which 12% of the bases had been modified with AAF, whereas, Fuchs et al.[40] and Levine et al.[30] studied samples that were much less heavily modified. Thus, the data obtained by Chang et al.[43] may apply only to extreme conditions (denatured and highly modified DNA) and probably do not relate to the orientation of the fluorene residue in DNA modified in vivo.

B. Localized Regions of Denaturation

The base displacement model predicts that AAF modification of double-stranded nucleic acids should produce a localized denaturation at the site of AAF modification. The distortion produced might result in a destabilization of double-stranded regions which could extend over a distance of several nucleotide residues adjacent to the modified G residue. Several different types of experimental studies support these predictions.

1. Heat denaturation

Heat denaturation studies indicate that AAF modification decreases the T_m of DNA.[30,40,44-47] For each 1% of the bases modified, there is an approximate 1.5°C decrease in T_m.[47]

The decrease in T_m might be explained if we assume that AAF substitution of G residues simply displaces these G residues, thereby breaking single G-C base pairs and thus decreasing the effective G-C content of the DNA sample. A comparison of the data with the nomogram of Marmur and Doty[48] relating T_m to G + C content, however, indicates that the observed decrease in T_m is greater than that predicted by this assumption. It appears, therefore, that the destabilizing effect of AAF modification of double-stranded DNA extends beyond the immediate G residue that has been substituted.

2. Viscosity

AAF modification causes a marked decrease in the intrinsic viscosity of the DNA.[30] The viscosity of DNA is a function of both its flexibility and the length of strands. Denaturation of native DNA is known to lead to a decrease in its intrinsic viscosity, whereas the noncovalent binding of acridines, Miracil D, or polycyclic hydrocarbons to DNA, via intercalation, results in an increase in intrinsic viscosity.[15,16,49,50] This is explained by the fact that localized regions of denaturation provide flexible elbows in the DNA strand. On the other hand, sites of drug intercalation have a decreased flexibility, and intercalation is also associated with a lengthening of the DNA strand.[16,50]

3. Formaldehyde Unwinding

In order to more accurately assess the extent of local denaturation in AAF-modified DNA, Fuchs and Daune[31,41] have applied the formaldehyde unwinding method of Utiyama and Doty[51] and von Hippel and Wong.[52] This method has the advantage of providing information about the dynamic structure of DNA and can be used to calculate the number of open base pairs. They measured the kinetics of unwinding of calf thymus DNA-AAF and found that the number of open base plates in the vicinity of a covalently bound fluorene residue was 12 to 13. This number was independent of the percentage of modified bases, within the range of 1.7 to 3.7% modification.[31,41]

4. S_1 Nuclease Digestion

The best evidence for localized regions of denaturation in double stranded DNA modified by AAF comes from studies on the susceptibility of AAF-modified DNA to digestion by S_1 nuclease, a single-strand specific endonuclease from *Aspergillus oryzae*.[53,54] When the kinetics of hydrolysis of AAF-modified calf thymus DNA by S_1 nuclease were measured, they were found to be intermediate between that of native and fully denatured DNA.[53] Moreover, by measurements at A_{305}, the material rendered acid-soluble during the digestion was shown to contain fluorene residues. Utilizing a similar approach, Yamasaki et al.[54] have estimated the number of base pairs destabilized by a single AAF modification. Purified duck reticulocyte DNA was modified with [14C]-N-acetoxy AAF yielding preparations in which 0.01 to 4% of the total nucleotides were modified. Evidence that AAF modification leads to localized regions of denaturation was obtained by incubating the modified DNAs with endonuclease S_1.[54] As shown in Figure 8, under the conditions of nuclease incubation, unmodified native DNA underwent less than 5% digestion; heat denatured DNA was, however, rapidly and completely hydrolyzed. With a sample of DNA in which 3% of the nucleotides were modified with AAF, over 60% of the nucleotides were digested. This was associated with the release of [14C]AAF residues, which occurred more rapidly than the release of total nucleotides, indicating that [14C]AAF nucleotides were preferentially removed.

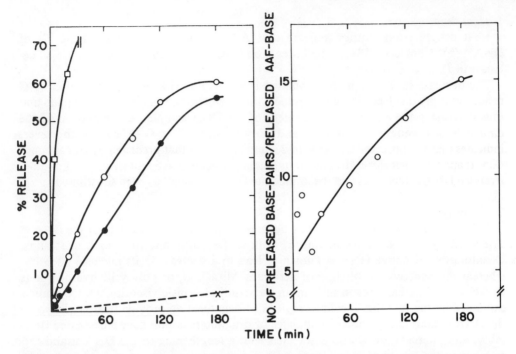

FIGURE 8.   Digestion of samples of DNA with S_1 nuclease. (A) Percentage of digestion of heat-denatured DNA (□), native unmodified DNA (X), and [^{14}C]AAF-modified native DNA (●), based on the release of ethanol-soluble A_{260} material; (○), the release of ethanol-soluble radioactivity S_1 nuclease was used at 5 × 10³ units/mℓ, and 3% of the bases were modified in the [^{14}C]AAF DNA. (B) The ratio of base pairs released per each [^{14}C]AAF residue released. (From Yamasaki, H., Leffler, S., and Weinstein, I. B., *Cancer Res.*, 37, 684, 1977. With permission.)

With a DNA sample in which only 0.5% of the nucleotides were modified by AAF, the reaction rate was slower and the total number of nucleotides released was smaller than that obtained with the 3% modified DNA. In the former case, only 15% of the DNA nucleotides were released.[54]

These results indicate that modification of native DNA by covalent attachment of AAF residues lead to localized regions of denaturation, since the modified regions were excised by S_1 nuclease. The estimated number of base pairs destabilized by a single AAF modification was in the range of 5 to 50 depending on the extent of modification of the DNA, the length of the nuclease digestion period, and the NaCl concentration during the digestion (Figure 8).[54] This value appeared to decrease when DNA samples were modified to an increasing extent with AAF. A possible explanation is that AAF-modified regions are preferentially further modified by AAF, because they were already denatured. This interpretation is consistent with the fact that denatured DNA is more susceptible to AAF modification than native DNA.[30] Thus, at high extents of modification, there is a tendency for clustering of AAF residues in denatured regions. The digestion of such regions by S_1 nuclease would lead to a lower ratio of released base pairs to released AAF residues than the digestion of more randomly dispersed AAF residues. Clustering is less likely to play an important role in vivo because of the extremely low extents of modification that occur under in vivo conditions.

C. Preferential Modification of Single-Stranded Regions

According to the base displacement model, attachment of AAF to G residues requires rotation of the base about the glycosidic bond. Because there is less hindrance to the rotation of bases in single-stranded than in double stranded regions, one would predict that G residues in single-strand regions will be more accessible to modification. The tRNAs are convenient molecules with which to test this possibility, since they have known sequences consisting of both single-strand or "loop" regions and double-strand or "stem" regions.[55] We found that when formylmethione tRNA from *Escherichia coli,* which contains 25 G residues, was reacted with [^{14}C]acetoxy-AAF, the carcinogen was bound only to the G residue at position 20 in the single-strand D loop.[56] Specificity was also observed with AAF modification of yeast tyrosine tRNA.[57] In the latter case, AAF was bound to two G residues in the D loop, and also to a G residue in the anticodon loop. X-Ray crystallography studies of yeast phenylalanine tRNA have provided information on the tertiary structure of tRNA molecules, which is entirely consistent with our results.[58,59] According to these studies, G^{20} in the D loop and bases in the anticodon loop of phenylalanine tRNA are in single-strand regions which are exposed on the exterior of the molecule.

Evidence that single-stranded regions of nucleic acids are more susceptible to AAF modification than double-stranded regions has also been obtained by comparing the reactivity of native and denatured calf thymus DNA with N-acetoxy-AAF. We have found that denatured DNA is approximately twice as susceptible to AAF modification as native DNA.[30] Media of high ionic strength are known to stabilize nucleic acid secondary structure, and an increase in ionic strength decreases the reactivity of native DNA with N-acetoxy-AAF.[30] A similar effect has been observed in the reaction of N-acetoxy-AAF with duplexes between synthetic polydeoxynucleotides.[60]

Harvan et al.[60] have studied the effects of base sequence and nucleic acid structure on the interaction of N-acetoxy-AAF with synthetic polydeoxynucleotides. They found that the alternating copolymer poly(dG-dC)·(dG-dC) was 1.5 to 3 times more reactive than the homopolymer complex poly(dG)·poly(dC), and 10 to 20 times more reactive than the A + T polymers. At an ionic strength at which the two guanine-containing polymers had equal thermal stability, the alternating copolymer was seven times as reactive as the homopolymer. They postulate that AAF attack on the alternating copolymer poly (dG-dC)·poly(dG-C) would generate by local denaturation two single-strand guanine-containing polymers that would be highly susceptible to further modification by AAF. On the other hand, with the homopolymer complex, localized denaturation due to initial attack by AAF would generate only one guanine-containing single-strand polymer. It is also likely that since G-G and G-AAF stacking interactions are much greater than those with G-C,[38] the C spacers in the alternating copolymer would provide a less rigid structure that is more susceptible to the conformational changes associated with AAF modification. It is possible, therefore, that in native DNA G residues flanked by C (or T) are more susceptible to AAF modification than those flanked by other G residues. Elsewhere, we have discussed the effects of base sequence on the structure and base-pairing properties of AAF-containing oligonucleotides (See Section II.D). Taken together, these findings suggest that during in vivo administration, specific regions of the genome may suffer preferential damage by this carcinogen.

D. Functional Consequences of the Base Displacement Model: Impairment of Base Pairing

The base displacement model enables one to make several predictions concerning the functional aspects of the modified nucleic acid. The model predicts that AAF-modified G residues will not participate in base pairing, since by rotation from *anti* to *syn*, they are displaced from their usual alignment with adjacent bases. This was tested in an in vitro translational system using triplet codons or polynucleotides containing AAF-modified G residues as messenger RNAs.[39,61] It was found (Figure 9) that the effects of modification were twofold. The first effect was that if the G residue to which

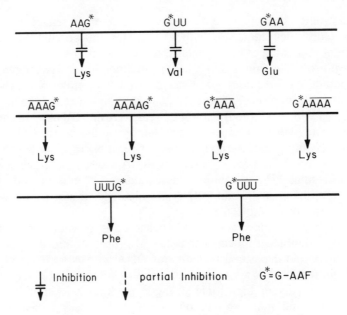

FIGURE 9.   Effect of AAF modification on codon function.

AAF was covalently bound was part of a codon, then that codon was inactive. This was the case with the lysine (Lys) codon, AAG; the valine (Val) codon, GUU; or the glutamic acid (Glu) codon, GAA. With these triplets, complete inactivation of their function and no miscoding was observed. The second effect was that if there was an A residue adjacent, either at the 5′ or 3′ side of the modified G, the codon containing the residue was partially impaired in terms of its ability to stimulate ribosomal binding of the corresponding aminoacyl-tRNA.[39,61] This was observed with the tetramers GAAA and AAAG in which modification of G residues with the carcinogen led to approximately a 50% reduction of the recognition of the AAA codon by lysyl-tRNA. This inhibition diminished when pentamers containing an additional A residue, GAAAA or AAAAG, were modified with AAF, suggesting that the inhibitory effect was limited mainly to the base immediately adjacent to the modified G residue. In contrast, the U residues adjacent to the modified G in GUUU and UUUG tetramers were not impaired in terms of their coding function. Both of these effects are entirely consistent with the CD, as well as with the PMR data,[38,39] which showed a strong interaction in oligonucleotides between the fluorene moiety and the adjacent A, but not the adjacent U residues.

If the base-pairing ability of modified G residues in oligonucleotides is blocked during translation, then similar effects might be observed during transcription of an AAF-modified DNA template. It has, indeed, been found that mammalian DNA modified with AAF is impaired in its template activity for bacterial RNA polymerase.[44,62] The transcription of AAF-modified bacteriophage T7 DNA by RNA polymerase is also markedly inhibited.[63] Analysis of the RNA products demonstrated that this inhibition is due to premature chain termination, probably because of failure of base pairing when, during chain elongation, the polymerase encounters AAF-modified G residues. The inhibition of rat hepatic nuclear RNA synthesis after in vivo administration of N-OH-AAF could also reflect impairment of nucleolar DNA template function.[64] As a result of AAF modification, direct effects on polymerase function may also be involved.[65-68]

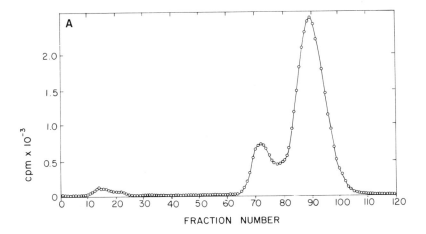

FIGURE 10. Sephadex® LH-20 column chromatography of a nucleoside hydrolysate of [^{14}C]AAF-modified DNA. One A$_{260}$ unit of DNA (equivalent to 150 nmol of nucleotide residues) containing 700 pmol of [^{14}C]AAF was completely hydrolyzed by a series of enzymes after heat denaturation, and a total hydrolysate was then applied to a Sephadex® LH-20 column. The column (0.8 × 20 cm) was eluted first with 50 mℓ of 10 mM (NH$_4$)$_2$CO$_3$ to elute unmodified nucleosides and then with 35% ethanol containing 10 mM (NH$_4$)$_2$CO$_3$. Fractions (1 mℓ) were collected, and radioactivity was measured in a liquid scintillation spectrometer. (From Yamasaki, H., Pulkrabek, P., Grunberger, D., and Weinstein, I. B., *Cancer Res.*, 37, 3756, 1977. With permission.)

E. Differences in Conformation Between the C⁸ and N² Guanosine Adducts

The modification of DNA by AAF in vivo and by N-acetoxy-AAF in vitro leads to the formation of two AAF-DNA adducts: the major adduct, N-(deoxyguanosin-8-yl)-AAF, accounts for about 80% and the minor adduct, 3-(deoxyguanosin-N²-yl)-AAF, accounts for about 20% of the covalently bound carcinogen.[35,69] It seemed probable that differences might exist between the conformational distortions in the DNA helix associated with these two different types of adducts because of differences in the steric aspects associated with the C⁸ and N² positions of G. Since earlier studies concentrated on the conformation of the C⁸ adduct, we have more recently examined possible differences with respect to the minor adduct, utilizing the technique of S₁ nuclease digestion.[70]

Figure 10 confirms previous studies[69] indicating that when DNA is modified in vitro with [^{14}C]-N-acetoxy-AAF and completely hydrolyzed enzymically, two radioactive peaks are resolved by Sephadex® LH-20 column chromatography. The first peak has been identified as 3-(deoxyguanosine-N²-yl)-AAF and the second peak as N-(deoxyguanosine-8-yl)-AAF.[69]

Figure 11 indicates that during the course of digestion with S₁ nuclease, under conditions which preferentially hydrolyze single-stranded regions, there is a change in the ratio of the AAF adducts in the S₁ nuclease-resistant fraction of the DNA. In these studies, AAF-modified DNA was exposed to S₁ nuclease for 0, 2, 4.5, or 6 hr. The undigested fraction was then reisolated, hydrolyzed completely, and the modified nucleosides separated on a Sephadex® LH-20 column. It is evident that during the 6-hr incubation with S₁ nuclease, there was a progressive and marked decrease in the amount of N-(deoxyguanosin-8-yl)-AAF in the S₁ nuclease-resistant fraction. Under the same conditions, however, there was little loss from the undigested fraction of the 3-(deoxyguanosin-N²-yl)-AAF residues. Thus, S₁ nuclease preferentially digests regions of the DNA containing N-(deoxyguanosin-8-yl)-AAF residues, whereas sites with 3-(deoxyguanosin-N²-yl)-AAF residues remained basically intact. To confirm that the

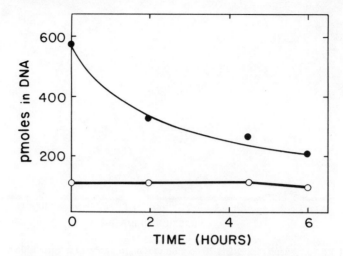

FIGURE 11.   The amount of G-AAF residues in the S_1 resistant
fractions of [^{14}C]AAF-DNA. One A_{260} unit of DNA (equivalent to
150 nmol of nucleotide residues) containing 700 pmol of [^{14}C]AAF
was incubated with 5×10^3 units of S_1 nuclease in 30 mM sodium
acetate buffer (pH 4.5), 50 mM NaCl, and 1 mM ZnSO$_4$ for either 0,
2, 4.5, or 6 hr at 37°C. In each case, the nondigested fraction of DNA
was precipitated and then completely hydrolyzed to nucleosides, and
the total hydrolysate was chromatographed on Sephadex® LH-20
columns, as in Figure 10. The ordinate indicates the number of pmol
of N-(deoxyguanosin-8-yl)-AAF (●), and 3-(deoxyguanosin-N^2-yl)-
AAF (○) remaining in the S_1 nuclease-resistant fractions obtained
from equivalent samples (1 A_{260} unit) of [^{14}C]AAF-modified DNA following various incubation times with S_1 nuclease. (From Yamasaki,
H., Pulkrabek, P., Grunberger, D., and Weinstein, I. B., *Cancer
Res.*, 37, 3756, 1977. With permission.)

oligonucleotides in single-stranded regions contain mainly N-(deoxyguanosin-8-yl)-
AAF, another single-strand specific endonuclease from *Neurospora crassa* was used.
Following incubation, the undigested fraction of the DNA was precipitated with cold
ethanol. This material and the released oligonucleotides present in the supernatant
fraction were then separately hydrolyzed completely to nucleosides and analyzed by
Sephadex® LH-20 column chromatography (Figure 12). The profile of the undigested
fraction of the DNA demonstrated a decrease in the ratio of the C^8 to N^2 AAF-guanine
adducts. In addition, the C^8 but not the N^2 AAF adduct was detected in the oligonucleotide fraction released by *N. crassa* enzyme. Thus, the latter enzyme, like the S_1
nuclease, recognizes the N-(deoxyguanosin-8-yl)-AAF-modified regions, but not the 3-
(deoxyguanosin-N^2-yl)-AAF-modified regions, as single-stranded regions on AAF-
modified DNA molecules.

It appears, therefore, that in contrast to the C^8 adduct, substitution of AAF on the
N^2 position of guanine does not produce a major change in conformation of the DNA
helix. Although the precise conformation of the helix at the latter sites has not been
determined, model-building studies indicate that the N^2 position, in contrast to the C^8
position, of guanine is readily susceptible to chemical modification, and the fluorene
residue could simply occupy the minor groove of the DNA helix. Thus, the base displacement model (see previous sections, this chapter) may apply only to the C^8 adduct
of AAF.

In terms of the in vivo significance of our results, it is of interest that Kriek[36] found
that the C^8 adduct is rapidly removed from rat liver in vivo (half-life, 7 days), whereas

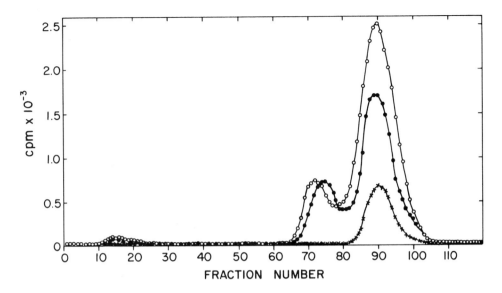

FIGURE 12. Sephadex® LH-20 column chromatography of nucleoside hydrolysates of the total, the *N. crassa* nuclease-digested fraction, and the *N. crassa* nuclease-resistant fraction of [¹⁴C]AAF-modified DNA. [¹⁴C]AAF-modified DNA was completely digested to nucleosides after heat denaturation. *N. crassa* nuclease digestion was performed in 10mM Tris-HCl (pH 7.9), 100 mM NaCl and 1 mM MgCl₃ for 3 hr at 37°C. The resistant fraction was precipitated with 2.5 volumes of ethanol, collected by centrifugation, and hydrolyzed to nucleosides. (O), total [¹⁴C]AAF-modified DNA; (●), *N. crassa* nuclease-resistaat fraction; (X) *N. crassa* nuclease digested fraction. (From Yamasaki, H., Pulkrabek, P., Grunberger, D., and Weinstein, I. B., *Cancer Res.*, 37, 3756, 1977. With permission.)

the guanine-N² adduct remained persistently bound to DNA (see Volume II, Chapter 1). Taken together with out in vitro results, this suggests that the DNA excision repair enzyme system preferentially recognizes and excises lesions associated with major distortions in conformation of the DNA helix. Assuming that the DNA excision repair system operates with high fidelity, persistent carcinogen substituents, such as adducts on the N² position of guanine, might be more significant in terms of carcinogenesis. In other words, carcinogen potency might be a function of two factors: (1) ability to bind to DNA and alter its template function, and (2) ability to bind in a form that does not produce a conformational distortion that is readily recognized and excised by DNA repair systems.

III. STRUCTURAL AND CONFORMATIONAL PROPERTIES OF NUCLEIC ACIDS MODIFIED WITH A BENZO[A]PYRENE DIOL-EPOXIDE (BPDE)

A. Structures of Nucleoside Adducts

Several studies have documented that the 7,8-dihydrodiol-9,10-oxide of benzo[a]pyrene (BPDE) is the major metabolic intermediate in the covalent binding of this polycyclic aromatic hydrocarbon to cellular nucleic acids.[71-75] It has also been established that in both RNA and DNA the major nucleoside adduct results from linkage of the 10 position of BPDE to the 2-amino (N²) group of guanine.[76-79]

Two stereoisomers of BP 7,8-dihydrodiol-9,10-oxide (BPDE) have been synthesized. In isomer I, the 7-hydroxyl and 9,10-oxide groups are on the opposite sides of the plane of the ring system. In isomer II, they are on the same side.[80,81] Each stereoisomer has two enantiomers.[82] In the 7R enantiomers, the 7-hydroxyl faces upward, and in the 7S enantiomer downward, with respect to the ring system (see Figure 13). In theory,

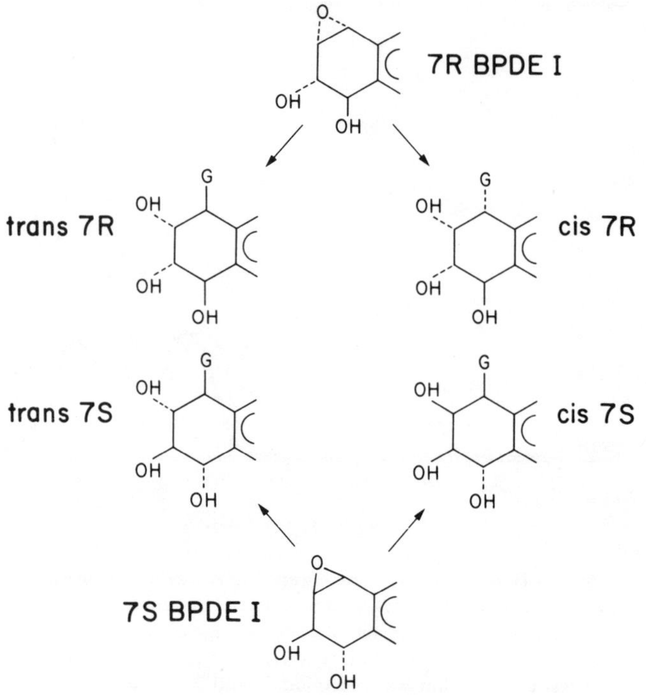

FIGURE 13.   Possible structures of N_2 guanosine adducts from *trans* and *cis* openings at C^{10} of 7R and 7S BPDE I.

each enantiomer could also generate two different forms of the guanine adduct, one resulting from a 9,10 *trans* addition of the guanine and the other from a 9,10 *cis* addition. Thus, it is possible for BPDE I to generate four different isomers of a BPDE-guanine adduct (Figure 13). Similarly, BPDE II can also generate four different isomeric guanine adducts. The structure and absolute stereochemistry of a guanine adduct resulting from 9,10 *trans* addition of the 7R enantiomer of BPDE I has been elucidated[76,83] and is depicted in Figure 14. This structure was found to be the major nucleic acid adduct found in RNA and DNA when human or bovine bronchial segments were incubated in vitro with [³H]-BP.[77-82] This specific isomer is also the major adduct formed when a racemic mixture of BPDE I is incubated with DNA at neutral pH in vitro.[108] CD spectroscopy has proved to be a valuable tool for identifying diastereoisomeric pairs of BPDE-nucleoside adducts. High-pressure liquid chromatographic (HPLC) methods have been developed for the separation of these adducts with high resolution.[84]

In the following discussion on conformations associated with BPDE modifications of nucleic acids, we will be concerned mainly with the specific structure and stereoisomer depicted in Figure 14. We must emphasize, however, that there is evidence that both BPDE isomers I and II are formed in vivo, although BPDE II is formed to a much lesser extent than BPDE I.[85-87] In addition, it appears that both the 7R and 7S enantiomers of BPDE I and II can be formed in vivo.[88] Studies in progress indicate that, in contrast to the relatively simple profile seen in human and bovine bronchial DNA, in certain rodent cell cultures and in mouseskin exposed to BP, the DNA may contain adducts derived from both BPDE isomers I and II, from both 7R and 7S enantiomers, and from both 9,10 *trans* and 9,10 *cis* additions to guanine residues.[86,88,89] The relative amounts of these other adducts varies considerably and their identification is tentative.

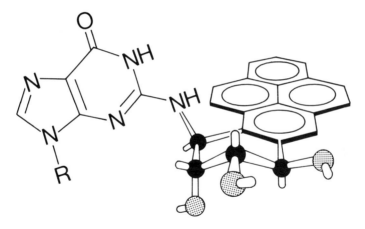

FIGURE 14.   Schematic representation of the quanosine-BP adduct formed from the reaction of BP-diol-epoxide isomer I with poly[G]. The 2-amino group of guanine is linked to the C^{10} position of the BP moiety. The solid black spheres designate carbons 10,9,8, and 7 on the saturated ring of BP. The shaded spheres designate OH residues on carbons 9,8, and 7. The R designates the ribose residue. The guanine residue is *trans* to the 9-OH, the 9- and 8-OH are *cis*, and the 8- and 7-OH are *trans*. (From Weinstein, I. B., Jeffrey, A. M., Jennette, K. W., Blobstein, S. H., Harvey, R. G., Harris, C., Autrup, H., Kasai, H., and Nakanishi, K., *Science*, 197, 592, 1977. With permission. Copyright 1977 by the American Association for the Advancement of Science.)

B. Circular Dichroism Spectra of Dinucleoside Monophosphates Modified with BPDE

To obtain information on how attachment of the bulky hydrocarbon residue of BP to the N^2 position of G residues might alter the tertiary structure of nucleic acids, we have used, as model compounds, dinucleoside monophosphates (dimers) modified with BPDE and analyzed their CD spectra.[90] The reaction of the dimer GpU with BPDE I (a racemic mixture of 7R and 7S) resulted in the formation of four products which were well resolved by HPLC (Figure 15). Analyses of their nucleoside composition and CD studies indicated that these represented four types of modified dimers with each type containing a different stereoisomer of the G-BPDE adduct: 7R 9,10 *cis*; 7S 9,10 *trans*; 7S 9,10 *cis*; and 7R 9,10 *trans* (see Figure 13). Figures 16A and B show the CD spectra of GpU and the G*pU compounds I through IV (G* designates BPDE-modified guanosine). It is apparent that BPDE modification markedly alters the CD spectra of GpU. The fact that the CD spectra of G*pU I and III are almost mirror images, and that the same relationship is true of G*pU II and IV, provides one type of evidence that the four modified dimers differ from each other by their content of different stereoisomers of G*.

The molar elipticity [θ] values of the modified dimers were 1.5 to 2-fold higher than those of the corresponding G* monomers. This suggested that there is a physical interaction between the BPDE residue and the adjacent uracil base. Since this type of interaction might be disrupted by organic solvents or by elevated temperatures, we further analyzed the CD spectra in a water-methanol mixture and also at 80°C (Table 1). The presence of methanol or heating produced a significant decrease in the [θ] values at 282 nm for all four compounds. The decrease varied from 27% for G*pU III to 50% for G*pU IV. When the four G*pU samples were dissolved in 50 or 100% methanol, the [θ] values were similar to those of the corresponding G* monomers dissolved in water. Thus, an organic solvent or heating diminishes interactions between the BPDE residue and the adjacent uracil base, but does not appear to change the basic conformation of a guanosine monomer adduct.

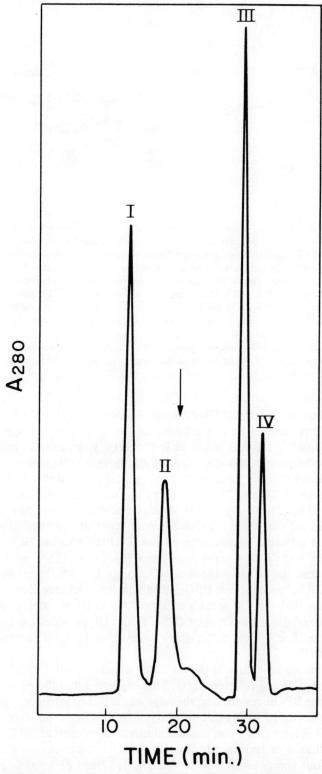

FIGURE 15.   HPLC profile of the G*pU adducts isolated from the Sephadex® LH-20 column. The arrow indicates the start of a linear gradient of 5 to 10% methanol in water. (Reprinted with permission from Pulkrabek, P., Leffler, S., Weinstein, I. B., and Grunberger, D., *Biochemistry*, 16, 3127, 1977. Copyright by the American Chemical Society.)

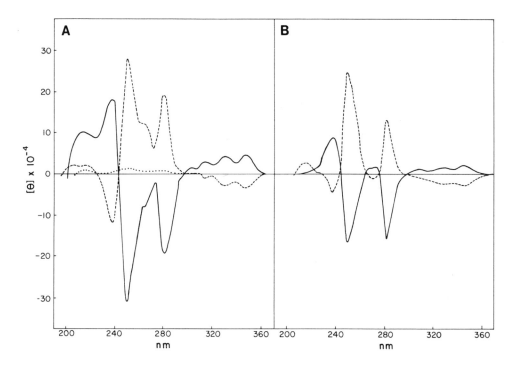

FIGURE 16.   CD spectra of GpU and G*pU adducts. Adducts were purified by HPLC prior to the CD measurements. Spectra were determined in water, and $[\theta]$ was based on $\varepsilon_{278} = 1.16 \times 10^4$ for GpU and $\varepsilon_{278} = 5.84 \times 10^4$ for G*pU. (A) G*pU I, —; G*pU III, ---; GpU, $\cdots$; (B) G*pU II, —; G*pU IV, ---. (Reprinted with permission from Pulkrabek, P., Leffler, S., Weinstein, I. B., and Grunberger, D., *Biochemistry*, 16, 3127, 1977. Copyright by the American Chemical Society.)

Possible explanations for the above results were sought with CPK space-filling models. A plausible model for G*pU II or G*pU IV, the two 9,10 *trans* products, is shown schematically in Figure 17. Starting with a dimer having the usual conformational parameters of RNA (see Section I), an alteration in conformation which maximizes stacking interaction between the pyrene ring system and the neighboring uracil was achieved, largely by rotating the guanine residue about 45° around its glycosidic bond. In this conformation, the plane of the pyrene ring is perpendicular to the long axis of the phosphate-sugar backbone, and the displaced guanine is no longer coplanar to the neighboring uracil. At the same time, the hydrophilic hydroxyls of the BPDE residue face the ribose of the modified G.

We must stress, however, that our CD data, while providing evidence for a physical interaction between the BPDE residue and an adjacent uracil, do not in themselves establish that this is a stacking interaction. In studies on dimers containing covalently bound AAF residues,[37,38] the changes in CD spectra were more pronounced than those seen with BPDE-modified dimers. It is possible, therefore, that whereas the AAF residue is actually stacked with the adjacent base, the BPDE residue interacts with the adjacent base, but is not actually coplanar to it. The latter would be the case if the BPDE residue resides in a position analogous to the minor groove of the helix (see Section III. C. 5). Definitive assignments of the conformations of the BPDE-modified dimers requires further studies, such as nmr spectroscopy and X-ray crystallography.

C. Conformation of DNA Modified with BPDE

To examine conformational changes in high-molecular-weight nucleic acids, we have reacted native calf thymus DNA with BPDE I in vitro under nondenaturing conditions

TABLE 1

Effects of Temperature and Solvent on the Molar Elipticity Values of G*pU Compounds ($[\theta]_{282}$ × 10^{-4})

Compound	Water		Methanol at 25°C	
	25°C	80°C	50%	100%
G*pU I	19.5	12.8	17.5	—
II	15.8	10.0	13.6	8.6
III	18.6	13.6	15.5	13.6
IV	13.1	9.2	9.8	6.4

*   For formulas, see Figure 16.

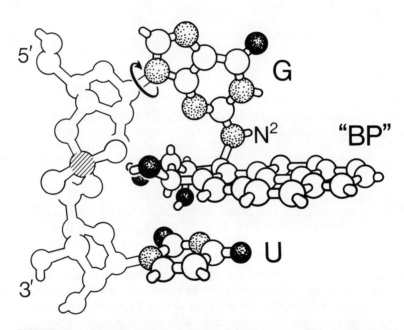

FIGURE 17.   Schematic representation of the proposed conformation of G*pU II and IV (*trans* adducts). The O designates oxygen, ◐ nitrogen, ● phosphorus, and "BP" the BPDE residue following its covalent attachment to the N² of G. The G residue has been rotated about its glycosidic bond to allow "insertion" of the "BP" residue coplanar to the adjacent U. (Reprinted with permission from Pulkrabek, P., Leffler S., Weinstein, I. B., and Grunberger, D., *Biochemistry*, 16, 3127, 1977. Copyright by the American Chemical Society.)

and then studied certain physical properties of the modified DNA molecules.[91] When the nucleoside composition of the modified DNA was analyzed, the only BPDE adduct detected was that depicted in Figure 14, thus simplifying the interpretation of our physical studies. The physical properties have included heat denaturation, formaldehyde unwinding, susceptibility to a single-strand specific endonuclease, sedimentation in cesium chloride and in neutral and alkaline sucrose gradients, electric dichroism, and fluorescense.

1. Heat Denaturation

Figure 18 shows that increasing extents of modification of native DNA with BPDE

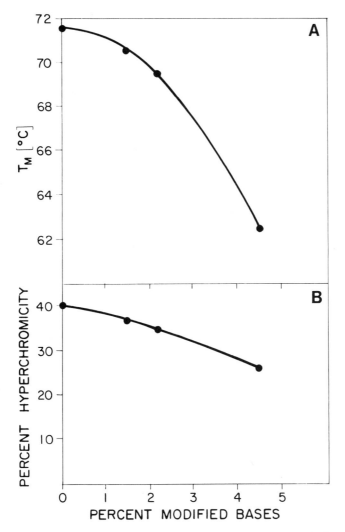

FIGURE 18. (A) Effect of modification of DNA on T_m and (B) hyperchromicity. Each DNA sample (1 A_{260}) in 0.042 M sodium borate (pH 9.0) was melted in a thermocell of a Gilford® Type 240 recording spectrophotometer equipped with Type 2527 Thermoprogrammer®. Temperature was increased at a rate of 1°C/min and absorption at 260 nm was recorded by a Gilford® Type 5040A recorder. Data were plotted against the percentage of modified bases. (Reprinted with permission from Pulkrabek, P., Leffler, S., Weinstein, I. B., and Grunberger, D., *Biochemistry*, 16, 3127, 1977. Copyright by the American Chemical Society.)

led to a progressive decrease in T_m during heat denaturation. The decrease in T_m was not linearly related to the percent of bases modified. When less than 1% of the bases were modified, no significant decrease in T_m could be detected (data not shown). In the range of 1 to 2% modification, the decrease in T_m was about 0.75°C per each 1% modification. In DNA with a 4.5% modification, the T_m was lowered by about 1.7°C for each 1% modification. The decrease in T_m was associated with a decrease in total hyperchromicity (Figure 18), suggesting that portions of the DNA duplex had undergone localized denaturation as a consequence of modification by BPDE.

2. Kinetics of Formaldehyde Unwinding

In order to more accurately assess the extent of denaturation in the BPDE-modified DNA samples, we applied the formaldehyde unwinding method of Utiyama and Doty[51] and of von Hippel and Wong.[52] Since formaldehyde reacts preferentially with bases in open regions of the helix, it can be used as a chemical probe for determining the number of open base pairs in double helical DNA at temperatures below the T_m of the DNA. Figure 19 plots the increase with time in absorbance at 251 nm, following the addition of formaldehyde to equal concentrations of various types of DNA. It is apparent that the formaldehyde reactivity increased with the level of DNA modification. The average number of open base plates calculated according to Utiyama and Doty was zero to one with the 1.5% modified sample, two to three with the 2.2% sample, and six to seven with the 4.5% modified sample. Thus, only with the highly modified sample did the binding of the BPDE derivative produce large regions of open base plates.

3. S_1 Nuclease Digestion

A very useful method to determine whether covalent binding of the BPDE derivative to native DNA produced localized single-strand regions in the DNA molecule was to incubate the DNA samples with S_1 endonuclease from *Aspergillus oryzae,* an enzyme which, under appropriate conditions, will cleave single but not double-stranded regions of DNA.[92] Figure 20 indicates that a sample of DNA that had been previously completely heat denatured was rapidly and almost completely digested during a 240 min incubation with S_1 nuclease. The BPDE-DNA sample that contained a 1.5% modification was identical to the control in its resistance to S_1 digestion, whereas that which contained a 2.2% modification was slightly more susceptible to S_1 digestion (15%

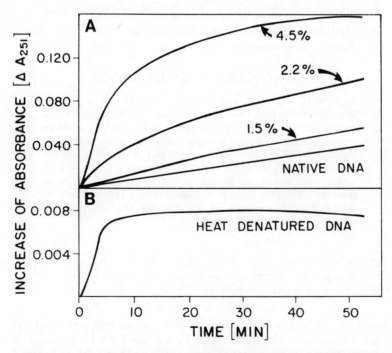

FIGURE 19.   Kinetics of formaldehyde unwinding of DNA samples. Increase in optical density of DNA at 251 nm was followed in reaction mixtures containing 0.042 *M* sodium borate (pH 9.0)-1 *M* formaldehyde. (A) Native, 1.5%, 2.2%, and 4.5% BPDE modified DNA; (B) Heat-denatured DNA.

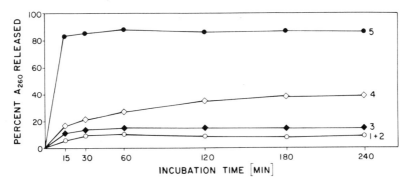

FIGURE 20.. Kinetics of hydrolysis of DNA samples by S_1 endonuclease from *Aspergillus oryzae*. The incubation mixtures contained (final volume 0.3 ml); 0.05 M sodium acetate (pH 4.6), 0.05 M NaCl, 1×10^{-3} M ZnSO$_4$, 0.1 mg of DNA, and 5 units of S_1 nuclease. Incubation was carried out at 45°C and terminated by chilling, then 0.25 mg of DNA was added as a carrier and nonhydrolyzed DNA was immediately precipitated with 0.6 ml of 10% perchloric acid. Samples were centrifuged and A_{260} was determined in supernatants. (O — O) Control DNA (1) and 1.5% BP-modified DNA (2); (◆ — ◆) 2.2% BP-modified DNA (3); (◇ — ◇) 4.5% BP-modified DNA (4); (● — ●) heat denatured DNA (5). (Reprinted with permission from Pulkrabek, P., Leffler, S., Weinstein, I. B., and Grunberger, D., *Biochemistry*, 16, 3127, 1977. Copyright by the American Chemical Society.)

digestion at 240 min). The 4.5% modified sample showed a marked increase in susceptibility to digestion with about 40% hydrolysis at 240 min.

4. Density Gradient Centrifugation

To establish whether the reaction of native DNA with BPDE introduced single- and/or double-strand breaks in the DNA molecules, we analyzed the modified DNA samples by sucrose density gradient centrifugation. The alkaline sucrose gradient profile of the 1.5 and 2.2% modified sample was identical with that of the control unmodified DNA (Figure 21). On the other hand, the 4.5% modified sample sedimented considerably slower, indicating that apparently all of the molecules had undergone chain scissions. These breaks are single-strand, or appear only after treatment with alkali, since neutral sucrose gradients (Figure 21B), which would reveal double-strand breaks, did not show differences in sedimentation profiles between the control and the 1.5% and 4.5% modified samples. There was no significant shift in buoyant density when the modified DNA samples were studied by cesium chloride density gradient centrifugation.[91]

Gamper et al.[93] have also presented evidence for single-strand scissions in DNA modified by BPDE, and these scissions may reflect modification of the DNA backbone (see Section D).

5. Orientation of the Pyrene Chromophore in the DNA Helix

Recent electric dichroism studies of BPDE-modified DNA performed by Geacintov et al.[94] indicate that, in contrast to covalently bound AAF residues and intercalated drugs which are oriented perpendicular to the long axis of double-strand DNA (see Reference 31 and Section II.A), the covalently bound pyrene chromophore occupies an angle of about 35° with respect to the long axis of the DNA helix. In addition, studies by Prusik et al.[95] on the ability of various compounds to quench the fluorescence of the pyrene chromophore provide evidence that it resides on the exterior surface of the DNA helix and is not inserted or intercalated within the base plates of the helix.

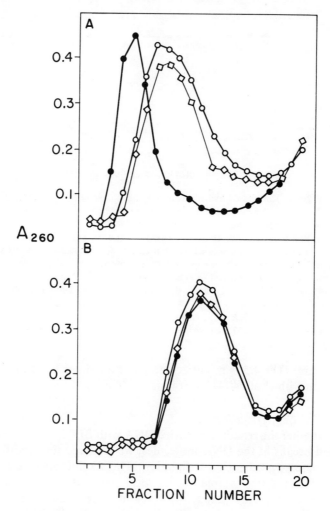

FIGURE 21.   Sucrose gradient centrifugations of DNA. (A) Alkaline gradient; 1 A_{260} unit of each DNA sample in 0.1 ml of 0.2 M NaOH was applied to the top of 5 to 20% sucrose gradient in 0.1 M NaOH and 0.9 M NaCl. Gradients were centrifuged in a Beckman® SW 41 rotor at 40,000 rpm for 240 min at 20°C. Fractions were collected from the top with a Buchler® Auto-Densi-Flow and A_{260} was measured on a Gilford® Type 240 spectrophotometer. (B) Neutral gradient: 1 A_{260} unit of each DNA sample in 0.1 ml was applied to the top of a 10 to 30% sucrose gradient in 0.01 M sodium cacodylate (pH 7.1), 0.1 M NaCl, and 1 × 10^{-3} M EDTA. Gradients were centrifuged in a Beckman® SW 41 rotor at 40,000 rpm for 300 min at 20°C and processed as above. (O — O) Control DNA; (◇ — ◇) 1.5% BP-modified DNA; (● — ●) 4.5% BP-modified DNA. (Reprinted with permission from Pulkrabek, P., Leffler, S., Weinstein, I. B., and Grunberger, D., *Biochemistry*, 16, 3127, 1977. Copyright by the American Chemical Society.)

6. The ''Minor Groove Model''

Table 2 contrasts the physical properties of *N*-acetoxy-AAF and BPDE-modified DNAs. It is apparent that the BPDE modification produces a less drastic distortion in the conformation of native DNA than that produced by AAF. This also appears to be the case with modified dimers (see Section III.B). In native DNA modified to low extents with BPDE, the regions of denaturation are considerably smaller than those

TABLE 2

Comparative Effects of Modification of C^8 and N^2 Positions of Guanosines in DNA with Activated Forms of AAF or BP[a]

	AAF	BP
Modification of G	C^8	N^2
Decrease in T_m	1.1°	0.75
Formaldehyde unwinding Relative fraction open base plates	0.172[b]	0.023
Average number open base plates per modified base	12—13[b]	0—1
S_1 nuclease digestion	15%	0
Orientation of the chromophore with respect to the long axis	80°[b]	35°
Conformation	Base displacement	Minor groove?

[a] Extrapolated to a 1% modification of the total bases.
[b] From data of Fuchs and Daune.[41]

associated with a comparable extent of AAF modification. The mean values are 0 to 1 destabilized base plates per BPDE-modified G vs. about 12 per AAF-modified G.

Examination of a model of double-stranded DNA with Watson-Crick geometry indicates that the N^2 group of G (in contrast to the C^8 position which is the major site of attack of AAF) is relatively exposed in the minor groove of the helix. It is likely, therefore, that BPDE can bind covalently to the N^2 residue with little distortion of the native DNA conformation (Figure 22). The S_1 nuclease digestion and formaldehyde denaturation data do suggest that there may be slight destabilization of the helix at sites of BPDE-modified G residues. This may be due to interference in the usual hydrogen bonding of the N^2 group of G to C, perhaps secondary to a slight distortion of the helix to fully accommodate the bulky BPDE residue in the minor groove.

The electric dichroism and fluorescence data[94,95] are also generally consistent with a model in which the covalently bound BPDE residue lies in the minor groove of the DNA helix. Specific aspects of the fluorescence quenching data suggest that the structure may be a dynamic one allowing for further exposure of the pyrene chromophore to the external environment of the DNA molecule.[95]

D. Alternative Sites of Attack and Structural Changes

A full consideration of the conformational changes in DNA modified by BPDE is complicated by the recent evidence that in certain cell systems various isomers of BPDE, in addition to BPDE I (7R), are formed and react with DNA (see Section III. A). It is likely that each type of modification is associated with subtle variations in conformation which could be of biologic significance. The problem is further complicated by the fact that, although guanine residues are the major nucleic acid targets, both isomer I and II of BPDE can also react with adenine and cytosine residues in vitro and perhaps also in vivo.[82,89,96,97] It seems likely that the attack is on the N^6 of adenine and the N^4 group of cytosine, although this remains to be established. These amino groups lie in the major rather than in the minor groove of the DNA helix and, therefore, the conformational aspects would be quite different from those associated with adducts on the N^2 group of guanine.

In this respect, the recent studies by Kakefuda and Yamamoto[98] are quite provocative. Superhelical double-stranded circular SV-40 or plasmid Col El DNA were modified with BPDE and subjected to stepwise degradation with endonuclease S_1 and

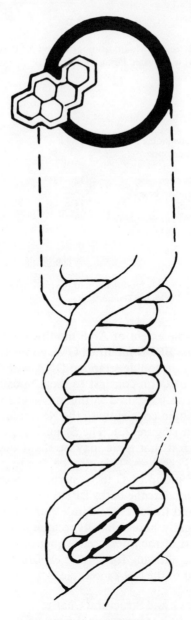

FIGURE 22.   Schematic representation of a double-stranded
DNA with covalently bound BP
residue residing in a minor groove.

DNase. Carcinogen modification of G residues was about tenfold greater than A residues. It appears, however, that S_1 nuclease preferentially excised the modified A residues, suggesting that the A modification produced a greater localized denaturation of the helix than the G modification. In addition, they found that although the synthetic double-stranded polymer poly (dG-dC)·(dG-dC) was modified to a greater extent with BPDE than poly (dA-dT)·(dA-dT), only the latter showed marked susceptibility to S_1 nuclease digestion following BPDE modification. These results provide evidence that BPDE modification of A residues produces a marked destabilization of A-T base pairs. Elucidation of the actual structure of the adenine adduct and its conformation may, therefore, be of considerable importance.

BPDE adducts in which the BPDE is attached to the exocyclic amino groups of the bases are chemically quite stable and, therefore, readily detected. Recent studies suggest that BPDE may also attack the N^7 position of guanine, but this adduct is readily lost from the DNA due to labilization of the glycoside bond and depurination.[99] Depurination can lead to spontaneous or enzymically mediated chain scissions and thus have major biologic consequences.[100]

An alternative mechanism of chain scissions could occur via the formation of phosphotriesters. Koreeda et al.[78] have presented indirect evidence for the formation of phosphotriesters in the reaction of BPDE with poly[G]. Gamper et al.[93] have detected single-strand scissions in superhelical *E. coli* plasmid DNA, and in RNA modified with BPDE. The strand scissions represented less than 1% of the DNA modification by the diol-epoxide. From the kinetics of DNA nicking, they inferred that BPDE forms phosphotriesters with DNA. They suggest that the C^9 hydroxyl group of the hydrocarbon then facilitates hydrolysis of the triester resulting in strand scission. Extensive phosphotriester formation is known to occur with the nitroso-alkylating agents,[101] but more direct evidence for its occurrence with BPDE remains to be obtained. It is apparent, therefore, that the modification of nucleic acids by BPDE can produce diverse types of structural and conformational changes.

E. Template Activity of BPDE-Modified DNA

To relate the structural and conformational changes of BPDE-modified DNA molecules to possible alterations in function, we have studied whether modification of DNA by BPDE affects its template acitvity during transcription by *E. coli* DNA-dependent RNA polymerase.[102] Transcription was assayed under two different conditions.[103] In one, RNA polymerase was allowed to recycle continuously on the DNA template, while in the other only a single round of initiation was permitted. In this way, the initiation and elongation phases of transcription are distinguishable.

When RNA synthesis was studied under nonreinitiating conditions, native and mock-modified DNA gave similar levels of incorporation, while BP-modified DNA showed a progressive inhibition of incorporation with increasing extents of modification (Table 3). A DNA sample of 0.2% modified bases showed approximately 25% inhibition of RNA synthesis when compared with native unmodified DNA. When the assays were performed under conditions which permitted multiple rounds of initiation, BP-modified samples were even more inhibited in their template capacities than in the nonreinitiating assay. Thus, under the former condition, the 0.2% modified sample showed about 40% inhibition, whereas under the latter condition, inhibition with the same template was only 25% (Table 3). These results are consistent with a model in which BPDE modification of DNA inhibits chain elongation, but not chain initiation during transcription. Presumably, movement of the polymerase along the DNA template is blocked when it encounters sites modified by BPDE, and the enzyme cannot recycle. Thus, chain elongation during transcription would be prematurely interrupted, yielding lower-molecular-weight products. Sucrose gradient centrifugation of the native DNA transcripts yielded products ranging in size from about 30 to 70S, with a broad peak at about 30S. On the other hand, transcripts obtained from samples containing a 0.5% modification showed a lower size distribution, ranging from about 25 to 7S, with a peak at approximately 14S; those obtained from DNA containing either 1.5 or 2.2% modification tended to be even smaller.[102] These results provide evidence that BPDE modification of DNA does interrupt chain elongation during transcription.

The impairment of chain elongation might reflect conformational distortions at sites of BPDE modification, preventing polymerase function and/or direct interference with the base-pairing capacity of the modified G residues in the DNA template. There is evidence that the interference with chain elongation during transcription also extends

TABLE 3

In Vitro Template Activity of Calf Thymus DNA Modified With BPDE

DNA	Modified bases (%)	No reinitiation incorporation relative to native DNA (%)	With reinitation incorporation relative to native DNA (%)
Native	0	100	100
Mock modified	0	92.5	114.9
BP-modified	0.2	74.8	59.3
BP-modified	0.5	55.8	46.5
BP-modified	1.5	45.3	26.7
BP-modified	2.2	26.0	14.7
BP-modified	4.5	11.0	3.2

Note: Incorporation of [³H]UTP with native DNA under nonreinitiating conditions was 298.8 pmol and under reinitiation conditions 756 pmol. For details see Reference 100.

to effects on replication of BPDE-modified DNA. Hsu et al.[104] have modified ΦX174 DNA with BPDE I and found that one molecule of bound BPDE is sufficient to inhibit in vivo replication of a single molecule of φ X DNA. When BPDE modified φX174 DNA was used as a template for DNA synthesis in vitro, the rate and extent of reaction were decreased. In addition, the propagation of new DNA strands was blocked so that incomplete, newly synthesized chains were detected. Interference with progression of the replicating fork during DNA synthesis in vivo may explain the action of BP and other polycyclic aromatic hydrocarbons as frame-shift mutagens in *Salmonella typhimurium*[105] and as inducers of phage production and "SOS" error-prone DNA synthesis in *E. coli.*[106,107]

IV. BIOLOGICAL SIGNIFICANCE

The studies described above were carried out largely with nucleic acids modified with carcinogens in vitro to a much higher degree than occurs in vivo. In addition, certain results were obtained with model compounds, such as oligonucleotides, and others with highly heterogeneous DNA modified in the naked state. The in vivo significance of these results is, therefore, highly speculative. In eukaryotic cells, the DNA exists as a nucleoprotein complex, chromatin. It is likely that this aspect of quarternary structure influences the accessibility of specific regions of the genome to carcinogen attack, as well as the types of structural and functional changes that result from *in situ* modification of DNA. It is possible, for example, that the association of specific regions of DNA with protein protects these regions from carcinogen attack. Alternatively, changes in the DNA associated with its packaging into the chromatin structure may render specific regions of the DNA more susceptible to carcinogen attack. Preliminary studies suggest that AAF and BP modification of DNA does not cause a gross distortion of nucleosome structure,[54] but the finer aspects of structure and function in chromatin that contains carcinogen-modified DNA remain to be studied.

The changes in nucleic acid conformation resulting from carcinogen modification may also relate to in vivo mechanisms by which DNA repair enzymes recognize and excise damaged regions of DNA. The studies with AAF suggest that AAF adducts on the C^8 position of guanine are repaired more efficiently than those on the N^2 position because the former are associated with a gross change in nucleic acid conformation, whereas the latter are not. It is possible, therefore, that the potency and tissue specificity of a carcinogen relate not only to its extent of cellular uptake, activation, and DNA binding, but also to its ability to bind to DNA with a conformation that minimizes recognition by DNA excision repair mechanisms and yet causes functional impairment of the DNA. An unresolved question is whether the critical functional impairment in carcinogen- modified DNA is impairment of template function during DNA replication, impairment during RNA transcription or impairment of the association of DNA with other molecules concerned with cell regulation and differentiation. Hopefully, further studies on the structural and functional changes in nucleic acids modified by chemical carcinogens will provide insights into the molecular mechanisms of carcinogenesis.

Acknowledgments

The authors wish to acknowledge the valuable roles played by K. Nakanishi, A. M. Jeffrey, P. Pulkrabek, S. Leffler, H. Yamasaki, K. Frenkel, and R. G. Harvey in these research studies. We are grateful to Dr. Lou Katz for performing the computer graphics in our studies. We express our appreciation to Ms. Sue A. Allen for her assistance in preparing the manuscript. We thank the Chemical Repository of the National Cancer Institute for making available samples of N-acetoxy-AAF and BPDE used in these studies.
This work was supported by DHEW Grant No. CA 21111.

REFERENCES

1. **Miller, J. A.**, Carcinogenesis by chemicals: an overview, G. H. A. Clowes Memorial Lecture, *Cancer Res.*, 30, 559, 1970.
2. **Weinstein, I. B.**, Types of interaction between carcinogens and nucleic acids. *Colloq. Int. C.N.R.S.*, 256, 2, 1976.
3. **Ward, D. C. and Reich, E.**, Relationship between nucleoside conformation and biological activity, in *Annual Reports in Medicinal Chemistry*, Cain C. K., Ed., Academic Press, New York, 1969, 272.
4. **Sundaralingam, M.**, *Structure and Conformation of Nucleic Acid and Protein-Nucleic Acid Interactions*, (Part 5), University Park Press, Baltimore, 1975, 487.
5. **Donohue, J. and Trueblood, K. N.**, Base pairing in DNA. *J. Mol. Biol.*, 2, 363, 1960.
6. **Arnott, S. and Hukins, D. W. T.**, Conservation of conformation in mono and poly-nucleotides, *Nature* (London), 224, 886, 1969.
7. **Haschemeyer, A. E. V. and Rich, A.**, Nucleoside conformations: an analysis of steric barriers to rotation about the glycosidic bond, *J. Mol. Biol.*, 27, 369, 1967.
8. **Suck, D. and Saenger, W.**, Molecular and crystal structure of 6-methyluridine. A pyrimidine nucleoside in the *syn* conformation, *J. Am. Chem. Soc.*, 94, 6520, 1972.
9. **Bugg, C. E. and Thewalt, V.**, Effects of halogen substituents on base stacking in nucleic acid components: the crystal structure of 8-bromoguanosine, *Biochem. Biophys. Res. Commun.*, 37, 623, 1969.
10. **Tavale, S. S. and Sobell, H. M.**, Crystal and molecular structure of 8-bromoguanosine and 8-bromoadenosine, two purine nucleosides in the *syn* configuration, *J. Mol. Biol.*, 48, 109, 1970.
11. **Crick, F. H. C. and Klug, A.**, Kinky helix, *Nature* (London), 255, 530, 1975.
12. **Sobell, H. M., Tsai, C-C, Jain, S. C., and Gilbert, S. G.**, Visualization of drug-nucleic acid interactions at atomic resolution. III. Unifying structural concepts in understanding drug-DNA interactions and their broader implications in understanding protein-DNA interactions. *J. Mol. Biol.*, 144, 333, 1977.
13. **Singer, B.**, The chemical effects of nucleic acid alkylation and their relation to mutagenesis and carcinogenesis, *Prog. Nucleic Acid Res. Mol. Biol.*, 15, 219, 1975.
14. **Nagata, C., Tagashira, Y., and Kodama, M.**, Metabolic activation of BP: significance of the free radical, *Chemical Carcinogenesis, Part A.*, Ts'o P. O. P. and DiPaolo, J. A., Eds., Marcel Dekker, New York, 1974, 87.

15. Carchman, R. A., Hirschberg, E., and Weinstein, I. B., Miracil D: effect on the viscosity of DNA, *Biochim. Biophys. Acta*, 179, 158, 1969.
16. Lerman, L. S., Acridine mutagens and DNA structure, *J. Cell. Comp. Physiol.*, 64 (Suppl. 1), 1, 1964.
17. Ts'o, P. O. P., Kondo, N. S., Schweizer, M. P., and Hollis, D. P., Studies of the conformation and interaction in dinucleoside mono- and diphosphates by proton magnetic resonance, *Biochemistry*, 8, 997, 1969.
18. Warshaw, M. M. and Cantor, C. R., Oligonucleotide interactions. IV. Conformational differences between deoxy- and ribodinucleoside phosphates, *Biopolymers*, 9, 1079, 1970.
19. Van Holde, K. E., Brahms, J., and Michelson, A. M., Base interactions of nucleotide polymers in aqueous solution, *J. Mol. Biol.*, 12, 726, 1965.
20. Kondo, N. S., Holmes, H. M., Stempel, L. M., and T'so, P. O. P., Influence of the phosphodiester linkage (3′ -5′, 2′ -5′, and 5′ -5′) on the conformation of dinucleoside monophosphate, *Biochemistry*, 9, 3479, 1970.
21. Chan, S. I. and Nelson, J. H., Proton magnetic resonance studies of ribose dinucleoside monophosphates in aqueous solution. I. The nature of the base-stacking interaction in adenylyl (3′ -5′) adenosine, *J. Am. Chem. Soc.*, 91, 168, 1969.
22. Hruska, F. E. and Danyluk, S. A., Conformational changes of the ribose group in dinucleoside mono- and diphosphates. Temperature dependence, *J. Am. Chem. Soc.*, 90, 3266, 1968.
23. Warshaw, M. M. and Tinoco, I., Jr., Absorption and optical rotary dispersion of six dinucleoside phosphates, *J. Mol. Biol.*, 13, 54, 1965.
24. Warshaw, M. M. and Tinoco, I., Jr., Optical properties of sixteen dinucleoside phosphates, *J. Mol. Biol.*, 20, 29, 1966.
25. Topal, M. D. and Warshaw, M. M., Dinucleoside monophosphates. I. Optical properties and conformation in solution with one base charged, *Biopolymers*, 15, 1755, 1976.
26. Chan, S. I., Schweizer, M. P., Ts'o, P. O. P., and Helmkamp, G. K., Interaction and association of bases and nucleosides in aqueous solutions. III. A nuclear magnetic resonance study of the self-association of purine and 6-methyl-purine, *J. Am. Chem. Soc.*, 86, 4182, 1971.
27. Gray, A. A., Smith, I. C. P., and Hruska, F. E., A model for the molecular conformation of α-pseudouridine from nuclear magnetic resonance data, *J. Am. Chem. Soc.*, 93, 1765, 1971.
28. Weinstein, I. B. and Grunberger, D., Structural and functional changes in nucleic acids modified by chemical carcinogens, in *Chemical Carcinogenesis, Part A*, Ts'o, P. O. P. and BiPaolo, J. A., Eds., Marcel Dekker, New York, 1974, 217.
29. Grunberger, D. and Weinstein, I. B., The base displacement model: an explanation for the conformational and functional changes in nucleic acids modified by chemical carcinogens, in *Biology of Radiation Carcinogenesis*, Yuhas, J. M., Tennant, R. W., and Regan, J. D., Eds., Raven Press, New York, 1976, 175.
30. Levine, A. F., Fink, L. M., Weinstein, I. B., and Grunberger, D., Effect of N-2-acetylaminofluorene modification on the conformation of nucleic acids, *Cancer Res.*, 34, 319, 1974.
31. Fuchs, R. and Daune, M., Physical basis of chemical carcinogenesis by N-2 fluorenylacetamide derivatives and analogs, *FEBS Lett.*, 34, 295, 1973.
32. Heidelberger, C., Chemical oncogenesis in culture, *Adv. Cancer Res.*, 18, 317, 1973.
33. Essigmann, J. M., Croy, R. G., Nadzan, A. M., Busby, W. F., Jr., Reinhold, V. N., Buchi, G., and Wogan, G. N., Structural identification of the major DNA adduct formed by aflatoxin B₁ *in vitro*, *Proc. Natl. Acad. Sci. U.S.A.*, 74, 1870, 1977.
34. Miller, E. C., Juhl, U., and Miller, J. A., Nucleic acid guanine: reaction with the carcinogen N-acetoxy-2-acetylaminofluorene, *Science*, 153, 1125,1966.
35. Kriek, E., Miller, J. A., Juhl, U., and Miller, E. C., (N-2-fluorenylacetamide)guanosine, an arylamidation reaction product of guanosine and the carcinogen N-acetoxy-N-2-fluorenylacetamide in neutral solution, *Biochemistry*, 6, 177, 1967.
36. Kriek, E., Persistent binding of a new reaction product of the carcinogen N-hydroxy-N-2-acetylaminofluorene with guanine in rat liver DNA *in vivo*, *Cancer Res.*, 32, 2042, 1972.
37. Grunberger, D., Nelson, J. H., Cantor, C. R., and Weinstein, I. B., Coding and conformational properties of oligonucleotides modified with the carcinogen N-2-acetylaminofluorene, *Proc. Natl. Acad. Sci. U.S.A.*, 66, 488, 1970.
38. Nelson, J. H., Grunberger, D., Cantor, C. R., and Weinstein, I. B., Modification of ribonucleic acid by chemical carcinogens. IV. Circular dichroism and proton magnetic resonance studies of oligonucleotides modified with N-2-acetylaminofluorene, *J. Mol. Biol.*, 62, 331, 1971.
39. Grunberger, D., Blobstein, S. H., and Weinstein, I. B., Modification of ribonucleic acid by chemical carcinogens. VI. Effect of N-2-acetylaminofluorene modification of guanosine on the codon function of adjacent nucleosides in oligonucleotides, *J. Mol. Biol.*, 82, 459, 1974.

40. Fuchs, R. P. P., Lefevre, J-F., Pouyet, J., and Daune, M. P., Comparative orientation of the fluorene residue in native DNA modified by N-acetoxy-N-2-acetylaminofluorene and two 7-halogeno derivatives, *Biochemistry*, 15, 3347, 1976.

41. Fuchs, R. P. P. and Daune, M. P., Dynamic structure of DNA modified with the carcinogen N-acetoxy-N-2-acetylaminofluorene, *Biochemistry*, 13, 4435, 1974.

42. Morris, H. P., Velat, C. A., Wagner, B. P., Dahlgard, M., and Ray, F. E., Studies of carcinogenicity in the rate of derivatives of aromatic amines related to N-2-fluorenylacetamide, *J. Natl. Cancer Inst.*, 24, 149, 1960.

43. Chang, C-T., Miller, S. J., and Wetmur, J. G., Physical studies of N-acetoxy-N-2-acetylaminofluorene-modified deoxyribonucleic acid, *Biochemistry*, 13, 2142, 1974.

44. Troll, W., Rinde, E., and Day, P., Effect on N-7 and C-8 substitution of guanine in DNA on T_m, buoyant density and RNA polymerase priming, *Biochim. Biophys. Acta*, 174, 211, 1969.

45. Kapuler, A. M. and Michelson, A. M., The reaction of the carcinogen N-acetoxy-2-acetylaminofluorene with DNA and other polynucleotides and its stereochemical implications, *Biochim. Biophys. Acta*, 232, 436, 1971.

46. Fuchs, R. P. P. and Daune, M., Changes of stability and conformation of DNA following the covalent binding of a carcinogen, *FEBS Lett.*, 14, 206, 1971.

47. Fuchs, R. P. P. and Daune, M., Physical studies on deoxyribonucleic acid after covalent binding of a carcinogen, *Biochemistry*, 11, 2659, 1972.

48. Marmur, J. and Doty, P., Determination of the base composition of DNA from its thermal denaturation temperature, *J. Mol. Biol.*, 5, 109, 1962.

49. Lerman, L. S., Structural considerations in the interaction of DNA and acridines, *J. Mol. Biol.*, 3, 19, 1961.

50. Lerman, S., The combination of DNA with polycyclic aromatic hydrocarbons in *Proc. 5th Natl. Cancer Conf.*, Lippincott, Philadelphia, 1964, 36.

51. Utiyama, H. and Doty, P., Kinetic studies of denaturation and reaction with formaldehyde on polydeoxyribonucleotides, *Biochemistry*, 10, 1254, 1971.

52. Von Hippel, P. H. and Wong, K. Y., Dynamic aspects of native DNA structure: kinetics of the formaldehyde reaction with calf thymus DNA, *J. Mol. Biol.*, 61, 587, 1971.

53. Fuchs, R. P. P., *In vitro* recognition of carcinogen induced local denaturation sites in native DNA by S$_1$ endonuclease from *Aspergillus oryzae*, *Nature* (London), 257, 151, 1975.

54. Yamasaki, H., Leffler, S., and Weinstein, I. B., Effect of N-2-acetylaminofluorene modification on the structure and template activity of DNA and reconstituted chromatin. *Cancer Res.*, 37, 684, 1977.

55. Cramer, F., Three dimensional structure of tRNA, *Prog. Nucleic Acid Res. Mol. Biol.*, 11, 391, 1971.

56. Fujimura, S., Grunberger, D., Carvajal, G., and Weinstein, I. B., Modifications of ribonucleic acid by chemical carcinogens. Modification of *Escherichia coli* formylmethionine transfer ribonucleic acid with N-acetoxy-2-acetylaminofluorene, *Biochemistry*, 11, 3629, 1972.

57. Pulkrabek, P., Grunberger, D., and Weinstein, I. B., Effects of the ionic environment on modification of yeast tyrosine transfer ribonucleic acid with N-acetoxy-2-acetylaminofluorene, *Biochemistry*, 13, 2414, 1974.

58. Kim, S. H., Quigley, G. J., Suddath, F. I., McPherson, A., Sneden, D., Kim, J. J., Weinzierl, J., and Rich, A., Three-dimensional structure of yeast phenylalanine transfer RNA: folding of the polynucleotide chain, *Science*, 179, 285, 1973.

59. Robertus, J. D., Ladner, J. E., Finch, J. T., Rhodes, D., Brown, R. S., Clark, B. F. C., and Klug, A., Structure of yeast phenylalanine tRNA at 3 Å resolution, *Nature* (London), 250, 546, 1974.

60. Harvan, D. J., Hass, R. J., and Lieberman, M. W., Adduct formation between the carcinogen N-acetoxy-2-acetylaminofluorene and synthetic polydeoxyribonucleotides, *Chem. Biol. Interact.*, 17, 203, 1977.

61. Grunberger, D. and Weinstein, I. B., Modifications of ribonucleic acid by chemical carcinogens. III. Template activity of polynucleotides modified by N-acetoxy-2-acetylaminofluorene, *J. Biol. Chem.*, 246, 1123, 1971.

62. Troll, W., Belman, S., Berkowitz, E., Chmielewicz, Z. F., Ambrus, J. L., and Bardos, T. J., Differential responses of DNA and RNA polymerase to modifications of the template rat liver DNA caused by action of the carcinogen acetylaminofluorene *in vivo* and *in vitro*, *Biochim. Biophys. Acta*, 157, 16, 1968.

63. Millette, R. L. and Fink, L. M., The effect of modification of T7 DNA by the carcinogen N-2-acetylaminofluorene: termination of transcription *in vitro*, *Biochemistry*, 14, 1426, 1975.

64. Grunberger, G., Yu, F. L., Grunberger, D., and Feigelson, P., Mechanism of N-hydroxy-2-acetylaminofluorene inhibition of rat hepatic ribonucleic acid synthesis, *J. Biol. Chem.*, 248, 6278, 1973.

65. Zieve, I. J., Effects of the carcinogen N-acetoxy-2-fluorenylacetamide on the template properties of deoxyribonucleic acid, *Mol. Pharmacol.*, 9, 658, 1973.

66. Glazer, R. I., Glass, L. E., and Menger, F. M., Modification of hepatic ribonucleic acid polymerase activities by N-hydroxy-2-acetylaminofluorene, *Mol. Pharmacol.*, 11, 36, 1975.

67. Herzog, J., Serroni, A., Briesmeister, B. A., and Farber, J. L., N-hydroxy-2-acetylaminofluorene inhibition of rat liver RNA polymerases, *Cancer Res.*, 35, 2138, 1975.

68. Yu, F. L. and Grunberger, D., Multiple sites of action of N-hydroxy-2-acetylaminofluorene in rat hepatic nuclear transcription, *Cancer Res.*, 36, 3629, 1976.

69. Westra, J. G., Kriek, E., and Hittenhauser, H., Identification of the persistently bound form of the carcinogen N-acetyl-2-aminofluorene to rat liver DNA *in vivo*, *Chem. Biol. Interact.*, 15, 149, 1976.

70. Yamasaki, H., Pulkrabek, P., Grunberger, D., and Weinstein, I. B., Differential excision from DNA of the C-8 and N^2 guanosine adducts of N-acetyl-2-aminofluorene by single-strand specific endonucleases, *Cancer Res.*, 37, 3756, 1977.

71. Borgen, A., Darvey, H., Castagnoli, N., Crocker, T. T., Rasmussen, R. E., and Wang, I. Y., Metabolic conversion of benzo[a]pyrene by Syrian hamster liver microsomes and binding of metabolites to deoxyribonucleic acid, *J. Med. Chem.*, 16, 502, 1973.

72. Daudel, P., Duquesne, M., Vigny, P., Grover, P. L., and Sims, P., Fluorescence spectral evidence that benzo[a]pyrene-DNA products in mouse skin arise from diol-epoxides, *FEBS Lett.*, 57, 250, 1975.

73. Ivanovic, V., Geacintov, N. E., and Weinstein, I. B., Cellular binding of benzo[a]pyrene to DNA characterized by low temperature fluorescence, *Biochem. Biophys. Res. Commun.*, 70, 1172, 1976.

74. Sims, P., Grover, P. L., Swaisland, A., Pal, K., and Hewer, A., Metabolic activation of benzo[a]pyrene proceeds by a diol-epoxide, *Nature (London)* 252, 326, 1974.

75. Grover, P. L., Hewer, A., Pal, K., and Sims, P., The involvement of a diol-epoxide in the metabolic activation of benzo[a]pyrene in human bronchial mucosa and in mouse skin, *Int. J. Cancer*, 18, 1, 1976.

76. Jeffrey, A. M., Jennette, K. W., Blobstein, S. H., Weinstein, I. B., Beland, F. A., Harvey, R. G., Kasai, H., Miura, I., and Nakanishi, K., Structure of guanosine adducts formed by reaction with a tetrahydrodiol epoxide of benzo[a]pyrene, *J. Am. Chem. Soc.*, 98, 5714, 1976.

77. Weinstein, I. B., Jeffrey, A. M., Jennette, K. W., Blobstein, S. H., Harvey, R. G., Harris, C., Autrup, H., Kasai, H., and Nakanishi, K., Benzo[a]pyrene diol-epoxides as intermediates in nucleic acid binding *in vitro* and *in vivo*, *Science*, 197, 592, 1977.

78. Koreeda, M., Moore, P. D., Yagi, H., Yen, J. C., and Jerina, D. M., Alkylation of polyguanylic acid at the 2-amino group and phosphate by the potent mutagen (±) -7α,8β-dihydroxy-9β,10β-epoxy-7,8,9,10-tetrahydrobenzo[a]pyrene, *J. Am. Chem. Soc.*, 98, 6720, 1976.

79. King, H. W. S., Osborne, M. R., Beland, F. A., Harvey, R. G., and Brookes, P., (±)-7α,8β-dihydroxy-9β,10β-epoxy-7,8,9,10-tetrahydrobenzo[a]pyrene is an intermediate in the metabolism and binding to DNA of benzo[a]pyrene, *Proc. Natl. Acad. Sci. U.S.A.*, 73, 2679, 1976.

80. Yagi, H., Hernandez, O., and Jerina, D. M., Synthesis of (±)-7β, 8α-dihydroxy-9β,10β-epoxy-7,8,9,10-tetrahydrobenzo[a]pyrene, a potential metabolite of the carcinogen benzo[a]pyrene with stereochemistry related to the antileukemic triptolides, *J. Am. Chem. Soc.*, 97, 6881, 1975.

81. Yagi, H., Akagi, H., Thakker, D. R., Mah, H. D., Koreeda, M., and Jerina, D. M., Absolute stereochemistry of the highly mutagenic 7,8-diol 9,10-epoxides derived from the potent carcinogen *trans*-7,8-dihydroxy 7,8-dihydrobenzo[a]pyrene, *J. Am. Chem. Soc.*, 99, 2358, 1977.

82. Jeffrey, A. M., Weinstein, I. B., Jennette, K. W., Grzeskowiak, K., Nakanishi, K., Harvey, R. E., Autrup, H., and Harris, C., Structures of benzo[a]pyrene nucleic acid adducts formed in human and bovine bronchial explants, *Nature (London)*, 269, 348, 1977.

83. Nakanishi, K., Kasai, H., Cho, H., Harvey, R. G., Jeffrey, A. M., Jennette, K. W., and Weinstein, I. B., Absolute configuration of a ribonucleic acid adduct formed *in vivo* by metabolism of benzo[a]pyrene, *J. Am. Chem. Soc.*, 99, 258, 1977.

84. Jeffrey, A. M., Blobstein, S. H., Weinstein, I. B., and Harvey, R. G., High-pressure liquid chromatography of carcinogen-nucleoside conjugates: separation of 7,12-dimethylbenzathracene derivatives, *Anal. Biochem.*, 73, 378, 1976.

85. Yang, S. K., Gelboin, H. V., Trump, B. F., Autrup, H., and Harris, C. C., Metabolic activation of benzo[a]pyrene and binding to DNA in cultured human bronchus, *Cancer Res.*, 37, 1210, 1977.

86. Shinohara, K. and Cerutti, P. A., Excision repair of BP-deoxyguanosine adducts in baby hamster kidney 21/C13 cells and in secondary mouse embryo fibroblasts C57BL/6J, *Proc. Natl. Acad. Sci. U.S.A.*, 74, 979, 1977.

87. Thakker, D. R., Yagi, H., Akagi, H., Koreeda, M., Lu, A. Y. H., Levin, W., Wood, W., Conney, A. H., and Jerina, D. M., Metabolism of benzo[a]pyrene. VI. Stereoselective metabolism of benzo[a]pyrene and benzo[a]pyrene 7,8-dihydrodiol to diol epoxide, *Chem. Biol. Interact.*, 16, 281, 1977.

88. Moore, P. D., Koreeda, M., Wislocki, P. G., Levin, W., Conney, A. H., Yagi, H., and Jerina, D. M., *In vitro* reactions of the diastereomeric 9,10-epoxides of (+) and (−)-*trans*-7,8-dihydroxy-7,8-dihydrobenzo[a]pyrene with polyguanylic acid and evidence for formation of an enantiomer of each diastereomeric 9,10-epoxide from benzo[a]pyrene in mouse skin, *Am. Chem. Soc. Symp. Ser.*, 44, 127, 1977.

89. Ivanovic, V., Geacintov, N. E., Yamasaki, H., and Weinstein, I. B., DNA and RNA adducts formed in hamster embryo cell cultures exposed to benzo[a]pyrene, *Biochemistry*, 17, 1597, 1978.

90. Frenkel, K., Grunberger, D., Boublik, M., and Weinstein, I. B., Conformation of dinucleoside monophosphates modified with benzo[a]pyrene diol epoxide as measured by circular dichroism, *Biochemistry*, 17, 1278, 1978.

91. Pulkrabek, P., Leffler, S., Weinstein, I. B., and Grunberger, D., Conformation of DNA modified with a dihydrodiol epoxide derivative of benzo[a]pyrene, *Biochemistry*, 16, 3127, 1977.

92. Vogt, V. M., Purification and further properties of single-strand specific nuclease from *Aspergillus oryzae, Eur. J. Biochem.*, 33, 192, 1973.

93. Gamper, H. B., Tung, A. S. C., Straub, K., Bartholomew, J. C., and Calvin, M., DNA strand scission by benzo[a]pyrene diol epoxides, *Science*, 197, 671, 1977.

94. Geacintov, N. E., Gagliano, A., Ivanovic, V., and Weinstein, I. B., Electric linear dichroism study on the orientation of benzo[a]pyrene-7,8-dihydrodiol 9,10-oxide covalently bound to DNA, *Biochemistry*, 17, 2552, 1978.

95. Prusik, T., Geacintov, N. E., Tobiasz, C., Ivanovic, V., and Weinstein, I. B., Fluorescence study of the physicochemical properties of a benzo[a]pyrene 7,8-dihydrodiol 9,10-oxide derivative bound covalently to DNA, *Photochem. Photobiol.*, 1978, in press.

96. Jennette, K. W., Jeffrey, A. M., Blobstein, S. H., Beland, F., Harvey, R. G., and Weinstein, I. B., Nucleoside adducts from the *in vitro* reaction of benzo[a]pyrene 4,5-oxide with nucleic acids, *Biochemistry*, 16, 932, 1977.

97. Meehan, T., Straub, K., and Calvin, M., Benzo[a]pyrene diol epoxide covalently binds to deoxyguanosine and deoxyadenosine in DNA, *Nature (London)*, 269, 725, 1977.

98. Kakefuda, T. and Yamamoto, H., Modification of DNA by the benzo[a]pyrene metabolite diolepoxide r-7, t-8-dihydroxy-t-9,10-oxy-7,8,9,10-tetrahydrobenzo[a]pyrene (I). *Proc. Natl. Acad. Sci. U.S.A.*, 75, 415, 1978.

99. Osborne, M. R., Harvey, R. G., and Brookes, P., The reaction of *trans*-7,8-dihydroxy *anti*-9,10 epoxy 7,8,9,10-tetrahydrobenzo[a]pyrene with DNA involves attack at N-7 position of guanine moieties, *Chem. Biol. Interact.*, 20, 123, 1978.

100. Ludlum, D. B., Alkylating agents and the nitrosoureas, in *Cancer, A Comprehensive Treatise*, Vol. 5, Becker, F. F., Ed., Plenum Press, New York, 1977, 285.

101. Singer, B., All oxygens in nucleic acids react with carcinogenic ethylating agents, *Nature (London)*, 264, 333, 1976.

102. Leffler, S., Pulkrabek, P., Grunberger, D., and Weinstein, I. B., Template activity of calf thymus DNA modified by a dihydrodiol epoxide derivative of benzo[a]pyrene, *Biochemistry*, 16, 3133, 1977.

103. Cedar, H. and Felsenfeld, G., Transcription of chromatin *in vitro*, *J. Mol. Biol.*, 77, 237, 1973.

104. Hsu, W. T., Lin, E. J. S., Harvey, R. G., and Weiss, S. B., Mechanism of phage φX174 DNA inactivation by benzo[a]pyrene-7,8-dihydrodiol-9,10-epoxide, *Proc. Natl. Acad. Sci. U.S.A.*, 74, 3335, 1977.

105. McCann, J., Spingarn, N. E., Kobori, J., and Ames, B. N., Detection of carcinogens as mutagens: bacterial tester strains with R factor plasmids, *Proc. Natl. Acad. Sci. U.S.A.*, 72, 979, 1975.

106. Moreau, P., Bailone, A., and Devoret, R., Prophage λ induction in *E. coli* K12 envA uvrB: a highly sensitive test for potential carcinogens, *Proc. Natl. Acad. Sci. U.S.A.*, 73, 3700, 1976.

107. Witkin, E. M., Ultraviolet mutagenesis and inducible DNA repair in *Escherichia coli, Bacteriol. Rev.*, 40, 869, 1976.

108. Pulkrabek, P., Unpublished studies, 1978.

Chapter 4

MUTAGENIC CONSEQUENCES OF CHEMICAL REACTION WITH DNA

Michael H. L. Green

TABLE OF CONTENTS

I. INTRODUCTION

A. General

Although the somatic mutation theory of cancer has had a long history (since 1914),[1,2] it has staged a spectacular renaissance in recent years. The long eclipse and recent restoration to favor are both closely related to progress in the field of chemical carcinogenesis. For many years it was known that some of the most potent chemical carcinogens were not mutagenic to lower organisms (mutagenesis experiments in mammals were at that time more or less impracticable). Gradually, however, the classic studies of the Millers and others[3,4] began to show that, although such carcinogens were chemically unreactive, they could be metabolized by mammalian tissues to compounds that would attack DNA and other cellular constituents. It was shown by Malling[5] that these active metabolites could be generated by a liver microsomal fraction and that they were then mutagenic to lower organisms. Ames and co-workers have built on these observations and developed a remarkably effective short-term test to detect chemical carcinogens, using a rat-liver microsomal fraction to provide metabolic activation and specific histidine-requiring strains of the bacterium *Salmonella typhimurium* to demonstrate mutagenesis.[6,7] The test has now been used with over 300 reference carcinogens and noncarcinogens,[8,9] and an extremely high correlation (perhaps greater than 90%) between carcinogenesis and mutagenesis has been shown to exist. It is now being used, in conjunction with other short-term tests, to determine whether new industrial products, and those already in use, are likely to be carcinogenic.

As a result of these developments, it must be recognized that a strong symbiotic relationship now exists between the study of chemical carcinogens, the somatic mutation theory of cancer, and the study of environmental mutagenesis and carcinogenesis. Somatic mutation provides a theoretical framework to explain the practical observations of reaction of chemical carcinogens with DNA. If the possibility exists that effects of this type, from chemicals present in the environment, might contribute significantly to human cancer, there is an outstanding case for pursuing all these lines of research. Fashions in cancer research do, of course, change and things are seldom as simple as at first sight. Although a cancer cell has undergone a relatively stable, heritable change, it would be surprising if the events leading to that change bore any very close relationship to the events leading to restoration of histidine biosynthesis in *Salmonella typhimurium*. Nor is it likely that the banning of a few ill-tested commercial products will lead to the abolition of human cancer. With these reservations however, it is still worthwhile to apply our present knowledge of mutagenesis to the study of carcinogenesis, and to use the short-term tests now available to see if we are giving ourselves cancer needlessly.

In this Chapter, the author will describe our current knowledge of DNA repair and mutation (mostly derived from bacterial studies) and then try to relate this to our current knowledge of how chemical carcinogens damage DNA. Also, it is hoped to show how measurement of DNA repair and mutation in bacteria can be used as a simple and sensitive way of obtaining a great deal of information about the mode of action of a chemical carcinogen. Any comments made in passing on the nature of mutagenesis or carcinogenesis in mammalian cells, are likely to be entirely speculative and can safely be disregarded.

B. Other Reviews

For more detailed reviews of different topics discussed in the Chapter, see the account of UV mutagenesis by Witkin,[10] the account of general mutagenesis by Drake and Baltz,[11] and the mutation-oriented review of DNA repair by Lehmann and Bridges.[12] Among other recent reviews of interest are those of Doudney on UV mutagenesis,[13] Strauss,[14] and Roberts[15] on repair of chemical damage, Grossman[16,17] and Friedberg et al.[18] on repair enzymology, and finally a comprehensive review by Swenson[19] on some of the less fashionable aspects of repair phenomenology.

Other contributors to this volume should provide an up-to-date account of reactions of chemical carcinogens with DNA, and Volume II, Chapter 5 by Maher and McCormick will cover mutagenesis in mammalian cell systems.

C. Types of Mutation

This chapter will not cover the variety of types of chromosomal alteration which can result in an altered phenotype in mammalian cells, but will be confined to the types of mutation detectable in bacteria.

1. Base-Pair Substitution Mutagenesis

The simplest genetic change leading to a recognizable mutation is alteration of a single base pair. A chemical may induce basepair-substitutions in one of three ways:

1. It may alter the coding properties of a base so that an incorrect base will be incorporated during DNA replication. Alkylation of the O^6 position of guanine appears to produce this effect.[20]
2. An agent may in theory interfere with normal polymerases or associated enzymes and reduce the fidelity of normal DNA replication. Although this has been suggested in other cases[21] as a possible mechanism of mutagenesis, the one reasonably well-established instance is the effect of certain metal cations on polymerase fidelity.[22]
3. The commonest result of chemical attack on DNA is simply to prevent the DNA from acting as a template for further replication. In addition to many different types of adduct which interfere with base pairing, there are lesions such as strand breaks and inter-strand DNA cross-links. Such types of damage must be repaired in order for the cell to survive and extremely efficient repair mechanisms have been found in all groups of organisms. Although most repair is highly accurate, it has been found in *Escherichia coli* and elsewhere that a minor error-prone repair pathway exists.[23] This pathway probably makes only a small contribution to overall repair,* but it is of extreme importance, since in its absence a number of carcinogens may not be detectably mutagenic. The existence of a similar pathway in mammalian cells is fairly likely but unproven.

---

* If the error-prone repair is of minor importance in determining survival, one may speculate teleologically as to why such a repair process exists at all. It has been suggested that its role may be to enable *E. coli* to raise its mutation rate under conditions of environmental stress. It is of interest that certain types of plasmid have the property of enormously increasing spontaneous and induced mutation in the host bacterium (see Section IV.B). Just as the normal bacterium is drug sensitive, but can rapidly acquire drug resistance through a plasmid, it appears that the normal bacterium has a very low mutation rate which can occasionally be greatly increased, either by a plasmid, or an insult to its DNA. One can speculate whether this might confer an evolutionary advantage.

2. Frameshift Mutagenesis

In frameshift mutagenesis, addition or deletion of (usually) a single base pair to the DNA causes the reading frame of the genetic code to go out of phase during translation. Considerably less is known about frameshift mutagenesis than about base substitution mutagenesis. This is unfortunate, since many polycyclic and aromatic amine carcinogens are specific frameshift mutagens in bacterial tests.

3. Deletion Mutagenesis

Even less is known about the mechanism of deletion mutagenesis, where a whole section of chromosome is lost. In bacteria, some, but by no means all, mutagens appear to induce deletions in addition to other changes.

4. Insertion Sequence Mutagenesis

Another type of event, which may in future prove to be of considerable importance, is mutagenesis by translocational elements. It is becoming increasingly clear that the chromosomes of bacteria and their plasmids contain sections of DNA that have the ability to translocate into fresh DNA, either at random or at a large number of potential sites.[24]

If insertion occurs into a gene, the gene may be inactivated. Translocating elements include the mutator bacteriophage Mu, insertion sequences, identifiable only by their inactivating effect, and transposons which carry identifiable genes. Many plasmid drug resistance genes are on transposons so that not only may resistance to a drug be transferred between bacteria on a plasmid, but it may be transferred between plasmids as part of a transposon. This natural genetic engineering is of considerable medical importance, and the mechanism is under active investigation. It does not seem related to conventional recombination. As well as the role of transposons in drug resistance, insertion sequences may be involved in such phenomena as bacterial conjugation and the unstable maize mutation systems examined in the classic studies of McClintock.[24]

It should be added that the author is not aware that insertion sequences have been identified in mammalian genomes, nor of evidence that their translocation is stimulated by chemicals. They should, however, be borne in mind as a possible area of future interest.

5. Variations in Mutagenesis

It is obvious that there are likely to be substantial differences between *E. coli* and mammalian cells in the frequency of different types of spontaneous and induced mutation. For one thing, there are fundamental differences between the structure of the prokaryotic and the eukaryotic gene. The size of the genome in many eukaryotes is very much greater than is required to code for its proteins. Unfortunately, although in a number of instances the working of the prokaryotic gene is well understood, the same cannot be said for the eukaryotic gene. Indeed, it may be that mutation will prove a valuable tool in elucidating this. For our purposes, on the assumption that the extra genetic material in eukaryotes has a function, one consequence will be that mutations affecting production of a protein indirectly will be much more frequent than mutations altering the protein itself.

Another possibility[25] is that small deletions will be very much more frequent in eukaryotes. Indeed, in eukaryotes repair involving deletion formation could conceivably constitute an additional error-producing repair mechanism[25] (see Section V.B). In this context, it is interesting that, in bacteria, ionizing radiation is a base substitution mutagen,[26] whereas in mammalian cells it may be a specific deletion mutagen,[25] (although base substitution at the level found in bacteria would probably not be detectable). This may be an extreme case, but it is likely to be generally true that chemicals will induce different types of mutation in different groups of organisms, both because of differences in repair mechanism and differences in the type of mutation likely to lead to a recognizable alteration in phenotype.

D. Outline

In order to understand how mutations arise, it is first necessary to consider the extremely efficient mechanisms by which the cell can prevent both spontaneous and induced mutation. The author will therefore start by describing ways in which the fidelity of normal DNA replication is ensured and ways in which damaged DNA may be accurately repaired. It will then be possible to consider the inaccurate error-prone DNA repair pathway of *E. coli*, and discuss how it may be regulated. Finally, the ways in which damage from a variety of mutagens and carcinogens may evade accurate repair and lead to mutation will be discussed.

II. SPONTANEOUS MUTATION

A. General

Although it is not certain that all spontaneous mutations arise as errors in DNA replication, it is clear that DNA replication itself must be an extraordinarily accurate process to achieve the low levels of spontaneous mutation found in an organism such as *E. coli* (less than one error per 10^9 base pairs per replication[26,27]). In *E. coli*, at least three different mechanisms appear to be involved. It is necessary to consider these mechanisms for two reasons. First, they are likely to modify the effects of chemical mutagens which act by causing errors in DNA replication. Second, the error-prone repair process involved in mutagenesis by agents such as UV appears to require the controlled suppression of these error-correcting processes, in order to allow DNA polymerization to continue past noncoding lesions.

B. Polymerase Fidelity

Reasonably enough, DNA polymerases tend to select the correct base, and mutations in the replication polymerase and associated enzyms which appear to decrease the accuracy of this process have been isolated both in *E. coli* and in bacteriophage T4.[11,28] However, the role (if any) of most *E. coli* mutator genes in DNA replication has not been established.*[29] The full mechanism for DNA replication in *E. coli* is complex and appears from in vitro studies to require at least thirteen components.[27,30] There is obviously considerable scope for mutations in any of these components to reduce the accuracy of polymerization.

C. Proofreading

In the case of *E. coli,* or its bacteriophage T4, the polymerase has an additional means of increasing the accuracy of replication through its 3′ to 5′ exonuclease activity. Although purified human polymerases do not possess 3′ to 5′ exonuclease activity, it is possible that such an activity is found in association with the enzyme.[31,32] This activity of the polymerase causes it to remove the base that it has just inserted. The backtracking has been called editing or proofreading and is significantly more likely to occur when an incorrect base has been inserted. Very elegant experimental evidence for the importance of this process has been obtained using a number of mutants of the bacteriophage T4 which are altered in DNA polymerase (gene 43). Both mutator and antimutator DNA polymerases may be altered in 3′ to 5′ exonuclease activity, which is revealed as a turnover of deoxynucleotide triphosphate during DNA replication.[33,34]

---

* Glickman[193] has recently obtained evidence that several mutator genes in *E. Coli* are in fact concerned with the mismatch correction process described in Section II.D.

D. Mismatch Correction

Recently it has been shown that in *E. coli* there exists an additional system for reducing spontaneous mutation. This third system operates by the correction of mismatches between the parental and newly replicated strand. Though evidence for mismatch correction is available (*uvrD* and *uvrE* mutants of *E. coli* are deficient in the process[35]), it has been hard to see how such a process could make DNA replication more accurate, unless the cell can distinguish the newly synthesized from the parental strand. Radman, Wagner, and Meselson[189] have now provided evidence that the newly synthesized strand may be recognized because it is undermethylated.

DNA in *E. coli* contains two naturally methylated bases, N^6 methyl adenine and 5-methyl cytosine. These methyl groups are added enzymically fairly slowly after the DNA is replicated. They are not formed by direct chemical methylation. Only 5-methyl cytosine appears to be found in human cells.[36] It is likely that the methylation enzymes recognize specific sequences so that a total of only about 1% of adenine residues and 0.4% of cytosine residues are methylated. Methylation of cytosine, and a small proportion of adenine, is concerned with restriction and modification, the process whereby *E. coli* can recognize and destroy foreign DNA, unless specific sequences are methylated. It appears, however, that most methylation of adenine is not concerned with this process. It is clearly important, nonetheless, since *dam* mutants of *E. coli* are partly deficient in methylation of adenine and show a range of altered properties.[37] Radman et al.[189] have now suggested a role for this methylation by showing that mismatch correction in reconstructed heteroduplexes of λ bacteriophage with one strand from a *dam* and one from a *dam⁺* host occurs with high efficiency in favor of the fully methylated strand.

This should provide an efficient final method of increasing the accuracy of DNA replication. Whether any similar process occurs in mammalian cells remains to be seen.

III. ACCURATE REPAIR OF DNA DAMAGE

A. General

It is not possible to consider chemical mutagenesis separately from DNA repair, because of the dual importance of repair in removing potentially mutagenic lesions from the DNA, and in converting such lesions into mutations. As a starting point, the author will try to describe our current knowledge of how DNA damage is accurately repaired by *E. coli*. Primarily, ultraviolet light (UV) induced damage will be discussed, and the responses of the bacterium to the whole spectrum of chemical carcinogens can then be considered as variations on a basic theme. UV is by far the most comprehensively investigated DNA damaging agent, and *E. coli* its most studied victim. As a reference agent, UV has several advantages, including easy administration, accurate dosimetry, and virtually instant treatment for kinetic studies. Moreover, the principal lesion is well characterized. Pyrimidine dimers are formed in which adjacent pyrimidines on the same DNA strand are joined by a cyclobutane type ring.[38] Formation of the cyclobutane structure saturates the 5,6-double bond in the pyrimidine ring, causing it to become nonplanar.

Much of our knowledge of repair processes in *E. coli* comes from the study of mutants deficient in DNA repair. For reference purposes, Table 1 gives a list of some *E. coli* genes associated with DNA repair and mutation. (See Clarke and Ganesan[39] for a similar list). The success of this approach has encouraged a search for repair-deficient human mutants, which at this stage shows considerable promise, and which will be discussed in Volume II, Chapter 5 by Maher and McCormick.

Although DNA repair processes in *E. coli* are complex because they may interact to form a whole network of repair pathways, it is possible that four main types of repair may be distinguished. Three of these are accurate and will be discussed now.

TABLE 1

A List of Some Genes in *E. coli* Associated with DNA Repair

Gene	Repair process	Comments	Ref.
phr	Photoreactivation	Photoreactivating enzyme	40,81
uvrA *uvrB* *uvrC*	endonuclease step of excision repair	jointly govern the endonuclease involved in dimer excision role of *uvrC* uncertain, *uvrB* cannot coexist with *polA*	42, 166
uvrD *uvrE*	Mismatch Correction	unknown function, possible alleles, *uvrD* is dominant, *uvrE* is a mutator, cannot coexist with *polA*.	35
polA	Exonuclease and DNA polymerase steps of excision repair and other gap-filling processes	polymerase 1 polymerase + 5′—3′ exonuclease activity	167, 168
lig	Strand rejoining	DNA ligase	169
recA	Completely deficient in recombinaton and error-prone repair	Gene product is protein X, possibly a specific protease possibly with other functions, protein X appears to control its own synthesis.	83, 170
tif *lexB* *zab*	Apparent alleles of *recA*	*tif* is a repair and recombination proficient co-dominant allele, constitutive for Rec-Lex functions at 42°, *lexB* and *zab* resemble *recA*, but are proficient in general recombination.	171, 172
recB *recC*	Deficient in general Recombination and recombination repair	Closely linked, jointly govern exonuclease V, proficient in error-prone repair	173
sbcA *sbcB* *rac* *xonA*	Suppressors of the defect in recB and recC	*sbcA* has acquired a novel exonuclease, *sbcB* and possibly *xonA* lack exonuclease 1	174
recF	Deficient in general recombination and recombination repair	Lacks the recombination ability found in *recB recC sbcB* mutants; *recB recC recF* mutants are virtually totally recombination-deficient but can perform error-prone repair	64
lexA	Deficient in error-prone repair and other *rec-lex* functions, but almost fully proficient in recombination repair and general recombination	Formerly *exrA*, *lexA* is dominant, possibly the protein X repressor, possibly an inhibitor of *rec-lex* functions	23, 90
tsl *rnmA* *spr* *lexC*	alleles of *lexA*	*tsl* and *rnm* are partial *lexA* revertants with some restoration of *rec-lex* functions; *tsl* strains filament at 42°; *spr* strains are constitutive for protein X production	88,98,175,176

TABLE 1 (Continued)

A List of Some Genes in *E. coli* Associated with DNA Repair

Gene	Repair process	Comments	Ref.
		and *rec-lex* functions; *lexC* (= *exrB*) resembles *lexA* except for hyper-filamentation	
lon	Lethal filamentation following DNA damage	Equivalent to *deg T* and affects control of a number of enzymes	177, 178
sul	Nonallelic suppressor of *lon*		10, 179
sfi	nonallelic suppressors of filamentation in *tif* strains	Several loci with differential effects on *rec-lex* functions	10
recGL	Other genes affecting recombination		174
ras	Miscellaneous	ntwA is the structural gene	39
ror	repair-deficient	for endonuclease 2, involved	
ntwA	mutants	in recognition of non-UV damage	

B. Photoreactivation

In the presence of light of 300 to 450 nm wavelength, an enzyme reverses the dimerization of pyrimidines and restores the DNA to its original configuration.[40] The process is entirely specific for pyrimidine dimers so that, provided care is taken to exclude certain artifacts, it is possible to use it as evidence that pyrimidine dimers have produced a given effect. Hart and Setlow, for instance, have used it to show that pyrimidine dimers induce tumors in a fish species.[41] It is also possible to use photoreactivation to study the kinetics of the lethal and mutagenic effects of UV by determining when the processes of killing or mutation can no longer be reversed by removal of the damage from the DNA.

Photoreactivation occurs in all groups up to marsupials. In humans, there is some evidence for a rather different type of photoreactivation, but the nature of this process and its biological relevance are still more than somewhat controversial.[18]

C. Excision Repair

In contrast to the high specificity of photoreactivation, almost all types of potentially mutagenic DNA damage appear to be subject to repair by some form of excision process in *E. coli*. The classical process by which pyrimidine dimers are excised, is shown in the left hand part of Figure 1.

The *E. coli* mutants *uvrA*, *uvrB*, and *uvrC* are deficient in the initial endonuclease step.[42] The defect in *uvrD* and *uvrE*, which are also deficient in excision of mismatched base pairs,[35] is quite unclear.

UvrA, *uvrB*, and *uvrC* are required for the recognition of a wide variety of bulky lesions, where damage to one strand is likely to cause a distortion of the double helix. It may be less essential for the lesion to affect the base pairing, since on the one hand, the genes do not appear to be involved in correction of mismatched bases,[35] and on the other hand, they may recognize lesions such as bulky O^6 alkylations of guanine which can participate in DNA replication.[43,44] It appears that the endonuclease can distinguish the damaged from the undamaged strand.

In a repair-proficient strain of *E. coli*, DNA polymerase 1 removes the damaged strand through its 5′ to 3′ exonuclease activity and at the same time replaces it through its polymerase activity. This is the main pathway in *E. coli*, and as far as can be judged, it is highly accurate. The patches formed are extremely short.[45,46] Occasionally in a

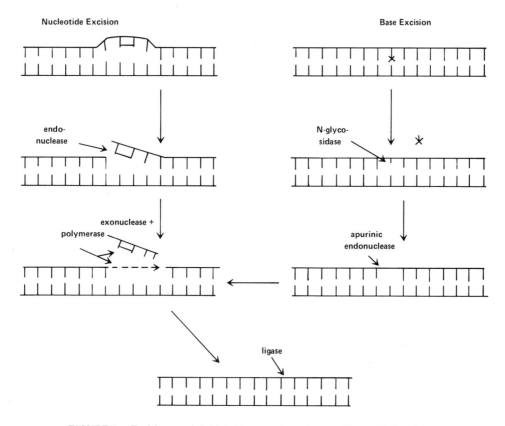

FIGURE 1.   Excision repair initiated by an endonuclease and by an N-glycosidase.

normal strain, the damaged region is removed by separate exonuclease attack and re-polymerization by DNA polymerase 3. This is the only system operating in a *polA* mutant (deficient in DNA polymerase 1) and for less obvious reasons it does not operate in a *recA* mutant (deficient in all recombination). The second process yields long patches (about 1000 bases).[45] Its accuracy is less certain and will be discussed later. The author is not aware of any controversy concerning the role of polynucleotide ligase in the final sealing of the patch.

The right-hand side of Figure 1 shows a more recently discovered variation in which the damaged base is recognized by an N-glycosidase which removes the base, leaving an apurinic (or apyrimidinic) site. Although such sites are alkali-labile and show up as discontinuities in alkaline sucrose gradients, the DNA backbone is intact in vivo. Apurinic sites, which can also form spontaneously, are recognized by an apurinic endonuclease, and the subsequent stages of repair are presumably identical to those of classical excision.[18]

The best characterized N-glycosidase specifically removes uracil from DNA.[18] Uracil is fairly readily formed by deamination of cytosine and would be expected to code as thymine.

A degree of controversy exists over the relative importance of endonuclease and N-glycosidase attack in the removal of damage by simple alkylating agents and also in the specificity of the enzymes involved.[18] One possibility is that there is a specific enzyme for each subtly altered base. The inducible repair system for N-methyl-N'-nitro-N-nitrosoguanidine damage, recently described by Samson and Cairns[47] may involve such enzymes.

Although the DNA repair defect in most patients with the human syndrome xeroderma pigmentosum bears a close superficial resemblance to the Uvr defect in *E. coli*, it would be unwise to extrapolate too readily. First, the evidence from existing repair-deficient human cell lines suggests a much greater level of specificity of repair enzymes than in *E. coli*. Second, extracts from xeroderma cells seem to be able to remove dimers from free DNA, although those from cells of some groups are unable to remove dimers from chromatin.[18] The defect in such cells may lie in a failure to make damaged DNA in chromatin available to the repair enzymes. This conclusion is supported by evidence that although xeroderma cells are hypersensitive to both UV and *N*-hydroxyacetamidofluorene, different enzymes appear to be involved in the recognition of the damage.[48,49]

D. Recombination Repair

Photoreactivation and excision repair remove the damage from the DNA. The other two processes in *E. coli,* recombination repair and error-prone repair, do not do this; instead they enable functional new DNA to be formed, despite the presence of damage in the template.

In *E. coli,* when the DNA is replicated, the polymerase appears to stop when it encounters a noncoding lesion such as a pyrimidine dimer and to restart further along the chromosome, probably at the next RNA primer site. As a result, large gaps are found in the newly synthesized strand.

These gaps appear to be filled by a process of strand exchanges with the sister duplex.[50,51] At one stage, it was believed that this process was inaccurate and led to mutation,[52] but a number of lines of evidence[53,54] suggest that a quite separate repair process is involved in mutagenesis.

In mammalian cells, gaps may be found in DNA synthesized immediately after UV irradiation. However, they are usually not formed at later times, even when there is evidence of persistence of damage in the parental DNA, and they are sometimes not found at all. Moreover, although gaps are filled, there is no definitive evidence that strand exchange is involved.[55] Even if strand exchanges are not found, it does not exclude the possibility that the opposite duplex is used in constructing DNA opposite noncoding lesions. A minor change of mechanism could result in the missing information being copied from the complementary newly synthesized strand. In Figure 2, for instance, recombination is initiated by a free 3' end of DNA pairing with its complementary strand in an intact duplex. There is some evidence for an initiating event of this type.[56,57] The author suggests that, in *E. coli,* endonucleolytic cleavage and rejoining of the invading strand and its homologue are likely, (Figure 2 D,E), whereas in mammalian cells, these events have a much lower probability (Figure 2H). In both cases, DNA polymerization will assist branch migration (Figure 2F and I), the only difference being that in mammalian cells the denatured region will also migrate. Joining of the free 3' and 5' ends will then generate a strand exchange in bacteria, but a "copy-choice" event in mammalian cells.

IV. INACCURATE DNA REPAIR

A. Error-Prone Repair as a Rec-Lex Function

One of the most significant observations on the mechanism of mutagenesis in bacteria was the demonstration by Witkin in 1967[23] that *exr* (now renamed *lex A*) strains of *E. coli* were immutable by UV. This was the initial evidence that the mutation induced by such agents occurred as part of a specific repair process and not by random errors in replication of damaged DNA.

The repair process joined a list of other effects associated with DNA damage, whose occurrence was shown to depend on the presence in the cell of the *recA*⁺ and *lexA*⁺

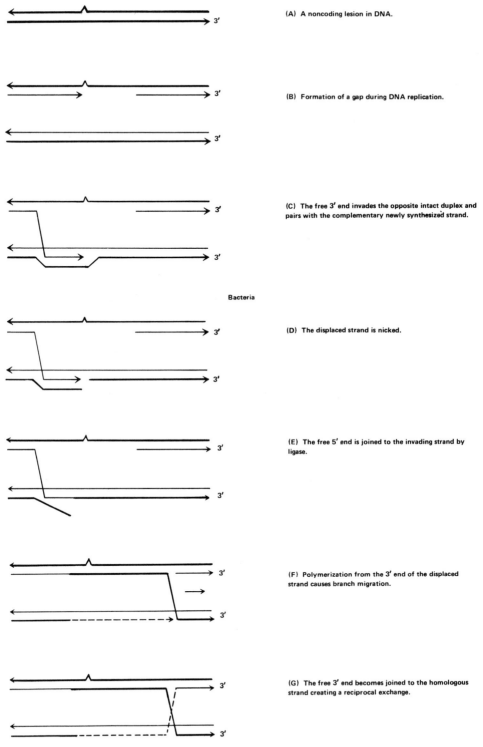

(A) A noncoding lesion in DNA.

(B) Formation of a gap during DNA replication.

(C) The free 3' end invades the opposite intact duplex and pairs with the complementary newly synthesized strand.

Bacteria

(D) The displaced strand is nicked.

(E) The free 5' end is joined to the invading strand by ligase.

(F) Polymerization from the 3' end of the displaced strand causes branch migration.

(G) The free 3' end becomes joined to the homologous strand creating a reciprocal exchange.

FIGURE 2.   A scheme for recombination repair in bacteria and mammalian cells.

gene products. Some of these Rec-Lex functions are listed in Table 2 (see Witkin[10] for a similar list).

A clue to the operation of error-prone repair came from the excessively renamed

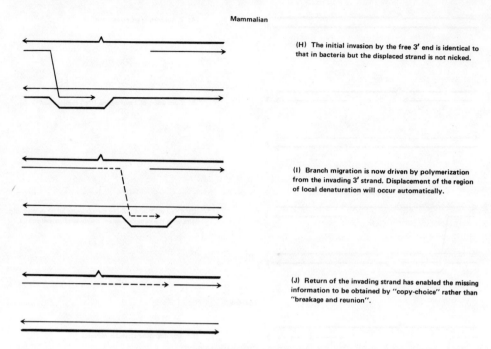

Mammalian

(H) The initial invasion by the free 3′ end is identical to that in bacteria but the displaced strand is not nicked.

(I) Branch migration is now driven by polymerization from the invading 3′ strand. Displacement of the region of local denaturation will occur automatically.

(J) Return of the invading strand has enabled the missing information to be obtained by "copy-choice" rather than "breakage and reunion".

FIGURE 2.   (continued)

TABLE 2

Some Rec-Lex Functions

Effect	Ref.
Induction of λ prophage	180—182
Filamentation induction in *lon* bacteria	183, 184
UV-induced mutation	23, 185
Weigle-reactivation and mutagenesis	59, 60
Protein X production	85
Control of DNA breakdown by exonuclease 5	186, 187
Inhibition of respiration through NAD depletion	188

phenomenon of UV-reactivation, Weigle-reactivation, W-reactivation or Induced reactivation. Weigle,[58.59] years previously, had shown that the survival of certain irradiated bacteriophages was increased if they infected a cell which itself had been lightly irradiated and that only under such conditions was there a high yield of bacteriophage mutants. It was subsequently shown that Weigle-reactivation belonged to the list of Rec-Lex functions,[60] and evidence was obtained that its mechanism did not involve recombination.[53] On the basis of Weigle-reactivation, Radman developed a hypothesis,[61] suggesting that Weigle-reactivation and bacterial mutagenesis were two manifestations of an inducible last-ditch repair process (SOS repair) which operated by permitting polymerization past noncoding lesions in the DNA. This elegant hypothesis has influenced all subsequent research into bacterial mutagenesis.

B. Is Error-Prone Repair Inducible?

Although Weigle reactivation shows the properties of an inducible error-prone repair system, not involving recombination, this does not necessarily imply that bacterial mutagenesis is inducible or that it does not involve recombination. At least four lines of evidence, however, suggest that bacterial mutations arise independently of recombination repair. First, bacterial mutagenesis can apparently occur in cells containing only one genome under conditions where recombination appears to be excluded.[62] Second, although *lexA* strains are not mutable by UV, they can recombine and fill gaps in newly synthesized DNA, at least at low doses.[63] Third, Eyfjord et al.[54] have shown that the kinetics of gap filling and of mutation formation after UV irradiation are different. Fourth, Kato, Rothman, and Clark[64] have found that *recB recF* double mutants show considerable UV mutagenesis despite being almost completely deficient in recombination.

The evidence for inducibility of bacterial error-prone repair has been summarized by Witkin.[10] Evidence less readily reconciled with inducibility has been summarized by Green,[65] who has suggested an alternative hypothesis that newly synthesized DNA may be temporarily immune to error-prone repair.

Two points deserve to be made. First, although DNA damage may induce increased levels of error-prone repair, it is likely that sufficient error-prone repair is constitutive to account for most mutagenesis in repair-proficient bacteria.[66] Second, the repair processes acting on bacteriophage DNA show considerable differences from those acting on the DNA of the *E. coli* cell itself. Among other differences, a process analogous to bacterial recombination repair does not appear to operate on irradiated bacteriophage DNA (although other types of repair involving recombination may occur[67]). When major differences exist between repair of different types of DNA within the same bacterial cell, any attempts to extrapolate inducible error-prone repair directly from bacteria to man would seem premature.

C. The Substrate for Error-Prone Repair

Although error-prone repair may be inducible, the question remains whether the rate-limiting step for mutation is a requirement for induction, or the availability of sites for error-prone repair. If error-prone repair occurs by polymerization past noncoding lesions in DNA where might this polymerization take place? When the frequency of Okazaki gaps in replicating DNA is related to spontaneous mutation, it is clear that error-prone repair must occur at these sites with negligible frequency.

The situation is less clear cut with the gaps found opposite pyrimidine dimers during DNA replication. Clearly such gaps, and indeed Okazaki gaps, may serve as sites for error-prone repair in certain circumstances, for instance in a *tif* strain (Table 1) at 42°,[68] or in a strain containing a particular type of mutation-enhancing plasmid.[69] (For this reason, McCann et al.[70] have followed a suggestion of MacPhee[71] and constructed hypersensitive *S. typhimurium* tester strains containing the plasmid pKM101.)

In other circumstances it seems likely that the majority of such gaps do not normally lead to mutation. A long-standing observation is that, especially in *E. coli* strains deficient in excision repair, UV-induced mutations arise according to the square of dose.[72] Bridges[73] suggested that this indicated the need for two lesions to generate a mutation. If this were so, only a dose-dependent minority of gaps opposite dimers could be substrate for error-prone repair in a normal strain. The concept of inducible error-prone repair allowed an alternative interpretation that the kinetics of mutation indicated a requirement to both induce error-prone repair and provide a substrate for it, although the evidence probably fits this model less readily. Sedgwick[75] has proposed a development of Bridge's hypothesis for excision-deficient bacteria, where the dimers which give rise to mutations are situated close to each other on opposite strands of DNA so that when the DNA is replicated, the gaps in the newly synthesized DNA will overlap. (Figure 3). It will then be impossible for recombination repair to be initiated

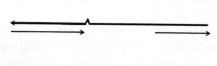

(A) Closely spaced noncoding lesions on opposite strands.

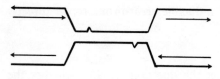

(B) On replication, lead to overlapping daughter strand gaps. Recombination cannot occur because no free end can pair with its complementary strand.

(C) In an excision-deficient strain errorprone polymerization past a dimer is the only possibility for repair.

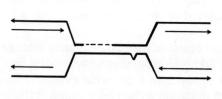

(D) Reannealing of the parental strands may occur.

(E) In an excision-proficient strain excision repair is now possible.

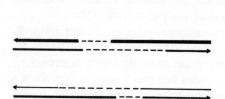

(F) The resulting structure is now capable of error-free repair.

FIGURE 3.   A model of *R*eannealing *A*nd *P*ost-replication *E*xcision.

by a free end pairing with its complementary strand (Figure 2), and unless error-prone repair occurs the double lesion will be lethal. A specific prediction of this model is that error-prone repair should only occur once at any given site. This prediction has been confirmed by Doubleday et al.[76] A second prediction is that all UV-induced mutations should arise in the first generation, even though dimers persist indefinitely in excision-deficient bacteria. Doubleday et al.[76] showed that although this prediction was fulfilled under some growth conditions, under other conditions, mutations arose over a period much longer than one generation after irradiation. It is, however, possible that DNA replication is stalled temporarily in potentially mutant cells, an extremely difficult thing to test.

Green et al.[77] in turn have extended the Sedgwick hypothesis to argue that in excision-proficient bacteria overlapping daughter strand gaps will not be a substrate for error-prone repair, since where gaps overlap, the parental strands will reanneal and allow further excision repair to occur (Figure 3). This hypothetical *Reannealing And Post-replicative Excision* (RAPE) conveniently explains a number of discrepancies between mutagenesis in excision-proficient and excision-deficient strains. As evidence, Green et al.[77] showed that, at a given dose of UV, the chance of daughter strand gaps (or overlapping gaps) giving rise to a mutation is very much lower in an excision-proficient than an excision-deficient strain. From this they concluded that an excision-dependent postreplication repair process must operate. On quite independent grounds (the properties of *recA tsl* double mutants (*tsl* is an allele of *lexA* (Table 1)), Mount et al. have reached a similar conclusion.[78] Green et al. went on to suggest that RAPE can be used to explain an obscure phenomenon in *E. coli* and *S. typhimurium* called Mutation Frequency Decline (MFD), which concerns mutation at certain *t*RNA suppressor loci.[79]

It now appears that in a normal repair proficient strain of *E. coli*, there is a most elegant coordination of repair processes which minimizes the chance of a dimer giving rise to a mutation. In the first instance, the dimer may be photoreactivated or excised, both efficient, accurate processes. If the dose of UV is high, DNA replication becomes stalled temporarily and restarts at the origin of replication.[80,81] This allows additional excision repair to occur. If a dimer is replicated, a gap is formed in the newly synthesized DNA that can be filled accurately by recombination repair. If gaps in daughter strands overlap, thus preventing recombination repair, Reannealing And Post-replication Excision occurs. It is only when all these processes fail that error-prone repair will be called into operation. In a repair proficient strain, this may well not be for a residuum of repair resistant damage, but for rare cases where conventional repair goes wrong.

Because of the extreme accuracy and efficiency of normal repair, there has been a tendency to study mutation in bacteria at sites (such as certain *t*RNA loci), where fully efficient repair may not occur or to use strains where repair or control processes are defective (such as excision deficient or *tif* strains). Although such approaches are valid and valuable, it must be remembered that they may give a distorted picture of normal mutagenesis.

D. Control of Rec-Lex Functions

Although the author has argued that the occurrence of induced mutations may be determined more by the presence of sites resistant to accurate repair, than by the need for induction of the error-prone repair system, this still implies the existence of an extremely strict control of error-prone repair. Since mutation is a Rec-Lex function, an obvious starting point for the understanding of this control is to consider the nature of the *recA*[+] and *lexA*[+] gene products themselves. There has recently been considerable progress in this direction. MacEntee et al.[82] have characterized the *recA*[+] gene product as a protein of MW 43,000, and it now appears[83] that it is identical with protein X, a protein of MW 40,000 initially isolated by Inouye.[84] Protein X is present constitutively in low amounts and is synthesized in large amounts following UV irradiation and other DNA damaging treatments.[85] It appears to regulate its own synthesis.[83] The most recent evidence is that it may be the specific protease that cleaves λ repressor.[85-88] A

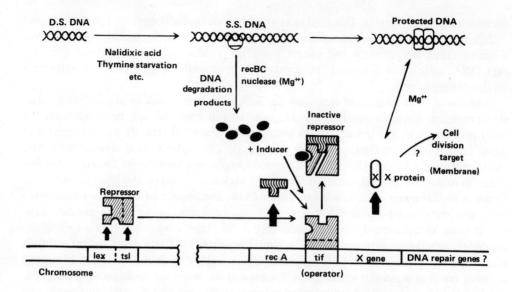

A feedback loop for control of DNA degradation. D.S. and S.S., double- and single-stranded, respectively.

FIGURE 4A.   The original model of Gudas and Pardee with *lexA* as a repressor. (From Gudas, L. J. and Pardee, A. B., *Proc. Natl. Acad. Sci. U.S.A.*, 72, 2330, 1975.)

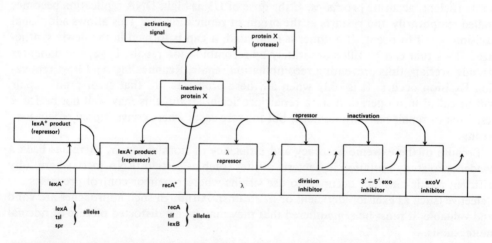

FIGURE 4B.   The model of Gudas and Pardee modified with *recA⁺* and *tif* allelic, *recA⁺* gene product protein X and *recA⁺* gene product an autoregulatory specific protease.[81,83,85,87]

specific protease would certainly be a plausible candidate for a highly pleiotropic gene, and there is evidence that the specific protease inhibitor antipain blocks a variety of *rec-lex* functions.[89] The most striking property of *lexA* is that it is dominant over *lexA⁺*.[90] This implies that the *lexA⁺* gene product is some form of repressor or inhibitor.

The first comprehensive model of *rec-lex* control was proposed by Gudas and Pardee[91] (Figure 4A) and modified by Gudas,[85] Mount,[88] and Emmerson and West[82] to take account of subsequent developments (Figure 4B). The distiguishing feature of all these models is that the *lexA⁺* gene product is a repressor for *rec-lex* functions. In Figure 4B, for instance, following a variety of DNA damaging treatments some sort of effector is produced which activates the proteolytic activity of the small amount of

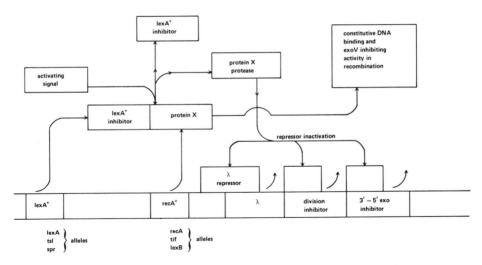

FIGURE 4C. The model of Morand et al.[92] *LexA* is an inhibitor of the *recA*[+] specific protease. *RecA*[+] gene product has an additional constitutive role in recombination.

protein X present constitutively so that it can cleave both its own repressor (*lexA*[+] gene product), and λ repressor.

In contrast to these models, Morand et al.[92] have suggested that the *recA*[+] gene product has a constitutive DNA binding function[93] involved in recombination, and a proteolytic function which is blocked by *lexA*[+] gene product and which can be activated by its release. In this case the *lexA*[+] gene product directly inhibits the *recA*[+] gene product, rather than repressing its synthesis (Figure 4C).

As yet another alternative, Witkin[10] has suggested that the *lexA*[+] gene product protects the sites which are sensitive to proteolytic attack (Figure 4D). In published form, this model does not account for the evidence that the *recA*[+] gene product is a specific protease, but it can be modified to do so (Witkin[190]).

Finally, Figure 4E shows yet another variant of the repressor model, in which the *lexA*[+] gene product represses several operons in addition to *recA*[+] (if it turns out to be a protease inhibitor, it could instead inhibit several proteases). This model is in a sense a compromise between the *lexA* repressor and the Witkin models.

There is insufficient evidence at present to choose among these various models. Since some Rec-Lex functions have been studied for up to 30 years, a considerable amount of phenomenology needs to be accommodated in any scheme. This creates several difficulties.

First, discrepancies between *lexA* and *recA* strains in their levels of residual Rec-Lex functions[94-96] suggest that the sole function of *lexA* cannot be to act as a repressor of *recA*. Witkin's model copes with this difficulty most satisfactorily, but it is possible to amend the other models (as in Figure 4E) so that *lexA* acts independently as a repressor of several Rec-Lex functions. However, it is fair to say that Witkin's model (Figure 4D) fits better than Figure 4E the observation that certain *sfi* (Table 1) mutations can differentially effect more than one Rec-Lex function.

A second problem is that it is unlikely that the *recA*[+] gene product is solely a protease. For one thing, far too much is formed, up to 4% of the total cell protein.[93] Gudas and Pardee[93] also showed that protein X bound specifically to single-stranded DNA, and it is possibly this property which enhances the survival of *uvr*[+] *recA tsl* mutants.[78,97] These mutants appear to produce constitutively an otherwise inactive *recA* gene product.[93] Further difficulties arise in reconciling the apparent constitutive

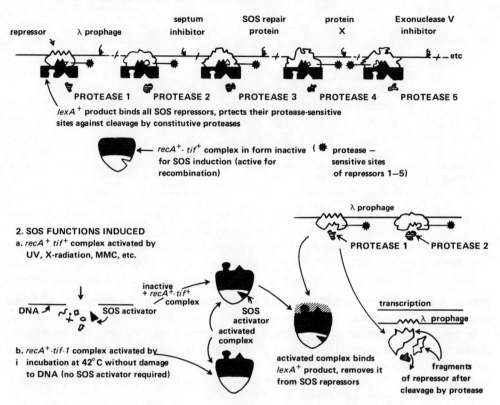

FIGURE 4D.   The model of Witkin. *LexA* protects sites subject to proteolytic cleavage. (From Witkin, E. M., *Bacteriol. Rev.*, 40, 892, 1976. With permission.)

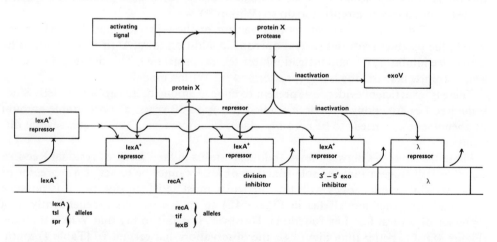

FIGURE 4E.   A remodified *lexA*-repressor model, in which lexA is the repressor for several *rec-lex* functions, in addition to repressing *recA*.

nature of recombination, with the apparent inducible nature of other *rec-lex* functions, and it is these considerations that have led Morand et al. to formulate their model.[92]

A third difficulty concerns the nature of the signal which activates *recA*[+] gene product. Since the original observation of Borek and Ryan[99] that UV-irradiated DNA in the form of an F factor when transferred into an unirradiated cell would induce λ bacteriophage, a considerable amount of work has been carried out in determining which Rec-Lex functions can be indirectly induced in this way and which types of irradiated DNA produce an effect (if all forms of irradiated DNA induced Rec-Lex functions, one could never demonstrate Weigle-reactivation, for instance). The situation is extremely complex and almost all the candidates for a low-molecular-weight effector to activate protein X are likely to be produced in high yield by types of transferred DNA which are not effective in indirect induction of Rec-Lex functions.[100-102]

E. The Mechanism of Error-Prone Repair

Some of the most significant efforts to determine the molecular mechanism of error-prone repair have come from Radman and co-workers.[103-105] It appears that the process involves some form of random polymerization past noncoding lesions since Radman et al.[104] have shown that, under Weigle-reactivation conditions, polymerization past dimers can occur in the single-stranded DNA bacteriophage ϕX174. This capability might be due to a novel inducible polymerase of low specificity or a terminal nucleotidyl transferase (which could add bases at random to a free end of DNA). Despite investigation, no evidence of either has been obtained in *E. coli*.

The most attractive hypothesis is that the fidelity of an existing polymerase (see Section II) is reduced under conditions of Weigle-reactivation and error-prone repair. The most direct evidence suggesting this comes from the work of Bridges and Mottershead,[106] who have used a temperature-sensitive mutant to show that DNA polymerase 3 is an essential enzyme for error-prone repair and that the effect on error-prone repair of a mutant DNA polymerase 3 shows greater temperature sensitivity than the effect on normal polymerizing ability.

Radman and co-workers have developed an in vitro assay for mutation.[104] The system involves a synthetic template (currently poly dC oligo dG, formerly poly dT oligo dA). If replication on the template occurs, only one type of base should be inserted. Insertion of A instead of G (or vice versa) gives a measure of the accuracy of replication. It is possible to add to the system a variety of cell extracts obtained under different conditions in order to look for evidence of an inducible error-prone polymerase activity. Since only two triphosphates are needed to assay correct and incorrect synthesis on the template, it is possible to omit the other triphosphates and reduce synthesis on residual DNA present in the extracts. Using this system, Radman et al.[107] obtained evidence of increased misincorporation using extracts of a *tif* strain prepared at elevated temperature. Recently, however, McGarva and Lehmann[108] have shown the presence of a DNA-dependent triphosphatase in such extracts,[27] which could cause serious artefacts, and the validity of this exciting in vitro approach to mutagenesis remains to be established.

On the assumption that error-prone repair is a modification of normal accurate polymerization, Radman and co-workers[104] have gone on to consider which of the mechanisms for ensuring fidelity of replication must be suppressed in order for error-prone repair to occur. They have found that when DNA containing noncoding lesions is used as a template for DNA polymerase, the polymerase does not simply stop, but converts triphosphate to monophosphate with high efficiency. This implies that a base is inserted opposite the noncoding lesion and then removed by 3' to 5' exonuclease activity. Hence it is not the fidelity of the polymerase, but its proofreading function which must be modified for error-prone repair to occur. Evidence that inhibition of 3' to 5' exonuclease activity by monophosphates leads to an increase in misincorporation has in fact been obtained by Byrnes et al.[109] To the knowledge of the author, mismatch correction has not been tested for its effect on error-prone repair, although it might be expected to produce an immunity of newly synthesized DNA to mutation as postulated by Green.[65] Certainly, considerable differences exist between mutation induction in newly synthesized and pre-existing DNA.[65]

Nevertheless, although it is entirely speculative, it is simplest to consider base substitution mutagenesis by agents such as UV as arising through suppression of the 3' to 5' exonuclease activity of DNA polymerase 3. This exonuclease suppression is under strict control and may be induced following DNA damage although a constitutive level is likely.[66]

V. VARIATIONS ON A REPAIR AND MUTATION THEME

A. DNA Cross-Linking Agents

Several groups of extremely cytotoxic agents have the property of forming interstrand DNA cross-links; these include bifunctional alkylating agents such as nitrogen mustard,[110] mitomycin C,[111] psoralens,[112] and pyrrolizidine alklaloids.[113] Structurally related compounds, which react with DNA but do not form cross-links, are much less toxic, suggesting that the cross-links are involved in cell killing.[114,115] Despite the problem of damage at virtually the same point in both strands, repair-proficient bacteria and human cells appear able to repair cross-links. (The release of cross-links can be followed by studying the rate of reannealing of denatured DNA. If the complementary strands are held together by a cross-link, reannealing is more rapid.)[110]

The most detailed study of the mechanism of repair has been made by Cole,[116] who used trimethylpsoralen and *E. coli*. Cole has shown that the basic repair process involves the coordinate action of excision and recombination repair. The process is shown in Figure 5. The initial step is recognition of the cross-link and an incision by *uvr* endonuclease. Next, a second incision releases the end of the cross-link. Possibly the 5' to 3' exonuclease activity of DNA polymerase 1 can perform this step, possibly an unknown enzyme is involved. Cole goes on to demonstrate that, although the resulting gap cannot be filled by simple polymerization, it appears to be filled by recombination with a preexisting intact duplex elsewhere in the cell. Whether excision-deficient bacteria can survive any cross-links is uncertain. Bacteria deficient in both excision and recombination repair are considerably more sensitive than the corresponding single mutants, but this difference could relate to repair of monoadducts.

Although the role of DNA cross-links in lethality seems clear, their role in mutagenesis is by no means clear. Some cross-linking agents such as nitrogen mustard, or 8-methoxypsoralen,[117] are relatively potent mutagens, whereas others are weakly mutagenic, like mitomycin C,[118] or apparently nonmutagenic, like monocrotaline.[119] Moreover, excision-deficient strains of bacteria show enhanced mutagenesis by nitrogen mustard (Table 3) or 8-meth oxypsoralen,[117] whereas excision-deficient bacteria have been reported not to be mutated at all by mitomycin C.[114]

The reason the author would suggest for these discrepancies is that, although cross-links are of major significance in determining survival, it is the nature of the monoadduct which primarily determines mutagenicity. Nitrogen mustard is considered to be a classical SN2-type alkylating agent and as such would be expected to resemble methyl methanesulfonate rather than ethyl methanesulfonate as a mutagen. It should therefore be rather weakly mutagenic, and the mutations would be expected to arise through error-prone repair. Surprisingly, experiments by W. J. Muriel and the author show that nitrogen mustard mutagenesis is entirely independent of error-prone repair (Table 3), since it occurs equally readily in a *lexA* strain of *E. coli*. This suggests that nitrogen mustard probably alkylates the O^6 position of guanine, and as such causes errors in replication. If a proportion of monoadducts are of this type, they will be highly mutagenic. Table 3 suggests that they are subject to uvr-dependent excision.

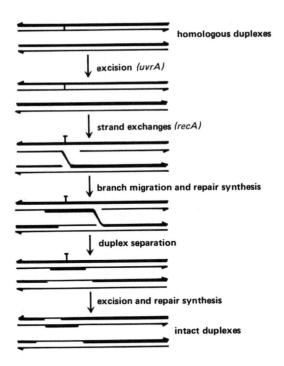

One possible mechanism for the repair of cross-linked DNA is shown here to illustrate the types of products and intermediates involved, and to indicate steps controlled by the *uvr* and *recA* genes. The sequence proceeds as follows: two incisions are first made near each cross-link. A nuclease then widens the gap, exposing a single-stranded region. Ensuing strand exchanges between homologous duplexes insert an intact base sequence complementary to the strand still carrying the partially excised cross-linking residue. When the twin helical DNA structure is restored, the remaining arm of the cross-link is excised. *Dashed lines* indicate regions of repair synthesis.

FIGURE 5. Repair of interstrand DNA cross-links. Model of R. S. Cole. (From Cole, R. S., *Proc. Natl. Acad. Sci. U.S.A.*, 70, 1064, 1973.)

TABLE 3

Characterization of the Mutagenicity of Nitrogen Mustard by Repair Deficient Strains of *Escherichia coli*

Strain	Concentration of nitrogen mustard (µg/ml)			
	0	0 · 01	0 · 1	1 · 0
	Tubes positive			
WP2 (UV resistant)	10	12	*24*	*35*
CM561 (lexA)	5	9	*16*	*25*
WP2 *uvrA*	8	*23*	*48*	*50*
CM611 *uvrA lexA*	4	*20*	*46*	*49*

Note: Protocol as in Green et al.[118] Values are mean numbers of tubes positive (out of 50) in 3 independent fluctuation tests. Values in italics are significantly higher than control (probability less than 0.001%). Experiments performed by W. J. Muriel.

In the case of the psoralens, mutagenesis appears to occur by error-prone repair, since it does not operate in a *lexA* strain.[117] However, the psoralen monoadduct is a product with some similarities to a pyrimidine dimer[112] and will prevent base pairing. Hence, every monoadduct will have the potential for causing mutation by a UV-like mechanism. As discussed previously, this type of mutation is disproportionately more likely in an excision deficient strain.

Murayama and Otsiji[114] have reported that mitomycin C is not mutagenic in excision-deficient bacteria although, at higher doses, related monofunctional compounds are mutagenic. Since the released cross-link consists of a gap opposite a noncoding lesion, an obvious explanation would be that these lesions were the main substrate for error-prone repair. The monoadducts would presumably be more weakly mutagenic, possibly neither altering nor preventing base pairing. Alkylation of the N^7 position of guanine might fit this description, but Iyer and Szybalski[111] on structural grounds argued that this was unlikely. The corroboration of this hypothesis would be a demonstration that at the same dose mitomycin C was more mutagenic to excision-proficient than to excision-deficient bacteria. The author has not been able to show this to date. At doses where mitomycin C mutates excision-proficient *E. coli*, excision-deficient strains are killed. The conclusion to date must be that, although interstrand DNA cross-links are of prime importance in determining cell survival, they may often be of no more than minor importance in mutagenesis.

It is possible that a similar situation might hold in mammalian cells. Cultured fibroblasts from patients with Fanconi's anemia show specific sensitivity to mitomycin C, and xeroderma pigmentosum cells show wild-type survival. However, xeroderma cells show increased frequencies of mitomycin C-induced sister chromatid exchanges.[120] (Fanconi's anemia cells show a slight reduction.[121]) The obvious interpretation is again that, although survival is related to cross-linking, monoadducts may be almost equally effective in determining other damage-related effects. It should be possible to use this type of situation where effects of an agent are mediated differentially by different lesions, to pinpoint much more closely the way in which DNA damage leads to mutation or cancer.

B. Ionizing Radiation

Ionizing radiation induces double-strand breaks, single-strand breaks and miscellaneous base damage.[122] A break in both strands of DNA at the same point would be thought likely to be even more harmful to the cell than a cross-link, and *E. coli* is thought not to be able to repair double-strand breaks.*[123] Other species of bacteria, and human cells, do however have this ability.[124,125] It is not certain that double-strand breaks are responsible for lethality in *E. coli*, since there are large effects of strain and culture conditions on survival. These factors would not be expected to affect the initial production of breaks, but they might influence the repair of breaks with a slight overlap.[126] The most readily studied lesions induced by ionizing radiation are single-strand breaks. The majority (over 90%) of these are repaired extremely rapidly by a process depending on DNA polymerase 1 (i.e., not occurring in *polA* strains).[127] Under most conditions, this process is complete before the DNA can be analyzed. A minority of breaks are repaired by a slow process involving the *lexA*+ and *recA*+ genes (i.e., not occurring in *recA* and *lexA* strains).[128,129]

One possibility is that the lesion requiring this type of repair consists of a strand break opposite a damaged base. In this case, repair might occur by the same mecha-

---

* Krasin and Hutchinson[194] have now shown that double strand breaks can be repaired in *E. coli*. This type of repair does not occur in *recA* strains, or in cells where a second genome is not present, suggesting that recombination between preexisting chromosomes may be involved.

nism as Cole[116] has suggested for DNA cross-linking agents. However, Bridges[62,130] used special growth conditions to produce cells containing less than two complete genomes and found that repair and mutation were essentially normal. This would preclude recombination of the type envisaged by Cole, and suggest that such lesions, like released cross-links, were likely to undergo error-prone repair with a high probability.

The contribution of base damage on its own to the lethality and mutagenicity of ionizing radiation is not known, but a crude indication can be obtained by comparing irradiation in the presence and absence of oxygen. Oxygen enhances the yield of strand breaks more than base damage, and the oxygen enhancement ratio for mutation is fairly low,[131] suggesting a possible role of base damage in mutagenesis.

Base-pair substitution mutagenesis by ionizing radiation is almost entirely lexA$^+$ and recA$^+$ dependent.

The human genetic disease ataxia telangiectasia confers hypersensitivity to ionizing but not to UV irradiation.[132] A defect in repair of base damage has been detected in some but not all cases,[133] but it is not certain that this is responsible for the enhanced sensitivity.[134] The patients show an increased frequency of immune-system tumors. Surprisingly, however, the cells may well show reduced mutation with ionizing radiation (C. F. Arlett[191]). Less surprisingly, UV mutagenesis is normal. It is possible that in mammalian cells, unlike bacteria, ionizing radiation may be predominantly a deletion mutagen. Ataxia telangiectasia cells could conceivably be deficient in a specific error-prone repair pathway that generates small deletions.[25] This pathway would represent too small a fraction of repair to be detected by existing biochemical techniques.[134]

C. O⁶ Akylation of Guanine

A large volume of work has followed the initial suggestion by Loveless[20] that the discrepancies in mutagenicity between simple alkylating agents might be accounted for by the ability of the agents to alkylate the O⁶-position of guanine. O⁶-alkylguanine would probably be expected to pair with both thymine and cytosine. Drake and Greening[135] have shown that antimutator strains of bacteriophage T4 show reduced mutability by the classic O⁶- alkylating agent Ethyl methane sulfonate (EMS), suggesting that slight discrimination of the polymerase in favor of cytosine may be possible.

There is now considerable evidence linking O⁶ alkylation of guanine with mutagenesis and carcinogenesis. First, comparison of agents which alkylate the O⁶ position of guanine with different efficiencies in general shows a fair correlation with both mutagenicity and carcinogenicity.[136,137] Second, a negative correlation exists between efficient removal of O⁶ alkylations and the site of tumor formation.[138] In opposition to this, it has been argued that agents which O⁶ alkylate guanine, such as EMS, are likely to be weak carcinogens,[139] and that agents which induce error-prone repair, such as UV, will be more effective carcinogens. In the case of EMS, it is quite possible that its carcinogenicity is not low when related to its low chemical reactivity.

Agents which cause O⁶ alkylation of guanine can be recognized by their ability to mutate recA and lexA strains of E. coli. In this way, inferential evidence can be obtained that unexpected compounds, such as nitrofurazone[140] (a nitrofuran) and nitrogen mustard (Table 3) may prove to O⁶ alkylate guanine. Although SN1-type agents with a low Swain-Scott factor are considered to be more likely to O⁶ alkylate guanine, the studies with bacteria may suggest that it is agents intermediate between SN1 and SN2 that are most specific in causing mutation by O⁶ alkylation. Agents with an extreme SN1 type mechanism may induce other lesions which are subject to error-prone repair.

Despite the subtlety of the modification in O⁶ alkylation, it is evident that the alkylated bases are subject to efficient excision repair. Lawley and Orr[141] showed specific excision of O^6-methyl guanine following treatment with N-methyl-N'nitro-N-nitroso-guanidine. There is recent evidence that this type of excision may be inducible.[47] Bulk-ier O^6 alkylations may be recognized by *uvr* endonuclease. O^6-ethylguanine seems mar-ginal in this respect,[136] but the lesions caused by volatile breakdown product of captan (possibly thiophosgene)[43] and sulfur half-mustard[44] appear to be readily *uvr* excisable, and to induce *lexA* independent mutations. Interestingly, O^6 alkylation of guanine is probably often not responsible for lethality,[43,136] this is particularly evident with sulfur half-mustard, where the lethal lesion is not uvr excisable, whereas the mutagenic lesion is.[44]

In mammalian cells, O^6 alkylation of guanine may be less important for in vitro mutagenesis, especially at high doses, since there is evidence at some loci that plots of mutation against survival for a number of mutagens, including N-methyl-N'-nitro-N-nitrosoguanidine and non-O^6 alkylating agents coincide.[142] This implies a role for po-tentially lethal damage in high dose mutagenesis. However, at low doses and other loci, O^6 alkylation of guanine might well be of greater significance.

A novel human mutant, diagnosed as light sensitive, shows increased killing by both UV and ethyl methanesulfonate.[143] Unlike xeroderma and xeroderma variants, which are ethyl methanesulfonate-resistant, no biochemical defect has been revealed to date. The cells show enhanced UV mutability (C. F. Arlett[191]) but ethyl methanesulfonate mutability has not yet been determined.

D. Other Base Modifications and Base Analogue Mutagenesis

Of the variety of possibilities, O^4-thymine is probably analogous to O^6-alkylguanine and might be expected to mispair. There is no evidence at present as to whether or not it contributes to overall mutagenesis. The proofreading function (3' to 5' exonuclease activity) of DNA polymerases and mismatch correction should tend to eliminate mis-coding through formation of unusual tautomeric forms of alkylated bases.

Another type of mutagenesis which will be strongly antagonized by repair is deami-nation of cytosine to form uracil. This will occur spontaneously and is induced by agents such as nitrous acid. However, the efficient removal of uracil by an N-glycosi-dase will greatly reduce the significance of this type of mutagenesis. One situation where such mutations will arise is where cytosine has been enzymically methylated to 5 methylcytosine. At these particular sites, deamination will lead directly to formation of thymine and such sites are indeed mutation hotspots.[195]

One of the arguments sometimes raised against the relevance of somatic mutation to cancer is that base analogues such as 5-bromouracil and 2-aminopurine are noncar-cinogenic, whereas they are potent mutagens. In fact, 5-bromouracil could never be considered a potent mutagen despite its efficient incorporation into DNA. Presumably it causes mutation by its higher frequency of change to the wrong tautomer. As already discussed, extremely efficient correction systems exist in *E. coli* to prevent errors from this type of effect and, in an elegant study, Rydberg[145] has shown that 5-bromouracil is only mutagenic to *E. coli* when greater than 10% overall substitution of bromouracil for thymine in the DNA has occurred. Presumably there is saturation of mismatch correction at these very high levels of substitution.

In contrast to 5-bromouracil, low concentrations of 2 aminopurine and 2,6-diami-nopurine are mutagenic to bacteria. The likeliest implication is that mispairings by these bases are for some reason not recognized as mismatches in *E. coli*, possibly be-cause they are ambiguous. 2-Aminopurine mutagenesis, however, does appear subject to correction by the 3' to 5' exonuclease activity of bacteriophage T4 polymerase.[146]

In the cases of deaminating agents, and base analogues, where some discrepancy is thought to exist between mutagenicity to bacteria and carcinogenicity to animals, it must be emphasized that extremely efficient repair processes may be in operation. If a

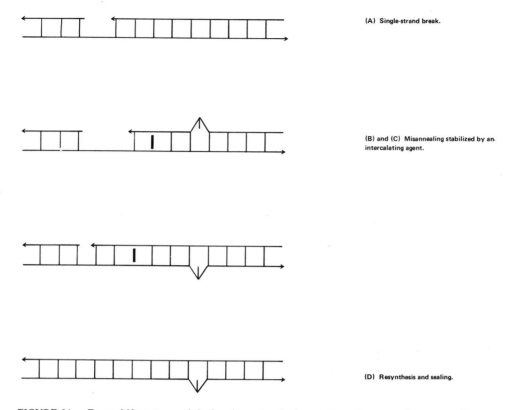

(A) Single-strand break.

(B) and (C) Misannealing stabilized by an intercalating agent.

(D) Resynthesis and sealing.

FIGURE 6A. Frameshift mutagenesis by looping out and misannealing of a repeated sequence of bases during excision type repair. (After Streisinger, G., Okada, Y., Emrich, J., Newton, J., Tsugita, A., Tarzaghi, E., and Inouye, M., Cold Spring Harbor Symp. Avant. Biol., 31, 77, 1966.)

discrepancy is eventually established, it will have to be between mutation in appropriate mammalian cells and carcinogenicity. The author is not aware of data on the mutagenicity of nitrous acid, 5-bromouracil, or 2-aminopurine or cultured mammalian cells.

E. Frameshift Mutagenesis

One of the puzzling features of frameshift mutagenesis is that two quite different types of agent appear to be specific frameshift mutagens in bacterial mutation tests. On the one hand, there are classical intercalating agents such as acridines. These agents are often weakly mutagenic even in the absence of covalent binding to the DNA.[147] They are likely to cause little distortion of the DNA, apart from an effect on supercoiling. In addition to this type of agent, many carcinogenic polycyclic hydrocarbons and aromatic amines are frameshift mutagens, but do not appear to be detectably mutagenic unless they bind covalently to DNA. As described in Volume II, Chapter 3, the covalent binding is likely to produce a lesion causing far greater distortion of the DNA than, for instance, a pyrimidine dimer.[148]

In fact, three types of mechanism for frameshift mutageneis have been proposed. Streisinger et al.[149] have suggested that frameshift mutations may arise through looping out of one or more bases in a repetitive sequence during DNA repair (Figure 6A). A difficulty with the model is that it would predict that a capacity to perform excision repair would be necessary to obtain frameshift mutagenesis, whereas frameshift mutation is greatly enhanced in the absence of excision repair.[150] The second suggestion is that frameshift mutations arise during recombination,[151,152] presumably when repet-

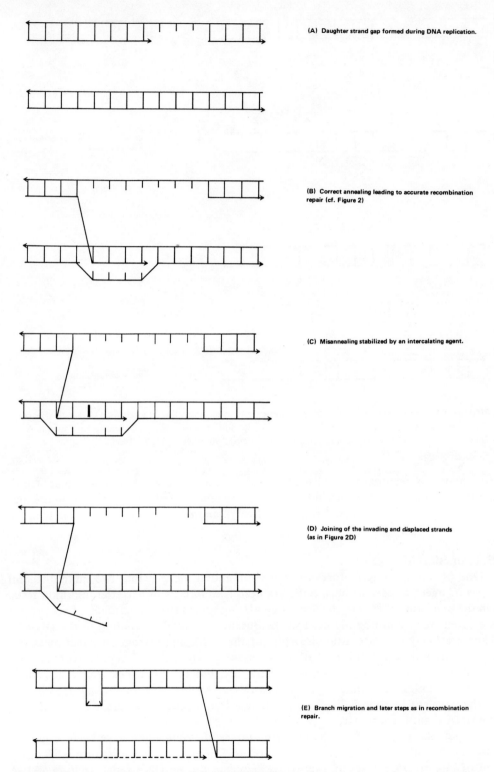

(A) Daughter strand gap formed during DNA replication.

(B) Correct annealing leading to accurate recombination repair (cf. Figure 2)

(C) Misannealing stabilized by an intercalating agent.

(D) Joining of the invading and displaced strands (as in Figure 2D)

(E) Branch migration and later steps as in recombination repair.

FIGURE 6B.   Frameshift mutation during recombination or recombination repair at a repeated sequence of bases.

itive sequences become incorrectly aligned (Figure 6B). This mechanism is more consistent with mutagenesis by intercalating agents, since they might be expected to make it more difficult for the incorrectly aligned bases to slip into the correct configuration.

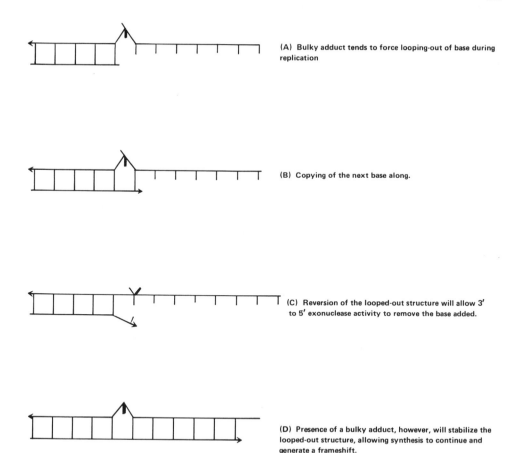

(A) Bulky adduct tends to force looping-out of base during replication

(B) Copying of the next base along.

(C) Reversion of the looped-out structure will allow 3' to 5' exonuclease activity to remove the base added.

(D) Presence of a bulky adduct, however, will stabilize the looped-out structure, allowing synthesis to continue and generate a frameshift.

FIGURE 6C. A model of frameshift mutation by bulky carcinogens in which adducts stabilize the looped-out configuration of bases during DNA polymerization and prevent error-correction by proofreading (3' to 5') exonuclease activity. (After Weinstein, I. B. and Grunberger, O., *Chemical Carcinogens,* T'so, P. O. P. and DiPaolo, A. J., Eds., Marcel Dekker, New York, 1974, 217.)

(In addition, by reducing supercoiling, they might shorten the potential recognition sequence).[57]

Although the suggestion of frameshift mutations arising through incorrect alignment of bases during recombination is probably the most satisfactory explanation for mutagenesis by intercalating agents such as acridines, neither this model, nor the Streisinger model provides a satisfactory explanation for mutagenesis by polycyclic hydrocarbons or aromatic amines. The most plausible model for this type of agent has been proposed by Weinstein and Grunberger[153] and is described in detail in Volume II, Chapter 3. They suggest that polycyclic hydrocarbons and aromatic amines produce frameshift mutations by increasing the probability of bases looping out during DNA replication (Figure 6C) (rather than during DNA repair as in the Streisinger model). Although an analogous mechanism has been proposed for spontaneous mutation,[154] it is possible that this type of frameshift mutation will be a very rare spontaneous event, because the looped out structure will revert and proofreading 3' to 5' exonuclease acitivity of polymerase will remove the incorrect base. However, the presence of a bulky adduct may stabilize the looped out structure and prevent proofreading from occurring. This model explains a number of observations:

1. Other base substitution mutagens such as UV would be expected to (and do) induce a detectable frequency of frameshift mutations.
2. Despite 8-methoxypsoralen being a classic intercalating agent, when covalently bound to DNA, it can act as a base substitution mutagen.[117] Presumably it does not distort the DNA sufficiently to enforce looping out.
3. Although polycyclic carcinogens are not necessarily planar, only those within a fairly well defined size range are active. Presumably only these molecules, when covalently bound can produce and maintain a configuration that enables premature replication of an adjacent base.
4. The enhancement of induced, but not of spontaneous, frameshift mutation by a plasmid such as pKM101[70,155] can be explained if looping out frameshifts are not normally generated spontaneously. On the other hand, since induced frameshift mutagenesis is enhanced, the model proposed here indicates a direct effect of the plasmid on the polymermase complex.

Two specific predictions of the model can be made. First, the process should be able to occur in the absence of error-prone repair in *lexA* and *recA* strains, although the effect might be smaller because of reduced repair. Second, the mechanism would preferentially generate deletions since, except immediately after treatment, the forced looping out process would have to occur in the parental strand.

This second prediction has in fact been tested, and Isono and Yourno[156] have in fact shown that certain polycyclic carcinogens specifically generate 2-base deletions. In contrast, a classic intercalating mutagen, ICR-191, generates a variety of frameshift types.*

A final point is that if this type of mechanism does operate, polycyclic hydrocarbons and aromatic amines will not necessarily be frameshift mutagens under all conditions. A number operate as base substitution mutagens in the presence of a plasmid,[70] and benzo [a] pyrene induces mutations to ouabain resistance in mammalian cells,[157] suggesting induction of base substitutions.

If intercalating agents do not induce frameshift mutation by looping out (Figure 6C) but by promoting errors during recombination (Figure 6B), the existence of two distinct mechanisms of frameshift mutagenesis may help to explain discrepancies in carcinogenicity between, on the one hand, polycyclic hydrocarbons and aromatic amines and, on the other hand, classical intercalating agents. Where different mechanisms of mutation operate, different mechanisms for error-correction will also be found. It could easily be that mammalian cells cope rather more readily than bacteria with intercalating agents, but rather less well with bulky adducts.

F. Deletion Mutagenesis

Very little is known about the mechanism of deletion mutagenesis, least of all by the author. At least three types of mechanism are possible and it is likely that more than one is involved.

The simplest mechanism would be loss of a section of chromosome by an illegitimate

---

* This observation raises a problem since one would predict that polycyclic and aromatic amine carcinogens would be relatively nonspecific in their site of action, whereas intercalating agents would only cause mutation at repetitive sequences. In fact mutagenesis by polycyclic and aromatic amine carcinogens appears even more sequence specific.[156] An explanation may come from the work of Glickman,[193] implicating a number of mutator genes in the process of mismatch correction (see Sections II.B. and II.D.). These mutator genes considerably increase the frequency of frameshift as well as base substitution mutation. The implication is that mismatch correction will normally prevent looping out frameshift mutagenesis with high efficiency. Mutations will therefore only occur at sites where for some reason mismatch correction does not occur with normal efficiency. Presumably the repetitive GC sequence in the Ames strains TA1538 and TA98 is such a site.

recombination event with itself. Such a mechanism, the Campbell model,[158] can be invoked to explain the formation of F primes (F factors containing chromosomal bacterial genes) and specialized transducing particles (bacteriophage particles which include bacterial genes). It can, however, hardly be general, since deletion mutagenesis occurs apparently normally in recombination deficient bacteria.[159]

The second possibility is that deletion mutations are generated by the unknown mechanisms involved in transposition of insertion sequences, and there is indeed some evidence for deletion associated with such sequences.[24] Again, although such a mechanism would be recA⁺ independent, it would mean that deletions were likely to occur at specific sites. This is certainly true in some cases,[160] but it is uncertain whether it is general.

A final simple and attractive mechanism for deletion mutagenesis would be random ligase activity joining free ends of DNA. There is evidence that ligase can act in this way with a low efficiency. Obviously if it did so with high efficiency the DNA would get tied in knots. Two items of circumstantial evidence are consistent with this model. First, mutants deficient in DNA polymerase 1 may show an excess frequency of deletion mutation.[161] Such mutants will have abnormally high numbers of free DNA ends because of the slow filling of Okazaki and repair gaps. Second, following UV irradiation, shorter deletions seem to be generated.[162] This would be consistent with free ends being generated on average closer to each other.

Whether more than one, or none, of the mechanisms suggested will operate is unresolved. Nor is it clear the extent to which any of these mechanisms might operate in mammalian cells, where deletion mutagenesis may be of much greater importance.

VI. CONCLUDING REMARKS

A. The Relevance of Bacterial Mutation to Cancer

In recent years, bacterial mutation tests have gained widespread acceptance as short-term methods for detecting potential carcinogens.[8,9] Not only are bacterial tests reasonably good, but it must be remembered that the classical approaches of experimental carcinogenesis and epidemiology are far from perfect methods of predicting human carcinogenicity.

Nevertheless, the arrival of effective short-term tests to predict carcinogenicity has led to a degree of cultural shock and difficulty in making best use of the data. For instance, it is not practical in terms of time and expense to repeat a properly constituted carcinogenesis experiment and the answer obtained is regarded as definitive. In contrast, bacterial tests by their nature should always be repeated, and judgments made on the basis of consistent results in several independent experiments. To do otherwise simply leads to wrong decisions.

Again, the ease of short-term tests enables existing results to be challenged with bewildering rapidity, creating alarm and confusion. One solution has been to accept the value of short-term tests for commercial products under development, but not for agents already present in our environment. (Although it is hard to see why the two types of agent should be thought to give rise to positive results by different mechanisms.)

What has happened is that now there is access to an enormous amount of new information, and it is necessary to learn to make sensible use of it in monitoring our environment. To start with, it is suggested that when bacterial mutation tests give a positive result one should:

1. Require the test to be of a high standard
2. Expect confirmation in other short-term systems

3. Attempt to determine effective exposure in pharmacokinetic and similar studies
4. Not ban everything in sight but genuinely attempt to assess the possible risk and balance it against benefit and convenience

Eventually, we should end up with a more confusing, but more realistic assessment of environmental hazards. One suspects that it is unlikely that a carcinogen-free environment could be created, and if it could, one suspects that it might well not be fit to live in.

B. Correlation of Mutagenicity and Carcinogenicity

The success of bacterial mutagen screening has led to a number of attempts to show a quantitative relationship between carcinogenic potency and bacterial mutagenicity.[163] These studies show a good correlation between carcinogenicity and mutagenicity, with a range of 10^6 between the most and the least efficient agents in the molarity required to produce a given effect. The principle exceptions probably relate to metabolism; compounds such as simple alkyl halides, and simple nitrosamines, may be activated less effectively in vitro, and nitrofurans and nitroimidazoles are activated more readily by bacterial than mammalian enzymes. (This is probably why they are effective antibacterial agents, but it is likely that they are also activated to some extent by mammalian cells in vivo.)

Despite the value of quantitative correlations in persuading people to believe in bacterial tests, this author has reservations. Such correlations take no account of genetic endpoint, pattern of metabolism, or pharmacokinetic considerations. They may be rather long-winded methods of showing that the efficiency of reaction of a compound with DNA in carcinogenesis experiments is about the same as its efficiency of reaction with DNA in mutation experiments.

On the other hand, if the enormous dose range of carcinogenicity/mutagenicity plots simply reflected the extent of reaction of the agent with DNA, it would lead to the conclusion that, in terms of carcinogenicity and mutagenicity, all types of DNA damage are equal. This author suspects that some are considerably more equal than others. Mutations arise mainly through the failure of accurate DNA repair, and it is damage which for some particular reason escapes accurate repair that is most likely to cause mutation, just as it is reactive metabolites which for some reason are not detoxified which are most likely to react with DNA. It would be surprising if the weak links in bacterial and mammalian DNA repair were always the same.

C. Bacterial Mutation as a Research Tool

The rather complex picture of mutagenesis that has been drawn suggests a role for bacterial mutation tests which will prove of increasing value in the future. By testing for lethality and mutagenesis in a series of strains, it should be possible not merely to designate a chemical as potentially carcinogenic, but also to define rather closely the type of DNA damage that it causes. Obvious examples are the detection of O^6 alkylation of guanine by the use of *lexA* and *recA* strains of bacteria and recognition of cases (such as nitrogen mustard or sulfur half-mustard)[44] where the lethal and mutagenic lesions may differ. It may be possible to characterize the electrophilicity and stability of active metabolites of some carcinogens by their relative effects on the *S. typhimurium* strains TA98 and TA100, or on strains with and without the *rfa* (deep-rough) mutation.

In the future, I believe that with the use of repair-deficient human cell lines in conjunction with agents where different lesions produce different genetic endpoints and pairs of agents producing different ratios of lesions, it will prove possible to characterize rather precisely the types of genetic damage most likely to lead to mutation and cancer.

A critical prediction of the somatic mutation theory of cancer is that the two events should be induced by the same types of damage. However, even within the limited repertoire of available mammalian cell mutation systems, remarkable mutagen specificity exists (A. M. Rogers[192]). If cancer can indeed originate through a somatic mutation, it will be interesting to see whether it is an event resembling mutation to thioguanine resistance, ouabain resistance, excess thymidine resistance, or cytosine arabinoside resistance.

D. Somatic Mutation and Cancer

It must be emphasized that the remarkable correlation found between mutagenicity and carcinogenicity does not in itself prove the somatic mutation theory of cancer, although more direct attempts at proof have been made[164] with some success. The author suspects, however, that within the next few years, it will be possible to establish fairly convincingly that chemical carcinogens induce cancer by reacting with DNA and causing mutation-like genetic changes. It is also suspected that such information will be of singularly little use without a knowledge of the processes that lead to somatic mutations becoming expressed. The two-stage model of chemical carcinogenesis, where initiation involves a mutation-like event, and promotion involves expression of the altered genotype, is an obvious approach to the problem.

A point perhaps worth making is that in *E. coli,* gene expression should only depend on an opportunity for dilution of preexisting gene product and an appropriate environment. In somatic mammalian cells, there may be an additional level of heritable control, if certain sets of genes may become locked off or locked on during early development. The interaction between a somatic mutation and a heritable control system which prevented its expression might lead to considerable complexity. Heritable control systems can, for instance, be subject to effects such as pseudomutation. (There is even a recondite example of this in *E. coli.*)[165] It is not certain that it is necessary to consider epigenetic effects and somatic mutation as mutually exclusive mechanisms in carcinogenesis, rather than as sequential steps with one or the other being rate-limiting in different model systems.

Acknowledgments

I would like to thank Dr. A. R. Lehmann, Professor B. A. Bridges, Dr. C. F. Arlett, Mr. D. McGarva, Dr. D. J. Sherratt, and Professor N. Symonds, all of whom I have continually pestered for information and in addition, Dr. L. J. Gudas and Dr. E. M. Witkin for permission to reproduce material and Dr. R. Devoret and Dr. M. Radman, for permission to quote material prior to publication. Miss W. J. Muriel performed the experiments described in Section V.A.

REFERENCES

1. **Boveri, T.,** *The Origin of Malignant Tumors,* Williams and Wilkins, Baltimore, 1929.
2. **Wolf, U.,** Theodor Boveri and his book "On the problem of the origin of malignant tumors", in *Chromosomes and Cancer,* German, J., Ed., John Wiley & Sons, New York, 1974, 3.
3. **Heidelberger, C.,** Chemical carcinogenesis, *Annu. Rev. Biochem.,* 44, 79, 1975.
4. **Maher, V. M., Curren, R. D., Ouellette, L. M., and McCormick, J. J.,** Role of DNA repair in the cytotoxic and mutagenic action of physical and chemical carcinogens, in *In Vitro Metabolic Activation in Mutagenesis Testing,* de Serres, F. J., Fouts, J. R., Bend, J. R., and Philpot, R. M., Eds., North-Holland, Amsterdam, 1976, 313.

5. **Malling, H. V.,** Dimethylnitrosamine; formation of mutagenic compounds by interaction with mouse liver microsomes, *Mutat. Res.,* 13, 425, 1971.

6. **Ames, B. N., Durston, W. E., Yamamasaki, E., and Lee, F. D.,** Carcinogens are mutagens: a simple test system combining liver homogenates for activation and bacteria for detection, *Proc. Natl. Acad. Sci. U.S.A.,* 70, 2281, 1973.

7. **Ames, B. N., McCann, J., and Yamasaki, E.,** Methods for detecting carcinogens and mutagens with the *Salmonella*/mammalian microsome mutagenicity test, *Mutat. Res.,* 31, 347, 1975.

8. **McCann, J., Choi, E., Yamasaki, E., and Ames, B. N.,** Detection of carcinogens as mutagens in the *Salmonella*/microsome test. Assay of 300 chemicals, *Proc. Natl. Acad. Sci. U.S.A.,* 72, 5135, 1975.

9. **McCann, J. and Ames, B. N.,** Detection of carcinogens as mutagens in the *Salmonella*/microsome test: assay of 300 chemicals: discussion, *Proc. Natl. Acad. Sci. U.S.A.,* 73, 950, 1976.

10. **Witkin, E. M.,** Ultraviolet mutagenesis and inducible DNA repair in *Escherichia coli, Bacteriol. Rev.,* 40, 869, 1976.

11. **Drake, J. W. and Baltz, R. H.,** The biochemistry of mutagenesis, *Annu. Rev. Biochem.,* 45, 11, 1976.

12. **Lehmann, A. R. and Bridges, B. A.,** DNA repair, *Essays Biochem.,* 13, 71, 1977.

13. **Doudney, C. O.,** Mutation in ultraviolet-light damaged microorganisms, in *Photochemistry and Photobiology of Nucleic Acids,* Vol. 2, Wang, S. Y., Ed., Academic Press, New York, 1976, 309.

14. **Strauss, B. S.,** Repair of DNA adducts produced by alkylation, in *Ageing, Carcinogenesis and Radiation Biology,* Smith, K. C., Ed., Plenum Press, New York, 1976, 287.

15. **Roberts, J. J.,** DNA repair and carcinogenesis, in *Scientific Foundations of Oncology,* Symington, T. S. and Carter, R. L., Eds., Heinemann, London, 1976, 319.

16. **Grossman, L., Braun, A., Feldberg, R., and Mahler, I.,** Enzymatic repair of DNA, *Annu. Rev. Biochem.,* 44, 19, 1975.

17. **Grossman, L.,** Enzymatic mechanisms capable of repairing damaged DNA, *Colloq. Int. CNRS,* 256, 129, 1977.

18. **Freidberg, E. C., Cook, K. H., Duncan, J., and Mortelmans, K.,** DNA repair enzymes in mammalian cells, *Adv. Radiat. Biol.,* 8, 1977, in press.

19. **Swenson, P. A.,** Physiological responses of *Escherichia coli* to far-ultraviolet irradiation, *Photochem. Photobiol. Rev.,* 269, 1976.

20. **Loveless, A.,** Possible relevance of 0-6 alkylation of deoxyguanosine to mutagenicity and carcinogenicity of nitrosamines and nitrosamides, *Nature (London),* 223, 206, 1969.

21. **Kondo, S.,** Evidence that mutations are induced by errors in repair and replication, *Genetics,* 73, 109, 1973.

22. **Sirover, M. A. and Loeb, L. A.,** Infidelity of DNA synthesis *in vitro:* screening for potential metal mutagens or carcinogens, *Science,* 194, 1434, 1976.

23. **Witkin, E. M.,** Mutation-proof and mutation-prone modes of survival in derivatives of *Escherichia coli* B differing in sensitivity to ultraviolet light, *Brookhaven Symp. Biol.,* 20, 17, 1967.

24. **Nevers, P. and Saedler, H.,** Transposable genetic elements as agents of gene instability and chromosomal rearrangements, *Nature (London),* 268, 109, 1977.

25. **Arlett, C. F., Turnbull, D., Harcourt, S. A., Lehmann, A. R., and Colella, C. M.,** A comparison of the 8-azaguanine and ouabain-resistance systems for the selection of induced mutant Chinese hamster cells, *Mutat. Res.,* 33, 261, 1975.

26. **Bridges, B. A., Dennis, R. E., and Munson, R. J.,** Mutation in *Escherichia coli* B/r WP2 try⁻ by reversion or suppression of a chain terminating codon, *Mutat. Res.,* 4, 502, 1967.

27. **Alberts, B. and Sternglanz, R.,** Recent excitement in the DNA replication problem, *Nature (London),* 269, 655, 1977.

28. **Hall, R. M. and Brammar, W. J.,** Increased spontaneous mutation rates in mutants of *E. coli* with altered DNA polymerase III, *Mol. Gen. Genet.,* 121, 271, 1973.

29. **Cox, E. C.,** Bacterial mutator genes and the control of spontaneous mutation, *Annu. Rev. Genetics,* 10, 135, 1976.

30. **Wickner, S. and Hurwitz, J.,** Conversion of φX 174 viral DNA to double-stranded form by purified *Escherichia coli* proteins, *Proc. Natl. Acad. Sci. U.S.A.,* 71, 4120, 1974.

31. **Loeb, L. A.,** Eucaryotic DNA polymerases, *Enzyme,* 10, 173, 1974.

32. **Radman, M., Spadari, S., and Villani, G.,** UV carcinogenesis, *J. Natl. Cancer Inst.,* 1977, in press.

33. **Muzyczka, N., Poland, R. L., and Bessman, M. J.,** Studies on the biochemical basis of spontaneous mutation. I. A comparison of the deoxyribonucleic acid polymerases of mutator, antimutator and wild-type strains of bacteriophage T4, *J. Biol. Chem.,* 247, 7116, 1972.

34. **Bessman, M. J., Muzyczka, N., Goodman, M. F., and Schnaar, R. L.,** Studies on the biochemical basis of spontaneous mutation. II. The incorporation of a base and its analogue into DNA by wild-type, mutator and antimutator DNA polymerases, *J. Mol. Biol.,* 88, 409, 1974.

35. Nevers, P. and Spatz, H.-C., *Escherichia coli* mutants *uvrD* and *uvrE* deficient in gene conversion of λ heteroduplexes, *Mol. Gen. Genet.*, 139, 233, 1975.

36. Lawley, P. D., Crathorn, A. R., Shah, S. A., and Smith, B. A., Biomethylation of deoxyribonucleic acid in cultured human tumor cells (HeLa). Methylated bases other than 5-methylcytosine not detected, *Biochem. J.*, 128, 133, 1972.

37. Marinus, M. G. and Morris, N. R., Pleiotropic effects of a DNA adenine methylation mutant (*dam-3*) in *Escherichia coli*, *Mutat. Res.*, 28, 15, 1975.

38. Setlow, R. and Setlow, J. K., Effects of radiation on polynucleotides, *Annu. Rev. Biophys. Bioeng.*, 1, 293, 1972.

39. Clark, A. J. and Ganesan, A., Lists of genes affecting DNA metabolism in *Escherichia coli*, in *Molecular Mechanisms for Repair of DNA*, Hanawalt, P. C. and Setlow, R. B., Eds., Plenum Press, New York, 1974, 431.

40. Harm, W., Rupert, C. S., and Harm, H., The study of photoenzymatic repair of UV lesions in DNA by flash photolysis, in *Photophysiology*, Vol. 6, Giese, A. C., Ed., Academic Press, New York, 1970, 279.

41. Hart, R. W. and Setlow, R. B., Direct evidence that pyrimidine dimers in DNA result in neoplastic transformation, in *Molecular Mechanisms for Repair of DNA*, Hanawalt, P. C. and Setlow, R. B., Eds., Plenum Press, New York, 1975, 719.

42. Seeberg, E. and Strike, P., Excision repair of ultraviolet-irradiated deoxyribonucleic acid in plasmolysed cells of *Escherichia coli*, *J. Bacteriol.*, 125, 787, 1976.

43. Bridges, B. A., Mottershead, R. P., Rothwell, M. A., and Green, M. H. L., Repair-deficient bacterial strains suitable for mutagenicity screening: tests with the fungicide captan, *Chem. Biol. Interact.*, 5, 77, 1972.

44. Gilbert, R. M., Rowland, S., Davison, C. L., and Papirmeister, B., Involvement of separate pathways in the repair of mutational and lethal lesions induced by a monofunctional sulfur mustard, *Mutat. Res.*, 28, 257, 1975.

45. Cooper, P. K. and Hanawalt, P. C., Role of DNA polymerase I and the *rec* system in excision-repair in *Escherichia coli*, *Proc. Natl. Acad. Sci.*, U.S.A., 69, 1156, 1972.

46. Cooper, P. K. and Hanawalt, P. C., Heterogeneity of patch size in repair replicated DNA in *Escherichia coli*, *J. Mol. Biol.*, 67, 1, 1972.

47. Samson, L. and Cairns, J., A new pathway for DNA repair in *Escherichia coli*, *Nature (London)*, 267, 281, 1977.

48. Ahmed, F. E. and Setlow, R. B., Different rate-limiting steps in excision repair of ultraviolet and *N*-acetoxy-2-acetyl-aminofluorene-damaged DNA in normal human fibroblasts, *Proc. Natl. Acad. Sci. U.S.A.*, 74, 1548, 1977.

49. Amacher, D. E., Elliott, J. A., and Lieberman, M. W., Differences in removal of acetylamino-fluorene and pyrimidine dimers from the DNA of cultured mammalian cells, *Proc. Natl. Acad. Sci. U. S. A.*, 74, 1553, 1972.

50. Rupp, W. D. and Howard-Flanders, P., Discontinuities in the DNA synthesized in an excision-defective strain of *Escherichia coli* following ultraviolet irradiation, *J. Mol. Biol.*, 31, 291, 1968.

51. Rupp, W. D., Wilde, C. E., III, Reno, D. L., and Howard-Flanders, P., Exchanges between DNA strands in ultraviolet-irradiated *Escherichia coli*, *J. Mol. Biol.*, 61, 25, 1971.

52. Bridges, B. A., Dennis, R. E., and Munson, R. J., Differential induction and repair of ultraviolet damage leading to true reversions and external suppressor mutations of an ochre codon in *Escherichia coli*B/r WP2, *Genetics*, 57, 897, 1967.

53. Blanco, M. and Devoret, R., Repair mechanisms involved in prophage reactivation and UV reactivation of UV-irradiated phage λ, *Mutat. Res.*, 17, 293, 1973.

54. Eyfjord, J. E., Green, M. H. L., and Bridges, B. A., Mutagenic DNA repair in *Escherichia coli*: Conditions for error-free filling of daughter strand gaps, *J. Gen. Microbiol.*, 91, 369, 1975.

55. Lehmann, A. R., Postreplication repair of DNA in mammalian cells, *Life Sci.*, 15, 2005, 1974.

56. Wilkins, B. M. and Howard-Flanders, P., The genetic properties of DNA transferred from ultravi-

57. Holloman, W. K. and Radding, C. M., Recombination promoted by superhelical DNA and the recA gene of *Escherichia coli*, *Proc. Natl. Acad. Sci. U.S.A.*, 73, 3910, 1976.

58. Weigle, J. J., Induction of mutations in a bacterial virus, *Proc. Natl. Acad. Sci. U.S.A.*, 39, 628, 1953.

59. Weigle, J. J. and Dulbecco, R., Induction of mutations in bacteriophage T3 by ultraviolet light, *Experientia*, 9, 372, 1953.

60. Defais, M., Fauquet, P., Radman, M., and Errera, M., Ultraviolet reactivation and ultraviolet mutagenesis of λ in different genetic systems, *Virology*, 43, 495, 1971.

61. Radman, M., SOS repair: an inducible mutagenic DNA repair, in *Molecular Mechanisms for the Repair of DNA*, Hanawalt, P. C. and Setlow, R. B., Eds., Plenum Press, New York, 1975, 355.

62. Bridges, B. A. and Mottershead, R. P., RecA⁺-dependent mutagenesis occurring before DNA replication in UV and γ-irradiated *Escherichia coli*, *Mutat. Res.*, 13, 1, 1971.

63. Bridges, B. A. and Sedgwick, S. G., Effect of photoreactivation on the filling of gaps in deoxyribonucleic acid synthesized after exposure of *Escherichia coli* to ultraviolet light, *J. Bacteriol.,* 117, 1077, 1974.

64. Kato, T., Rothman, R. H., and Clark, A. J., Analysis of the role of recombination and repair in mutagenesis of *Escherichia coli* by UV irradiation, *Genetics,* 1977, in press.

65. Green, M. H. L., On the possible immunity of newly-synthesized DNA to error-prone repair, *Mutat. Res.,* 44, 161, 1977.

66. Bridges, B. A. and Mottershead, R. P., Mutagenic DNA repair in *Escherichia coli* VII Constitutive and inducible manifestations, 1977, in preparation.

67. Devoret, R., Mechanisms involved in the recovery of phage λ from ultraviolet damage, in *Molecular Mechanisms for the Repair of DNA,* Hanawalt, P. C. and Setlow, R. B., Eds., Plenum Press, New York, 1975, 155.

68. Witkin, E. M., Thermal enhancement of ultraviolet mutability in a *tif-1 uvrA* derivative of *Escherichia coli* B/r: evidence that ultraviolet mutagenesis depends on an inducible function, *Proc. Natl. Acad. Sci. U.S.A.,* 71, 1930, 1976.

69. Walker, G. C., Plasmid (pKM101)-mediated enhancement of repair and mutagenesis: dependence on chromosomal genes in *Escherichia Coli* K-12, *Mol. Gen. Genet.,* 152, 93, 1977.

70. McCann, J., Spingarn, N. E., Kobori, J., and Ames, B. N., Detection of carcinogens as mutagens: bacterial tester strains with R factor plasmids, *Proc. Natl. Acad. Sci. U.S.A.,* 72, 979, 1975.

71. MacPhee, D. G., *Salmonella typhimurium his* G46 (R-Utrecht) - possible use in screening mutagens and carcinogens, *Appl. Microbiol.,* 26, 1004, 1973.

72. Witkin, E. M., Post-irradiation metabolism and the timing of ultraviolet-induced mutations in bacteria, *Proc. 10th Int. Congr. of Genetics, Montreal,* Vol. 1, 280, 1958.

73. Bridges, B. A., A note on the mechanism of UV mutagenesis in *Escherichia coli, Mutat. Res.,* 3, 273, 1966.

74. Sedgwick, S. G., Genetic and kinetic evidence for different types of post-replication repair in *Escherichia coli* B, *J. Bacteriol.,* 123, 154, 1975.

75. Sedgwick, S. G., Misrepair of overlapping daughter strand gaps as a possible mechanism for UV-induced mutagenesis in *uvr* strains of *Escherichia coli:* a general model for induced mutagenesis by misrepair (SOS repair) of closely spaced DNA lesions, *Mutat. Res.,* 41, 185, 1976.

76. Doubleday, O. P., Bridges, B. A., and Green, M. H. L., Mutagenic DNA repair in *Escherichia coli.* II. Factors affecting loss of photoreversibility of UV-induced mutations, *Mol. Gen. Genet.,* 140, 221, 1975.

77. Green, M. H. L., Bridges, B. A., Eyfjörd, J. E., and Muriel, W. J., An error-free excision-dependent mode of post-replication repair in *Escherichia coli, Colloq. Int. CNRS,* 256, 227, 1976.

78. Mount, D. W., Walker, A. C., and Kosel, C., Effect of *tsl* mutations in decreasing radiation sensitivity of a *recA⁻* strain of *Escherichia coli* K-12, *J. Bacteriol.,* 121, 1203, 1975.

79. Green, M. H. L., Bridges, B. A., Eyfjörd, J. E., and Muriel, W. J., Mutagenic DNA repair in *Escherichia coli.* V. Mutation frequency decline and error-free post-replication repair in an excision-proficient strain, *Mutat. Res.,* 42, 33, 1977.

80. Billen, D., Replication of the bacterial chromosome: location of new initiation sites after irradiation, *J. Bacteriol.,* 97, 1169, 1969.

81. Kelner, A., Growth, respiration and nucleic acid synthesis in UV-irradiated and in photo-reactivated *Escherichia coli, J. Bacteriol.,* 65, 252, 1953.

82. McEntee, K., Hesse, J. E., and Epstein, W., Identification and radio-chemical purification of the *recA* protein of *Escherichia coli, Proc. Natl. Acad. Sci. U.S.A.,* 73, 3979, 1976.

83. Emmerson, P. T. and West, S. C., Identification of protein X of *Escherichia coli* as the *recA⁺/tif⁺* gene product, *Mol. Gen. Genet.,* 155, 77, 1977.

84. Inouye, M., Pleiotropic effect of the *recA* gene of *Escherichia coli:* uncoupling of cell division from deoxyribonucleic acid replication, *J. Bacteriol.,* 106, 531, 1971.

85. Gudas, L. J., The induction of protein X in DNA repair and cell division mutants of *Escherichia coli, J. Mol. Biol.,* 104, 567, 1976.

86. Roberts, J. W., Roberts, C. W., and Mount, D. W., Inactivation and proteolytic cleavage of phage λ repressor *in vitro* in an ATP dependent reaction, *Proc. Natl. Acad. Sci. U.S.A.,* 74, 2283, 1977.

87. Roberts, J. W., *Proc. Society General Microbiol., September, 1977.*

88. Mount, D. W., A mutant of *Escherichia coli* showing constitutive expression of lysogenic induction and error-prone DNA repair pathways, *Proc. Natl. Acad. Sci. U.S.A.,* 74, 300, 1977.

89. Meyn, M. S., Rossman, T., and Troll, W., A protease inhibitor blocks SOS functions in *Escherichia coli:* antipain prevents λ repressor inactivation, ultraviolet mutagenesis, and filamentous growth, *Proc. Natl. Acad. Sci. U.S.A.,* 74, 1152, 1977.

90. Mount, D. W., Low, K. B., and Edmiston, S. J., Dominant mutations (*lex*) in *Escherichia coli* which affect radiation sensitivity and frequency of ultraviolet-light induced mutation, *J. Bacteriol.,* 112, 886, 1972.

91. Gudas, L. J. and Pardee, A. B., Model for regulation of *Escherichia coli* DNA repair functions, *Proc. Natl. Acad. Sci. U.S.A.*, 72, 2330, 1975.

92. Morand, P., Goze, A., and Devoret, R., Complementation pattern of *lexB* and *recA* mutations in *Escherichia coli* K-12, mapping of *tif-1*, *lexB* and *recA* mutations, *Mol. Gen. Genet.*, in press, 1977.

93. Gudas, L. J. and Pardee, A. B., DNA synthesis inhibition and induction of protein X in *Escherichia coli*, *J. Mol. Biol.*, 101, 459, 1976.

94. Bridges, B. A., Mottershead, R. P., and Green, M. H. L., Cell division in *Escherichia coli* B$_{r-12}$ is hypersensitive to deoxyribonucleic acid damage by ultraviolet light, *J. Bacteriol.*, 130, 724, 1977.

95. Green. M. H. L., Gray, W. J. H., Sedgwick, S. G., and Bridges, B. A., Repair of DNA damage produced by gamma-radiation in *Escherichia coli* K-12 and a radiation sensitive *exrA* derivative during inhibition of protein synthesis and normal DNA replication by chloramphenicol, *J. Gen. Microbiol.*, 77, 99, 1973.

96. Donch, J. J., Green, M. H. L., and Greenberg, J., Conditional induction of λ prophage in *exrA* mutants of *Escherichia coli*, *Genet. Res.*, 17, 161, 1971.

97. Mount, D. W., Kosel, C. K., and Walker, A., Inducible error-prone DNA repair in *tsl recA* mutants of *E. coli*, *Mol. Gen. Genet.*, 146, 37, 1976.

98. Mount, D. W., Walker, A. C., and Kosel, C., Suppression of *lex* mutations affecting deoxyribonucleic acid repair in *Escherichia coli* K-12 by closely linked thermosensitive mutations, *J. Bacteriol.*, 116, 950, 1973.

99. Borek, E. and Ryan, A., The transfer of a biologically active radiation product from cell to cell, *Biochim. Biophys. Acta*, 41, 67, 1960.

100. Rosner, J. L., Kass, L. R., and Yarmolinsky, M. B., Parallel behaviour of F and P1 in causing indirect induction of lysogenic bacteria, *Cold Spring Harbor Symp. Quant. Biol.*, 33, 785, 1968.

101. Kerr, T. L. and Hart, M. G. R., Effects of the *recA lex* and *exrA* mutations on the survival of damaged λ and P1 phages in lysogenic and non-lysogenic strains of *Escherichia coli* K-12, *Mutat. Res.*, 18, 113, 1976.

102. George, J., Devoret, R., and Radman, M., Indirect ultraviolet reactivation of phage λ, *Proc. Natl. Acad. Sci. U.S.A.*, 71, 144, 1974.

103. Radman, M., On the mechanism and genetic control of mutation: an approach to carcinogenesis, *Colloq. Int. CNRS*, 256, 293, 1977.

104. Radman, M., Villani, G., Boiteux, S., Defais, M., Caillet-Fauquet, P., and Spadari, S., On the mechanism and genetic control of mutagenesis due to carcinogenic mutagens, in *Origins of Human Cancer*, Hiatt, H., Watson, J. D., and Winsten, J. A., Eds., Cold Spring Harbor Laboratory, 1977, in press.

105. Radman, M., Inducible pathways in deoxyribonucleic acid repair, mutagenesis and carcinogenesis, *Biochem. Soc. Trans.*, 5, 1194, 1977.

106. Bridges, B. A., Mottershead, R. P., and Sedgwick, S. G., Mutagenic DNA repair in *Escherichia coli*. III. Requirement for a function of DNA polymerase III in ultraviolet light mutagenesis, *Mol. Gen. Genet.*, 144, 53, 1976.

107. Radman, M., Caillet-Fauquet, P., Defais, M., and Villani, G., The molecular mechanism of induced mutations and an *in vitro* biochemical assay for mutagenesis, in *Screening Tests in Chemical Carcinogenesis*, Montesano, R., Bartsch, H., Tomatis, L., and Davis, W., Eds., I.A.R.C. Publication No. 12, International Agency for Research on Cancer, Lyon, France, 1976, 537.

108. McGarva, D., Lehmann, A. R., and Bridges, B. A., DNA dependent triphosphatase activity in cell-free extracts of *Escherichia coli*, its effect on DNA misincorporation assays, *Proc. Soc. Gen. Microbiol.*, 4, 134, 1977.

109. Byrnes, J. J., Downey, K. M., Que, B. G., Lee, M. Y. W., Black, V. L., and So, A. G., Selective inhibition of the 3′ to 5′ exonuclease activity associated with DNA polymerases, a mechanism of mutagenesis, *Biochemistry*, 16, 3740, 1977.

110. Geiduschek, E. P., "Reversible" DNA, *Proc. Natl. Acad. Sci. U.S.A.*, 47, 950, 1961.

111. Iyer, V. N. and Szybalski, W., A molecular mechanism of mitomycin action: linkage of complementary DNA strands, *Proc. Natl. Acad. Sci. U.S.A.*, 50, 355, 1964.

112. Cole, R. S., Light-induced cross-linking of DNA in the presence of furocumarin (psoralen): studies with phage λ, *Escherichia coli* and mouse leukaemia cells, *Biochim. Biophys. Acta*, 217, 30, 1970.

113. Mattocks, A. R., Toxicity and metabolism of Senecio alkaloids, in *Phytochemical Ecology*, Harbourne, J. B., Ed., Academic Press, London, 1972, 179.

114. Murayama, I. and Otsuji, N., Mutation by mitomycins in the ultraviolet light sensitive mutant of Escherichia coli, *Mutat. Res.*, 18, 117, 1973.

115. Ashwood-Smith, M. J., Grant, E. L., Heddle, J. A., and Friedman, G. B., Chromosome damage in Chinese hamster cells sensitized to near-ultraviolet light by psoralen and agelicin, *Mutat. Res.*, 43, 377, 1977.

116. Cole, R. S., Repair of DNA containing interstrand crosslinks in *Escherichia coli*: sequential excision and recombination, *Proc. Natl. Acad. Sci. U.S.A.*, 70, 1064, 1973.

117. **Igali, S., Bridges, B. A., Ashwood-Smith, M. J., and Scott, B. R.,** Mutagenesis in *Escherichia coli.* IV. Photosensitization to near ultraviolet light by 8-methoxypsoralen, *Mutat. Res.,* 9, 21, 1970.

118. **Green, M. H. L., Muriel, W. J., and Bridges, B. A.,** Use of a simplified fluctuation test to detect low levels of mutagens, *Mutat. Res.,* 38, 33, 1976.

119. **Green, M. H. L. and Muriel, W. J.,** Use of repair-deficient strains of *Escherichia coli* and liver microsomes to detect and characterize DNA damage caused by the pyrrolizidine alkaloids heliotrine and monocrotaline, *Mutat. Res.,* 28, 331, 1975.

120. **Wolff, S., Rodin, B., and Cleaver, J. E.,** Sister chromatid exchanges induced by mutagenic carcinogens in normal and xeroderma pigmentosum cells, *Nature (London),* 265, 347, 1977.

121. **Latt, S. A., Stetton, G., Juergens, L. A., Buchanan, G. R., and Gerald, P. S.,** Induction by alkylating agents of sister chromatid exchanges and chromatid breaks in Fanconi's anaemia, *Proc. Natl. Acad. Sci. U.S.A,,* 72, 4066, 1975.

122. **Town, C. D., Smith, K. C., and Kaplan, H. S.,** Repair of X-ray damage to bacterial DNA, *Curr. Top. Radiat. Res. Q.,* 8, 351, 1973.

123. **Bonura, T., Town, C. D., Smith, K. C., and Kaplan, H. S.,** The influence of oxygen on the yield of DNA double-strand breaks in X-irradiated *Escherichia coli* K-12, *Radiat. Res.,* 63, 567, 1975.

124. **Burrell, A. D., Feldschreiber, P., and Dean, C. J.,** DNA-membrane association and the repair of double breaks in X-irradiated *Micrococcus radiourans, Biochim. Biophys. Acta,* 247, 38, 1971.

125. **Lehmann, A. R. and Stevens, S.,** The production and repair of double strand breaks in cells from normal humans and from patients with ataxia telangiectasia, *Biochim. Biophys. Acta,* 474, 49, 1977.

126. **Tomizawa, J.-I. and Ogawa, H.,** Breakage of DNA in *rec⁺* and *rec⁻* bacteria by radiophosphorus atoms in DNA and possible cause of pleiotropic effects of *recA* mutation, *Cold Springs Harbor Symp. Quant. Biol.,* 33, 243, 1968.

127. **Town, C. D., Smith, K. C., and Kaplan, H. S.,** DNA polymerase required for the rapid rejoining of X-ray induced DNA strand breaks *in vivo, Science,* 172, 851, 1971.

128. **Kapp, D. S. and Smith, K. C.,** Repair of radiation-induced damage in *Escherichia coli.* II. Effect of *rec* and *uvr* mutations on radiosensitivity, and repair of X-ray induced single strand breaks in deoxyribonucleic acid, *J. Bacteriol.,* 103, 49, 1970.

129. **McGrath, R. A. and Williams, R. W.,** Reconstruction *in vivo* of irradiated *Escherichia coli* deoxyribonucleic acid; the rejoining of broken pieces, *Nature (London),* 212, 534, 1966.

130. **Bridges, B. A.,** RecA⁺-dependent repair of gamma-ray damage to *Escherichia coli* does not require recombination between existing homologous chromosomes, *J. Bacteriol.,* 108, 944, 1971.

131. **Bridges, B. A. and Munson, R. J.,** Temperature, time and X-ray mutagenesis in *Escherichia coli, Mutat. Res.,* 1, 362, 1964.

132. **Taylor, A. M. R., Harnden, D. G., Arlett, C. F., Harcourt, S. A., Lehmann, A. R., Stevens, S., and Bridges, B. A.,** Ataxia telangiectasia, a human mutant with abnormal radiation sensitivity, *Nature (London),* 258, 427, 1975.

133. **Paterson, M. C., Smith, B. P., Lohman, P. H. M., Anderson, A. K., and Fishman, L.,** Defective excision repair of gamma-ray-damaged DNA in human (ataxia telangiectasia) fibroblasts, *Nature (London),* 260, 444, 1976.

134. **Lehmann, A. R.,** Ataxia telangiectasia and the lethal lesion produced by ionizing radiation, in *DNA Repair Processes,* Nichols, W. W. and Murphey, D., Eds., Symposia Specialists, Miami, 1977, in press.

135. **Drake, J. W. and Greening, E. O.,** Suppression of chemical mutagenesis in bacteriophage T4 by genetically modified DNA polymerases, *Proc. Natl. Acad. Sci. U.S.A.,* 66, 823, 1970.

136. **Lawley, P. D.,** Some chemical aspects of dose response relationships in alkylation mutagenesis, *Mutat. Res.,* 23, 283, 1976.

137. **Frei, J. V. and Lawley, P. D.,** The distribution and mode of DNA methylation in mice by methyl methanesulphonate and *N*-methyl-*N'*-nitro-*N*-nitrosoguanidine: lack of thymic lymphoma induction and low extent of methylation of target tissue DNA at O^6 of guanine, *Chem. Biol. Interact.,* 13, 215, 1976.

138. **Goth, R. and Rajewsky, M. F.,** Persistence of O^6 ethyl guanine in rat-brain DNA: correlation with nervous system-specific carcinogenesis by ethylnitrosourea, *Proc. Natl. Acad. Sci. U.S.A.,* 71, 639, 1974.

139. **Moreau, P. and Devoret, R.,** Potential carcinogens tested by induction and mutagenesis of prophage λ in *Escherichia coli* K-12, in *Origins of Human Cancer,* Hiatt, H., Watson, J. D., and Winsten, J. A., Eds., Cold Springs Harbor Laboratory, 1977, in press.

140. **Green, M. H. L., Rogers, A. M., Muriel, W. J., and McCalla, D. R.,** Use of a simplified fluctuation test to detect and characterize mutagenesis by nitrofurans, *Mutat. Res.,* 44, 139, 1977.

141. **Lawley, P. D. and Orr, D. J.,** Specific excision of methylation products from DNA of *Escherichia coli* treated with *N*-methyl-*N'*-nitro-*N*-nitrosoguanidine, *Chem. Biol. Interact.,* 2, 154, 1970.

142. Anderson, D. and Fox, M., The induction of thymidine- and IUdR-resistant variants in P388 mouse lymphoma cells by X-rays, UV and mono- and bi-functional alkylating agents, *Mutat. Res.*, 25, 107, 1974.

143. Arlett, C. F., Lehmann, A. R., Giannelli, F., and Ramsay, C. A., A human subject with a new defect in repair of ultraviolet damage, *J. Invest. Dermatol.*, 1978, in press.

144. Scarano, E., Tosi, L., and Granieri, A., Enzymic modifications of DNA, a model for the molecular basis of cell differentiation, in *The Biochemistry of Adenosyl methionine*, Salvatore F., Borek, E., Zappia, V., Williams-Ashman, H. G., Schlenk, F., Eds., Columbia University Press, New York, 1977, 369.

145. Rydberg, B., Bromouracil mutagenesis in *Escherichia ia coli*, evidence for involvement of mismatch repair, *Mol. Gen. Genet.*, 152, 19, 1977.

146. Drake, J. W. and Allen, E. F., Antimutagenic DNA polymerases of bacteriophage T4, *Cold Springs Harbor Symp. Quant. Biol.*, 33, 339, 1968.

147. Zampieri, A. and Greenberg, J., Mutagenesis by acridine orange and proflavin in *Escherichia coli* strain S, *Mutat. Res.*, 2, 552, 1965.

148. Daune, M. P. and Fuchs, R. P. P., Structural modification of DNA after covalent binding of a carcinogen, *Colloq. Int. CNRS*, 256, 83, 1977.

149. Streisinger, G., Okada, Y., Emrich, J., Newton, J., Tsugita, A., Terzaghi, E., and Inouye, M., Frameshift mutations and the genetic code, *Cold Spring Harbor Symp. Quant. Biol.*, 31, 77, 1966.

150. Ames, B. N., Lee, F. D., and Durston, W. E., An improved bacterial test system for the detection and classification of mutagens and carcinogens, *Proc. Natl. Acad. Sci. U.S.A.*, 70, 782, 1973.

151. Lerman, L. S., The structure of the DNA-acridine complex, *Proc. Natl. Acad. Sci. U.S.A.*, 49, 94, 1963.

152. Sesnowitz-Horn, S. and Adelberg, E. A., Proflavin treatment of *Escherichia coli*: generation of frameshift mutations, *Cold Spring Harbor Symp. Quant. Biol.*, 33, 393, 1968.

153. Weinstein, I. B. and Grunberger, D., Structural and functional changes in nucleic acids modified by chemical carcinogens, in *Chemical Carcinogenesis*, (Part A), T'so, P. O. P., and DiPaolo, J. A., Eds., Marcel Dekker, New York, 1974, 217.

154. Fowler, R. G., Degnen, G. E., and Cox, E. C., Mutational specificity of a conditional *Escherichia coli* mutator *mut D5*, *Mol. Gen. Genet.*, 133, 179, 1974.

155. Mortelmans, K. E. and Stocker, B. A. D., Ultraviolet light protection, enhancement of ultraviolet light mutagenesis and mutator effect of plasmid R46 in *Salmonella typhimurium*, *J. Bacteriol.*, 128, 271, 1976.

156. Isono, K. and Yourno, J., Chemical carcinogens as frameshift mutagens: *Salmonella* DNA sequence sensitive to mutagenesis by polycyclic carcinogens, *Proc. Natl. Acad. Sci. U.S.A.*, 71, 1612, 1974.

157. Newbold, R. F., Wigley, C. F., Thompson, M. H., and Brookes, P., Cell-mediated mutagenesis in cultured Chinese hamster cells by carcinogenic polycyclic hydrocarbons: nature and extent of the associated hydrocarbon: DNA reaction, *Mutat. Res.*, 43, 101, 1977.

158. Campbell, A. M., Episomes, *Adv. Genet.*, 11, 101, 1962.

159. Inselburg, J., Formation of deletion mutations in recombination deficient mutants of *Escherichia coli*, *J. Bacteriol.*, 94, 1266, 1967.

160. Itikawa, H. and Demerec, M., Ditto deletions in the cysC region of the *Salmonella* chromosome, *Genetics*, 55, 63, 1967.

161. Berg, C. M., Auxotroph accumulation in deoxyribonucleic acid polymeraseless strains of *Escherichia coli* K-12, *J. Bacteriol.*, 106, 797, 1971.

162. Ishii, Y. and Kondo, S., Comparative analysis of deletion and base change mutabilities of *Escherichia coli* β strains differing in DNA repair capacity (wild-type, *uvrA*, *polA*, *recA*) by various mutagens, *Mutat. Res.*, 27, 27, 1975.

163. Meselson, M. and Russell, K., in *Origins of Human Cancer*, Hiatt, H., Watson, J. D., and Winsten, J. A., Eds., Cold Spring Harbor Laboratory, 1977, 1473.

164. Bouck, N. and di Majorca, G., Somatic mutation as the basis for malignant transformation of BHK cells by chemical carcinogens, *Nature (London)*, 264, 722, 1976.

165. Novick, A. and Weiner, M., Enzyme induction as an all-or-none phenomenon, *Proc. Natl. Acad. Sci. U.S. A.*, 43, 553, 1957.

166. Howard-Flanders, P., Boyce, R. P., and Theriot, L., Three loci in *Escherichia coli* K-12 that control the excision of thymine dimers and certain other mutagen products from host or phage DNA, *Genetics*, 53, 1119, 1964.

167. De Lucia, P. and Cairns, J., Isolation of an *E. coli* strain with a mutation affecting DNA polymerase, *Nature (London)*, 224, 1164, 1969.

168. Kornberg, A., *DNA synthesis*, Freeman, San Francisco, 1974, 304.

169. Pauling, E. C., The role of polynucleotide ligase in normal DNA replication, *Cold Springs Harbor Symp. Quant. Biol.*, 33, 148, 1968.

170. **Clark, A. J. and Margulies, A. D.**, Isolation and characterization of recombination-deficient mutants of *E. coli* K-12, *Proc. Natl. Acad. Sci., U.S.A.*, 53, 451, 1965.

171. **Witkin, E. M.**, Thermal enhancement of ultraviolet mutability in a *tif-1* uvrA derivative of *Escherichia coli* B/r: evidence that ultraviolet mutagenesis depends on an inducible function, *Proc. Natl. Acad. Sci. U.S.A.*, 71, 1930, 1974.

172. **Castellazzi, M., Morand, P., George, J., and Buttin, G.**, Prophage induction and cell division in *E. coli*. V. Dominance and complementation analysis in partial diploids with pleiotropic mutation (*tif, recA zab* and *lexB*) at the *recA* locus, *Mol. Gen. Genet.*, 153, 297, 1977.

173. **Wright, M., Buttin, G., and Hurwitz, J.**, The isolation and characterization from *Escherichia coli* of an adenosine triphosphate-dependent deoxyribonuclease directed by *recBC* genes, *J. Biol. Chem.*, 246, 6543, 1971.

174. **Clark, A. J.**, Recombination deficient mutants of *E. coli* and other bacteria, *Annu. Rev. Genetics*, 7, 67, 1973.

175. **Volkert, M. R., George, D. L., and Witkin, E. M.**, Partial suppression of the *lexA* phenotype by mutations (*rnm*) which restore ultraviolet resistance, but not ultraviolet mutability to *Escherichia coli* B/r, *Mutat. Res.*, 36, 401, 1976.

176. **Greenberg, J., Berends, L. J., Donch, J., and Green, M. H. L.**, *ExrB*, a *malB* linked gene in *Escherichia coli* B involved in sensitivity to radiation and filament formation, *Genet. Res.*, 23, 175, 1974.

177. **Witkin, E. M.**, Genetics of resistance to radiation in *Escherichia coli*, *Genetics*, 32, 221, 1947.

178. **Shineberg, B. and Zipser, D.**, The *lon* gene and degradation of B galactosidase nonsense fragments, *J. Bacteriol.*, 116, 1469, 1973.

179. **Johnson, B. F., and Greenberg, J.**, Mapping of *sul* the suppressor of *lon* in *Escherichia coli*, *J. Bacteriol.*, 122, 570, 1975.

180. **Brooks, K. and Clarke, A. J.**, Behavior of λ bacteriophage in a recombination deficient strain of *Escherichia coli*, *J. Virology*, 1, 283, 1967.

181. **Fuerst, C. R. and Siminovitch, L.**, Characterization of an unusual defective lysogenic strain of *Escherichia coli* K-12 (λ), *Virology*, 27, 449, 1965.

182. **Donch, J., Greenberg, J., and Green, M. H. L.**, Repression of induction by UV of λ phage by *exrA* mutants of *Escherichia coli*, *Genet. Res.*, 15, 87, 1970.

183. **Donch, J., Green, M. H. L., and Greenberg, L.**, Interaction of the *exr* and *lon* genes in *Escherichia coli*, *J. Bacteriol.*, 96, 1704, 1968.

184. **Green, M. H. L., Greenberg, L., and Donch, J.**, Effect of a *recA* gene on cell division and capsular polysaccharide production in a *lon* strain of *Escherichia coli*, *Genet. Res.*, 14, 159, 1969.

185. **Witkin, E. M.**, The mutability toward ultraviolet light of recombination-deficient strains of *Escherichia coli*, *Mutat. Res.*, 8, 9, 1969.

186. **Howard-Flanders, P. and Boyce, R. P.**, DNA repair and genetic recombination studies on mutants of *Escherichia coli* defective in these processes, *Radiat. Res. Suppl.*, 6, 156, 1966.

187. **Pollard, E. C. and Randall, E. P.**, Studies on the inducible inhibitor of radiation-induced DNA degradation of *E. coli*, *Radiat. Res.*, 55, 265, 1973.

188. **Swenson, P. A. and Schenley, R. L.**, Respiration, growth and viability of repair-deficient mutants of *Escherichia coli* after ultraviolet irradiation, *Int. J. Radiat. Biol.*, 25, 51, 1974.

189. **Radman, M., Wagner, and Meselson**, personal communication, 1977

190. **Witkin, E. M.**, personal communication, 1977.

191. **Arlett, C. F.**, personal communication, 1977.

192. **Rogers, A. M.**, personal communication, 1977.

193. **Radman, M., Villani, G., Boiteux, S., Kinsella, A. R., Glickman, B. W., and Spadari, S.**, Replicational fidelity: mechanisms of mutation avoidance and mutation fixation, *Cold Spring Harbor Symp. Quant. Biol.*, 43, 1978, in press.

194. **Krasin, F. and Hutchinson, F.**, Repair of DNA double-strand breaks in *Escherichia coli*, which requires *recA* function and the presence of a duplicate genome, *J. Mol. Biol.*, 116, 1977, 81.

195. **Coulondre, C., Miller, J. H., Farabaugh, P., and Gilbert, W.**, Molecular basis of base substitution hotspots in *Escherichia coli*, *Nature (London)*, 274, 1978, 775.

Chapter 5

DNA REPAIR AND CARCINOGENESIS

Veronica M. Maher and J. Justin McCormick

TABLE OF CONTENTS

I. INTRODUCTION: DNA AND THE ORIGIN OF CANCER*

It is clear from the extensive research which has been reported in the preceding chapters in this volume that, during the past 10 years, attention has focused ever more intensely on DNA as the critical cellular target for the action of chemical carcinogens. For many years this was not the case. A combination of factors has contributed to our present understanding of the relationship between the interaction of carcinogens with DNA and the carcinogenesis process. It had been suggested by Boveri[1] as early as 1914 that carcinogens could bring about the transformation of a normal cell into a tumorigenic one by introducing a mutational event, an alteration in the hereditary material. This was a logical explanation for why there are so many different kinds of tumors and why the progeny cells derived from a tumor are themselves tumorigenic. Although the hypothesis was intellectually satisfying, it received little experimental support in the years following because well-recognized and potent carcinogens examined for their mutagenic action proved to be either nonmutagenic or only weakly so. When Burdette reviewed the situation in 1955,[2] he came to the conclusion that there was no correlation between carcinogens and mutagens. Similarly, when Kaplan in 1959 summarized the evidence for the various mechanisms that might be responsible for cancer, he left little room for involvement of somatic mutations in this process. He cited as evidence data showing that polycyclic hydrocarbons do not even enter the nucleus of cells.[3] Needless to say, these reviews did little to encourage further investigation into the role of carcinogen-DNA interaction or of somatic cell mutations in bringing about oncogenic transformation.

However, at that time, little was understood about the need for the majority of chemical carcinogens to be metabolically activated into reactive forms capable of interacting with cellular macromolecules.[4] The majority of the test systems used for assaying mutagenicity lacked the necessary activating enzymes for carcinogens and so gave negative results even with very powerful compounds. Remarkable progress has been made during the past 15 years in the area of metabolic activation, and it is now recognized that, if the need for activation is properly provided for, the majority of, if not all, chemical carcinogens are mutagenic. This important insight into the common action of a very diversified series of chemicals was obtained not only because signifi-

---

* Abbreviations used are (1) N-AcO-AAF, N-acetoxy-2-acetylaminofluorene, (2) MMS, methyl methane-sulfonate, (3) 7-BrMeBA, 7-bromomethylbenz[a]anthracene, (4) MNNG, N-methyl-N'-nitro-N-mitroso-guanidine, (5) MMC, mitomycin-C, (6) 4NQO, 4-nitroquinoline-1-oxide, (7) DMBA, 7,12-dimethylbenz[a]anthracene, (8) MNU, N-methyl-N-nitrosourea, (9) ENU, N-ethyl-N-nitrosourea, (10) DMN, dimethylnitrosamine, (11) O^6-MeG, O^6-methylguanine, (12) XP, xeroderma pigmentosum, (13) AT, ataxia telangiectasia, (14) FA, Fanconi's anemia; BUdR, bromodeoxyuridine; UV, ultraviolet light of 254 nm wavelength.

cant progress has been made in unraveling the intricacies of metabolic activation, but also because equally remarkable progress has been made in developing test systems[5] suitable for quantitating the induction of mutations in microorganisms[6] and in cultured mammalian cells,[7] including diploid human cells in culture.[8,9]

The purpose of this chapter is to examine evidence that cellular DNA repair processes play a role in the carcinogenesis process. To accomplish this, we will begin by presenting an overview of various forms of DNA repair operating in mammalian cells. We will then go on to consider evidence that DNA repair can alter the frequency (1) of somatic cell mutation induced by carcinogens, (2) of oncogenic transformation of cells in culture by these agents, and finally (3) of tumor induction in animals and in man.

II. TYPES OF DNA REPAIR PROCESSES

During the past 20 years since the first radiation-sensitive strain of bacteria was isolated,[10] a great deal has been discovered concerning the complex enzymatic processes by which procaryotic and eucaryotic cells deal with damage introduced into their DNA following attacks by radiation or chemical carcinogens or mutagens. An extensive overview of the molecular mechanisms for repair of DNA was summarized in 1975 in a two-volume text,[11] and this has been followed by a series of excellent reviews on the subject of DNA repair in bacteria[12,13] and in mammalian cells.[14,15] A review by Witkin deals principally with the role of inducible DNA repair in causing mutations in *Escherichia coli* by UV radiation.[13] Obviously, it is beyond the scope of this chapter to go into detail concerning the various pathways of enzymatic repair processes which are known or presumed to exist in various living organisms, such as bacteria, yeast, and molds. Some of these are dealt with in the preceding chapter. However, we will very briefly review the general categories of DNA repair processes in order to be in a position to discuss their role in mutagenesis.

A. Photoreactivation of Pyrimidine Dimers
Photoreactivation is the name given to the process by which a specific photoreactivating enzyme binds to the intrastrand cyclobutane-type dimer formed between adjacent pyrimidines by UV radiation, monomerizes it *in situ* with the energy of photoreactivating light (wave lengths of 310 to 500 nm), and thus, restores the DNA to its original undamaged state (Figure 1A). It has been shown to be completely specific for pyrimidine dimers and to prevent the lethal and mutagenic consequences of UV irradiation. Photoreactivating enzymes have been detected in both procaryotes and eucaryotes, including human cells. (See References 16 to 21 for an overview of this form of repair.) Because these enzymes are completely dependent upon the presence of visible light for their monomerizing action, their function in cells which are inaccessible to light is unexplained. Nevertheless, since they have such a specific substrate, these enzymes serve an important function in distinguishing which biological effects can be attributed to the presence of unrepaired pyrimidine dimers in the DNA of UV-irradiated cells (see below).

B. Excision Repair of DNA Damage
In contrast to photoreactivation, excision repair does not require the presence of light, is not limited to action on pyrimidine dimers, and instead of chemically reversing the damage, physically removes the damaged portion of the DNA from the rest of the strand and replaces the damaged section. A generalized schema for excision repair following recognition of the specific type of damage present in the DNA is diagrammed in Figure 1B. Excision repair requires four steps: (1) incision by an endonuclease near the site of the lesion, (2) excision by an exonuclease of the damaged nucleotide (or

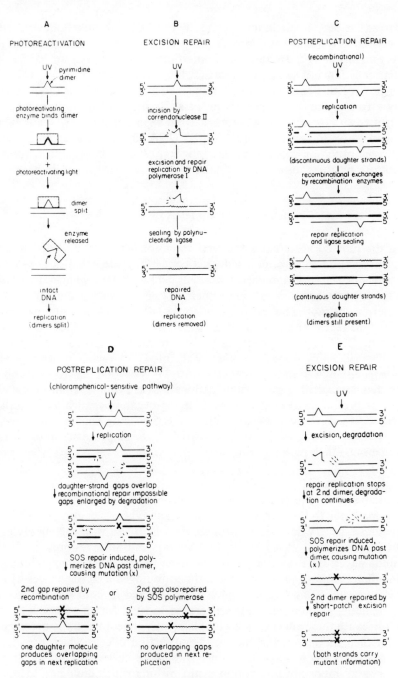

FIGURE 1.   Generalized diagram of pathways of enzymatic repair of damage to DNA. Photoreactivation (A) is specific UV-induced pyrimidine dimers. The other processes diagrammed here and discussed in the text can be considered as operating on various forms of DNA damage (represented by‑⌒‑). The heavy lines represent newly synthesized daughter DNA, the light lines represent parental DNA, the wavy lines represent DNA polymerized during repair replication. X indicates a mutation (i.e., altered base sequence). (This figure combines diagrams taken from Witkin, E. M., *Bacteriol. Rev.*, 40, 869, 1976. With permission.)

nucleotides) as well as additional neighboring nucleotides, the number depending upon the type of damage being excised, (3) filling in of the excision gap by a DNA polymerase (repair replication) using the intact opposite strand as a template, and (4) sealing of the phosphate-sugar linkage by polynucleotide ligase. Not unexpectedly, the excision repair replication process which replaces nucleotides using an undamaged strand of DNA as a template has been shown in bacteria[22] to be accurate, i.e., not to introduce mutations. We have recently been able to demonstrate that this is also true of diploid human cells in culture.[23,24]

1. Methods of Detecting Excision Repair

Excision repair of damage in parental DNA strands can be detected by various techniques. For example, loss of the lesion itself is detected by measuring loss of labeled pyrimidine dimers[25] or of covalently bound radioactive carcinogen residues,[26-28] or loss of endonuclease sensitive sites.[29] Repair synthesis (the incorporation of nucleotides into parental DNA rather than into daughter strands) can be detected by measuring the incorporation of ^{3}H-nucleotides into DNA when cells are not in S-phase, or when S-phase DNA synthesis is blocked. Such repair synthesis is most commonly detected by autoradiography, and is frequently referred to as "unscheduled DNA synthesis."[30,31] Other techniques for detecting excision repair include: (1) allowing incorporation of bromodeoxyuridine (BUdR) and radioactively labeled DNA precursor, and then physically separating the parental from the newly synthesized, daughter strands by alkaline density gradient centrifugation, and measuring incorporation of label into parental strands (light density)[32], or (2) allowing incorporation of BUdR followed by photolysis of DNA by 313-nm radiation, and measuring the size of the resulting DNA segments.[33]

2. Two Forms of Excision Repair in Human Cells

Much of our knowledge of the various steps and enzymes involved in excision repair has been obtained by the judicious use of mutant strains of bacterial cells which have lost a particular repair function. Considerably less is known about the excision repair enzymes in mammalian cells, and one of the reasons for this is the scarcity of repair-deficient, mutant strains of mammalian cells, and the almost complete lack of chemicals which can specifically inhibit particular DNA repair processes in such cells.[34-36] However, it is now known that cells from patients with such inherited cancer-prone syndromes as xeroderma pigmentosum (XP),[37,38] ataxia telangiectasia (AT)[39,40], and Fanconi's anemia (FA)[41-43] are deficient in various repair capabilities and can serve as repair-defective, mutant strains. Comparative investigations of the functions of the repair mechanisms in human cells is currently underway in many laboratories throughout the world using these strains of mutant human cells.

From comparative studies involving normal (repair-proficient) human cells in culture, and classical XP cells deficient in the first step of excision of UV-induced damage, it has been determined that the type of damage initially inserted into the DNA determines the kind of excision repair which will take place. For example, Stich and co-workers used normal human cells and classical XP cells to test a series of chemical and physical carcinogens for their ability to stimulate excision repair replication.[44] They found that some stimulated excision repair in both kinds of cells, while others resulted in repair replication in the normal cells, but not in the XP. This showed that the XP were defective in excision of that particular kind of damage. Similarly, Regan and Setlow, using their BUdR-313 nm photolysis technique,[45] divided a series of physical and chemical carcinogens into two types, viz., those resulting in long or "UV-like" repair and those causing short or "X-ray-like" repair, depending upon the approximate number of nucleotides inserted into the parental DNA of normal human cells during excision repair replication, and the length of time required. The former agents, e.g., N-acetoxy-2-acetylaminofluorene, (N-AcO-AAF) stimulate excision of a relatively large number of nucleotides, and the cells continue to carry out excision repair for a relatively long time (long repair). It is this kind of "UV-like" repair which is defective or absent in classical XP cells. The agents causing "X-ray-like" damage, e.g., methyl methane sulfonate (MMS), on the contrary, stimulate both sets of cells to carry out an excision repair process which adds a much smaller number of nucleotides, and is completed sooner (short repair).

We demonstrated that inability of XP cells to carry out repair of DNA damage inflicted by a particular agent can cause those cells to be significantly more sensitive to the killing action of that agent than are normal human fibroblasts,[46,47] and that the degree of sensitivity reflects the degree of inhibition in rate of repair. Thus, by comparing the percent survival of the colony-forming ability of normal and classical XP cells, one can determine which agents are repaired by the "UV-like" repair system. Taking advantage of such differential cytotoxicity, Heflich et al.[48] gained insight into the recognition signal for long-repair excision by showing that a series of directly acting carcinogens, or reactive derivatives of carcinogens which cause a significantly greater cytotoxic effect in XP cells than in normal human cells, e.g., 7-bromomethylbenz[a]-anthracene (7-BrMeBA), also result in significant distortion of the native structure of DNA, rendering it susceptible to the action of an S_1 nuclease specific for single-stranded DNA. In contrast, agents which do not cause a greater cytotoxic effect in XP cells than in normal, e.g., N-methyl-N'-nitro-N-nitrosoguanidine (MNNG), do not cause the formation of these single-stranded regions. These studies support the hypothesis that the recognition site for the action of long repair is not a specific lesion, but rather a particular degree of distortion in the DNA helix. They strengthen the concept that repair systems monitor the DNA for damage introduced by various agents and lessen their harmful biological consequences.

3. Loss of Individual Bases Followed By Excision Repair

Evidence has recently been obtained in *E. coli*,[49] for two forms of glycosylase which can break the glycosyl bond between the sugar and a damaged base, and cause the loss of a single base (depurination or depyrimidination). Chemical rather than enzymatic depurination can bring about a similar result. Such DNA is then susceptible to an endonuclease which has been shown to attack DNA specifically at such apurinic or apyrimidinic sites, introducing a single-strand break. This incision is followed by a limited amount of excision and repolymerization using the opposite strand as template.[49-52] Whether this is the same process as the "short repair" observed in mammalian cells is not known, but it can be expected to restore DNA to its undamaged state if an intact template is available for accurate repolymerizing of the excised region. Of course, if the particular segment on the opposite DNA strand itself contains damaged, noninstructive bases, (e.g., a pyrimidine dimer as shown in Figure 1E), then none of these excision-repair replication processes can be expected to function properly in their usual "error-free" manner. Therefore, in these particular instances, mutations might be introduced by as yet unidentified processes which the cell uses to take care of such special situations.

C. "Tolerance Repair" or "Postreplication By-Pass" Repair
1. Constitutive Tolerance Repair in Bacteria

It has been demonstrated in UV-irradiated *E. coli* that the presence of pyrimidine dimers which are neither photoenzymatically split nor excised from DNA will block DNA replication, but that synthesis can be reinitiated at some point beyond the dimer. Rupp and co-workers[53,54] presented evidence that gaps are formed in newly synthesized daughter-strand DNA which are approximately 1000 nucleotides in length and occur in proportion to the number of dimers present in the parental DNA strand. (Figure

1C). They suggest that these gaps are formed when a noninstructive lesion (a dimer in this case) passes through a replication fork. Exactly how *E. coli* cells handle the resulting gaps or discontinuities in daughter-strand DNA is not completely understood, but it is clear that replication of DNA containing such noninstructive pyrimidine dimers does take place, and that genetic exchange (recombination) between DNA strands occurs (Figure 1C) which frequently results in pyrimidine dimers being transferred into daughter strands.[55] In principle, one would not expect recombination to cause mutations, since the process does not involve replication of DNA from a noninstructive template. To examine this question, Kato et al. (quoted in Reference 13) constructed mutant strains of *E. coli (uvr⁺, recB⁻, recC⁻, recF⁻,* or *uvr⁻, recB⁻, recC⁻, recF⁻)* deficient in recA-dependent processes involved in recombination and "postreplication repair", and compared them with wild type cells for the frequency of UV-induced mutations. They found nearly normal levels, suggesting that mutagenic enzymes can act effectively even in the absence of the recA-dependent recombination processes. However, recent studies by Howard-Flanders and his colleagues on the effect of various gene products needed for repair and recombination in *E. coli* on the frequency of genetic exchanges (recombination) between superinfecting lambda phage treated with cross-linking agents and lambda prophage indicate that genetic recombination can take place with almost normal frequency even in a *recB⁻, recC⁻, recF⁻, sbcB⁻* quadruple mutant.[56,151] This result suggests that in the experiments of Kato et al.,[153] recombination was not altogether prevented.

2. Inducible "Tolerance Repair" in Bacteria

If a replication gap formed in one daughter strand should overlap a similar gap formed in the opposite daughter strand, (Figure 1D), recombination would not be possible, and nucleotides would somehow have to be inserted directly across from a noninstructive template. This situation can be expected to cause mutations. Evidence drawn from studies on the kinetics of UV mutagenesis in specially-constructed DNA-repair-deficient strains of *E. coli*[57-65] as well as biochemical evidence from studies employing protein synthesis inhibitors, points to the existence in this microorganism of an inducible protein factor (or enzyme), not constitutively present in the cell, but synthesized when a particular signal is perceived, which directly or indirectly makes it possible for the cell to insert nucleotides opposite such lesions. This insertion allows the cell to tolerate what otherwise might be a lethal event caused by the presence of unrepaired damage, but does so at the cost of introducing mistakes (mutations) into the DNA with a frequency characteristic of the particular lesion involved. Because some of the evidence suggests that the presence of particular lesions in DNA (e.g., a delay in DNA synthesis or the presence of persistent gaps) acts as a signal to induce the synthesis of such a protein, Radman designated the process "SOS repair".[59] Arguments that the factor is constitutive and does not require induction have recently been put forward by Bridges.[68] Regardless of the inducible nature of the process, it remains clear that in *E. coli* (and in *Salmonella* strains[69] as well as in *Haemophilus*[70]) there can be no mutagenesis by a number of carcinogenic and mutagenic agents — UV, X-ray, MMS, mitomycin C (MMC), 4-nitroquinoline-1-oxide (4NQO) — if the genes responsible for this process (*recA, lexA*) are absent. Thus, postreplication or tolerance repair (as that term is here applied to a factor or process which allows intact daughter strand DNA to be generated from parental DNA which contains unexcised damage) plays a crucial role in the induction of mutations in these *E. coli* cells. What is, however, of greater importance to the present discussion is whether similar factors or processes (inducible or constitutive) play a role in the induction of mutations in mammalian cells, and in human cells in particular.

3. "Postreplication" Repair in Mammalian Cells
a. Evidence of Gap-Filling

There is evidence in mammalian cells that DNA, newly synthesized from parental strand templates soon after exposure to UV or to X-irradiation, is made in shorter segments than are produced in unirradiated cells. Lehmann[72] suggested that in mouse lymphoma cells this low molecular weight DNA is physically converted into large molecular weight DNA by *de novo* synthesis. Buhl et al.[73] reported similar results following UV irradiation of normal human fibroblasts and those from XP patients. Fujiwara[74] showed that alkylating agents, e.g., MMS and methylnitrosourea (MNU), can cause this phenomenon in mouse L cells, and Koerner et al.[75] found that the size of the DNA newly synthesized in X-irradiated Chinese hamster cells was inversely related to the dose administered. Lehmann et al.[38] showed that fibroblasts derived from the class of XP patients called XP variants (i.e., persons who have all the clinical manifestations of the disease, but exhibit normal rates of excision repair[76]) are abnormally slow at making this conversion of small DNA, synthesized from UV irradiated templates, into normal-sized molecules. Maher and McCormick reported that DNA synthesized in human cells exposed to the 5,6-oxide of 7,12-dimethylbenz[a]anthracene (DMBA) is made in small segments. They showed that XP-variant cells take abnormally long to convert the small DNA into normal sized molecules.[24,47]

In these experiments DNA, newly synthesized during semiconservative replication, is labeled by a short pulse soon after exposure to the agent, and its initial size is determined. Then DNA synthesis is allowed to continue for several hours in the absence of label (chase), and the original pulse-labeled DNA is again examined for size using alkaline sucrose gradients or similar techniques. Pulse-labeled DNA is eventually found to reach the size of the DNA from untreated cells. Since there is good evidence in bacteria that daughter strands of DNA made from UV-irradiated templates contain gaps (Figure 1C), Lehmann suggested that in UV-irradiated mammalian cells similar gaps are left in daughter strands when the DNA polymerase encounters a blocking lesion.[72] The fact that the smaller DNA eventually reaches the size of DNA from unirradiated control cells suggests that during the chase such gaps are filled in some way. He[72] and others[73,74,77] could find no evidence that the gaps were filled by physical exchange between parental strands and daughter strands, and suggested, rather, that *de novo* synthesis is involved. If radioactive, pulse-labeled, low-molecular-weight DNA is chased in the presence of BUdR and then the DNA is subjected to 313-nm photolysis, its size is reduced once again to the original low molecular weight. This supports the hypothesis that the original shorter segments were interrupted by gaps which got filled by *de novo* synthesis utilizing the BUdR.

Some have questioned this model because they found that newly synthesized DNA in excision-defective cells some time after UV-irradiation (e.g., 18 hr in XP cells) was no longer smaller than that made in unirradiated cells,[75-81] indicating that the blocking lesions have somehow been removed, altered or "by-passed". Further investigation of these phenomena are called for. We have shown that if XP cells representing complementation groups C and D as well as XP variants are prevented from replicating for a period of time after lethal doses of UV, they exhibit 100% survival, suggesting that lesions that would otherwise have been lethal were removed.[82] We are currently examining the size of newly made DNA after many different periods of time, postirradiation.

b. Evidence of Recombination

In an attempt to detect genetic recombination as a form of postreplication repair in mammalian cells, Koerner and Malz[77] prelabeled parental DNA of Chinese hamster cells with BUdR, and then X-irradiated the cells and allowed DNA synthesis to occur

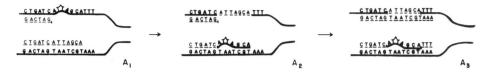

A. RECOMBINATION REPAIR: (TRANSFER of SEGMENT INTO DAUGHTER STRAND)

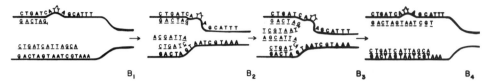

B. REPLICATION REPAIR: (STRAND DISPLACEMENT and BRANCH MIGRATION)

FIGURE 2. Diagram of two cellular processes (models) which can be proposed to explain how a cell which is replicating DNA containing unexcised damage might "by-pass" block, noninstructive bases in parental DNA without having to make use of the damaged section as a template. The second model (B) was originally proposed for mammalian cells by Higgins et al.[86]

in the presence of radioactive label. Then, 313-nm photolysis was used to see if labeled daughter DNA strands had received DNA sections containing BUdR by genetic exchange with parental strands. If they had, the daughter strands would be broken by the 313 nm radiation. No evidence of exchange was found.[83] However, it is likely that the length of material exchanged in mammalian cells is too small for this technique to be successful. A much more sensitive technique consists of determining whether UV-endonuclease-sensitive sites can be detected in daughter strands of UV-irradiated mammalian cells.[83-85] Using this technique, it has been possible to detect the loss of endonuclease-sensitive sites from parental strands in XP cells (which are totally incapable of excision) and the concomitant introduction of approximately the same number of sites in the daughter strands.[85] This suggest that genetic recombination occurs in the vicinity of at least a certain proportion of the lesions (See Diagram, Figure 2A).

c. Strand Displacement and Branch Migration

A different explanation for the low-molecular-weight DNA of pulse-labeled daughter strands which eventually reaches a larger size was suggested by Higgins et al.[86] and independently confirmed by Fujiwara and Tatsumi.[87] Their studies suggest that the production of low-molecular-weight DNA following UV irradiation reflects the fact that DNA synthesis is blocked by the presence of a lesion (i.e., dimer or some other configuration). They propose that when this smaller DNA is eventually chased into higher molecular-weight DNA segments (which contain the original, pulse-labeled, short sections), it merely reflects a drastically slower form of continuous DNA replication which eventually takes place around these blocks by making use of the temporarily displaced opposite-daughter strand as a coding template (see diagram Figure 2B). Biochemical as well as elctron microscopic evidence supports this model. However, such an explanation probably does not hold for X-ray induced lesions since, in the experiments of Koerner and Malz,[77] the rate of DNA synthesis was normal even though the DNA synthesized during thee first few hours following irradiation was made in short segments.

d. Inducibility of a "Rejoining Factor"

Recent physical evidence indicates that if V79 Chinese hamster cells are preirradiated with UV light or treated with N-AcO-AAF, and a few hours later given a second exposure to a higher dose of the agent and examined for the size of newly synthesized

DNA, the rejoining or conversion of smaller size DNA into larger size DNA takes place more rapidly than if only a single UV exposure is employed.[88] A similar effect was observed in XP variant human cells. This observation has been attributed to the induction by the DNA damaging agent of some kind of "facilitating factor," and it is easy to speculate that what is responsible for this effect is similar to the inducible "bypass" repair factor in *E. coli* described above. Trosko and his associates have observed that exposing V79 Chinese hamster cells to a low dose of UV followed a few hours later by a larger dose decreases slightly the expected killing effect of the two doses combined.[89] However, if this low dose induces an "error-prone" SOS factor in V-79 cells, similar to that proposed for mutation induction in UV-irradiated *E. coli* cells,[13] there is no experimental evidence of a biological effect on mutation frequency even though the question has been investigated in some detail.[89]

D. Other Forms of DNA Repair

1. Repair of Interstrand Cross-Links

Bifunctional alkylating agents such as nitrogen mustard and sulfur mustard, as well as many other agents with more than one reactive group which are capable of interacting with DNA, form intra-strand lesions as well as interstrand cross-links in the macromolecule. In mutant bacteria, which are completely unable to repair such damage, it has been found that a single cross-link in the genome constitutes a lethal event. However, repair proficient bacterial cells[90] as well as human cells[42] can remove such damage from DNA. However, the repair process for removing cross-links from human cell DNA is different from that seen in *E. coli*. In the latter species, the repair process requires the function of the endonuclease which begins the excision of pyrimidine dimers, whereas, in human, classical XP cells it is found that even those totally lacking in ability to excise dimers are not significantly more sensitive than normal cells to agents known to cause interstrand cross-links (e.g., MMC).[42] Cells derived from Fanconi's anemia patients, on the other hand, are incapable of removing cross-links, but have little difficulty excising UV dimers.

2. X-irradiation- and UV-irradiation-Induced Base Damage Other Than Dimerization

Hariharan and Cerutti[91] have demonstrated that a major DNA lesion produced by ionizing radiation consists of a monomeric, ring-saturated thymine product of the 5,6-dihydroxydihydrothymine type, and that such damage is also produced to a much lesser degree by UV radiation. They found that extracts derived from sonicated nuclei of normal human cells and from XP cells can excise such damage (designated t') from irradiated bacteriophage DNA (the excision was determined from loss of t' from acid-precipitable DNA). Recently Paterson et al.[40] reported that cell strains derived from certain ataxia (AT) patients are deficient in excision repair of such nonpyrimidine dimer damage. Cerutti and his co-workers however, using a different test system, found that sonicates of AT cells were normal in this kind of repair,[92] but that cells derived from Fanconi's anemia patients are defective.[43] Since many AT strains show increased sensitivity to the killing effect of X-rays, but fail to exhibit any difficulty rejoining strand breaks,[39] the finding that they may have a defect in excision of this particular kind of base damage is potentially important. The defect may occur in an enzyme similar to, or identical to, that recently isolated from human tissue.[93]

3. Repair of Single Strand Breaks and Double Strand Breaks

It is known that, within 30 to 60 min, mammalian cells can repair (rejoin) the single strand breaks caused by ionizing radiation.[94,95] This has also been shown for normal human cells and cells derived from XP, AT, and FA patients. One report has appeared,[96] which shows that cells from patients with Hutchinson-Progeroid syndrome are defective in such strand rejoining, but an accompanying report could not confirm this.[97] Bradley et al.[98] also report that progeroid as well as aging human cells exhibit completely normal rejoining of strand breaks. Much less is known about the kinetics of rejoining of double strand breaks in mammalian cells, but dose-dependent rejoining has been demonstrated to occur in Chinese hamster cells,[99] and in human fibroblasts.[39]

III. EVIDENCE THAT DNA REPAIR CAN ALTER THE FREQUENCY OF MUTATION INDUCED BY CARCINOGENS

A. Photoreactivation Decreases the Frequency of UV-Induced Mutations

As soon as the mechanism of enzymatic photoreactivation was recognized,[17] the process was used to determine whether the presence of nonphotoreactivated pyrimidine dimers was principally responsible for the cytotoxic or mutagenic effect of UV radiation in biological systems.[100,101] When cells which possess photoreactivating enzyme are UV-irradiated and subsequently either exposed to wavelengths suitable for the monomerization of dimers, or shielded from such light, comparison of the two sets of cells shows that the former treatment decreases both the killing action of UV and the frequency of mutations. Photoreactivation has been referred to as the epitome of "error-free" repair, since it opens the dimers without requiring excision, etc. However, because it eliminates the major lesions formed in UV-irradiated DNA, photoreactivation necessarily makes other cellular, enzymatic-repair processes, which operate on pyrimidine dimers as well as on other forms of damage, more available for repairing these other minor forms of damage. Thus, even though photoreactivation dramatically lowers the mutation frequency in UV-irradiated cells (presumably by removing pyrimidine dimers, which are premutagenic lesions, before they can be "fixed" by other cellular processes) there is always at least the possibility, as suggested by Witkin,[13] that the mutations decrease as a result of the action of other repair mechanisms, which have been rendered more efficient by its action. Nevertheless, photoreactivation clearly eliminates UV-induced mutagenesis.

B. Excision Repair Can Decrease the Frequency of Mutations

1. In bacteria

There is now overwhelming evidence that the excision repair processes operating in microorganisms are able to decrease both the cytotoxic and the mutagenic effect of exposure to carcinogenic agents such as UV, X-rays, alkylating agents, polycyclic aromatic hydrocarbons, aromatic amides, 4NQO, MMC, etc. When populations of excision-proficient *(uvr⁺)* and excision-deficient *(uvr⁻)* E. coli are exposed to UV radiation at doses low enough so that there is just slight cell killing in the *uvr⁺* strain, no increase in mutagenesis in the excision-proficient strain is seen, but the *uvr⁻* strain exhibits greatly reduced survival and a high frequency of mutations among the survivors examined.[71,101-103] A remarkably similar result is observed when 4NQO is substituted for UV radiation.[71] Indeed, the survival curves and the mutagenicity curves for the two agents are superimposable for the particular strains tested, suggesting that these two agents are repaired by a common mechanism which is deficient in the *uvr⁻* strain. Such data demonstrates that unexcised lesions in DNA are much more mutagenic than are products of excision repair, and that the process by which such lesions are excised is virtually "error-free".

2. In Mammalian Cells

Recent evidence from our laboratory demonstrates that this is also true in human cells. When excision-repair-proficient human fibroblasts derived from the skin of normal persons, and excision-repair-deficient fibroblasts derived from classical XP patients are exposed to equal low doses of UV radiation, there is neither a cytotoxic nor

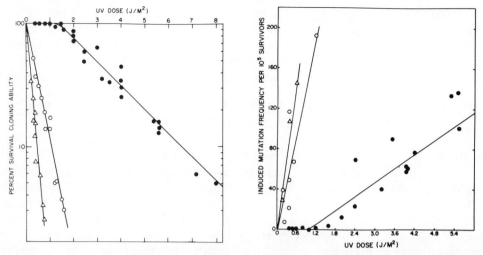

FIGURE 3.   Cytotoxic and mutagenic effect of ultraviolet radiation in strains of diploid human skin fibroblasts with different rates of excision repair. Normal cells,●: XP2BE from complementation group C with an excision rate of ∼ 16% of normal, 0: XP12BE from group A with no measureable excision repair capacity, △. Methods of procedure for these experiments have been published.[24,47,108,110] The genetic marker employed was resistance to 8-azaguanine.

a mutagenic effect in the normal cell strain, but a drastic decrease in survival in the XP strain. This is accompanied by a dramatic increase in induced mutation frequency among the surviving colonies[23,24,104] (see Figure 3). Significantly, cells derived from XP2BE (complementation group C), which is reported to carry out excision repair of UV-induced lesions at a rate approximately 16% of normal,[105] are slightly less sensitive to the killing and mutagenic effect of UV than are XP12BE cells (group A), which are totally lacking in such excision repair. These data indicate that the excision process in diploid human cells which dramatically decreases the cytotoxicity of UV is virtually "error-free", i.e., does not increase the mutation frequency. We,[106] as well as Simons and co-workers,[107] have demonstrated that if diploid human cells are not allowed to divide, but are permitted to carry out excision repair, the cytotoxic and mutagenic effects caused by UV radiation are decreased at a rate directly related to the rate of excision repair in the particular strain tested.

Studies comparing the frequency of mutations induced in repair-proficient and repair-deficient cells of other mammalian species are hampered by a lack of suitable strains which differ in repair capacities and also by the absence of chemicals which specifically inhibit excision repair in mammalian cells. However, comparative mutagenicity studies similar to those which we have reported with XP cell strains and normal strains exposed to UV radiation have been, and are currently being, carried out with ionizing radiation in cells derived from AT patients.[152] Data on the frequencies of mutation induced in the AT cells by ionizing radiation indicate that these are less than background, or at least not higher than that of normal human cells.

C. "Tolerance Repair" Can Increase the Frequency of Mutations
1. In Bacteria

As discussed above, evidence indicates that the process responsible for mutations in *E. coli* following exposure to a large series of carcinogens is completely dependent upon the presence of the recA, lexA gene products which are involved in tolerance of unexcised lesions in DNA. With the availability of an impressive battery of DNA repair deficient mutants in *E. coli*, it has been possible to test various hypotheses concerning the nature of the lesion (or process) which results in a mutation following exposure to carcinogenic agents, such as UV. For example, Sedgwick presents evidence that the mutagenic lesion consists of a daughter-strand gap which partially overlaps another daughter-strand gap in the opposite strand.[64] It is obvious from Figure 1D that this constitutes a special kind of damage. It cannot be patched by means of the recombination followed by repair replication which is diagrammed in Figure 1C. A somewhat comparable situation can result if excision repair of a lesion in a parental strand (Figure 1E) produces an excision gap large enough to overlap a noninstructive base on the opposite, parental strand. Evidence that such gaps which overlap noninstructive lesions, or gaps on the opposite strand, are repaired by an error-producing, gap-filling process in bacteria has been reviewed in detail.[13] If this particular repair process is absent or prevented, cell killing is greatly increased, but among the few survivors there is no increase in mutation frequency.

2. In Mammalian Cells

During replication, mammalian cells may handle unexcised damage: (1) by somehow directly inserting nucleotides across from noninstructive bases (direct misreplication), and then continuing on; (2) by temporarily stopping replication on the damaged strand before coming to the lesion while continuing it on the opposite strand for a short distance, and then, by means of strand displacement, using the newly replicated copy from the undamaged strand as a template (as in Figure 2B) to supply the information which was not available and continuing on; (3) by physically exchanging the damaged portion of the parental strand for the corresponding newly synthesized, intact, daughter strand — using a process similar to genetic recombination (see Figure 4 for a diagram of the model we propose for this process) which would eliminate the block and allow synthesis to continue; and (4) by interrupting synthesis near the lesion and reinitiating it at a subsequent site, leaving a gap in the daughter strand in the vicinity of the damaged site which could subsequently be filled by either *de novo* synthesis or by recombination between daughter and parental strand. Note that only in the fourth model would actual gaps or discontinuities be present in daughter DNA.

Which of these proposed processes is likely to be responsible for the production of mutations? The first is expected to introduce errors, e.g., base pair changes or frame shifts, since a noninstructive template is used for synthesis. The second ought to be

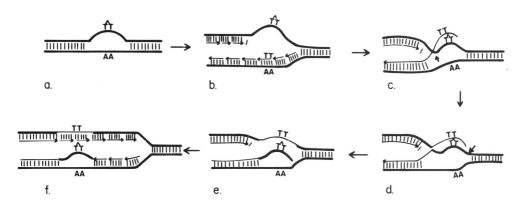

FIGURE 4.   Diagram of a proposed model by which human cells could "by-pass" unexcised damage during DNA replication without the need to form a gap or discontinuity in the daughter DNA. This model assumes that because of the lesion blocking replication, synthesis is prevented on the damaged parental strand, but that the corresponding portion on the opposite parental strand does get replicated. Because the lesion (dimer) distorts the DNA, base pairing is not normal, and we suggest that the newly replicated daughter strand could get displaced as indicated. The nicking action of an endonuclease is represented by the arrows. As a result of this endonucleolytic action, followed by ligation, an intact portion of the strand is exchanged for the portion of the parental strand which contains the dimer. The end result of this exchange is that DNA replication is no longer blocked and can proceed until it is blocked by another distorting lesion.

"error-free", since an undamaged template is substituted for the damaged one, but nothing is yet known about the fidelity on the polymerase(s) involved in carrying out the proposed replication from the displaced daughter strand or about other factors that may be necessary in this model. Since the third model involves endonucleases and ligases and does not depend upon accurate base pairing, it could result in the loss of small amounts of DNA (deletion mutations) or even larger amounts (chromosome aberrations). Neither the second nor the third model would operate efficiently in situations similar to those diagrammed in Figure 1D, i.e., situations believed to be responsible for the majority of the UV-induced mutations in *E. coli*. The fourth model, i.e., leaving gaps which must be filled *de novo*, or by recombination, holds obvious potential for the production of mutations—either by substituting incorrect bases across from the noninstructive lesion or by the loss of genetic information during recombination. While there is physical evidence for all four processes, there is no definitive evidence as to which of them results in mutations in mammalian cells.

To distinguish between the various processes, it would be useful to possess mutant cell strains which are incapable of one or more of these processes, or to identify chemicals which would inhibit or interfere with them. Unfortunately, a mammalian cell equivalent of a recA⁻, lexA⁻, UV-nonmutable, bacterial strain has not yet been identified, and, at present, the one chemical commonly used to block postreplication repair, viz., caffeine, has multiple effects. Furthermore, it is not effective in blocking excision repair processes in normal human cells. In order to examine the question indirectly, we selected nonmalignant cells from cancer-prone XP-variant patients because, although their cells have normal rates of excision repair, they are abnormally slow in replicating DNA from damaged templates and make use of a caffeine-sensitive process. We compared these cells with normal, human cells for the cytotoxic and mutagenic effect of UV.[108,109] Although both strains excise dimers at an equal rate, the XP-variant cells proved more sensitive to the killing action of UV and significantly more sensitive to its mutagenic action (Figure 5). At low doses of UV (e.g., less than 1 J/m²), there was no cytotoxic effect in either strain, but there was a significant increase in mutations over background in the XP variant; in contrast, there was no measurable increase in the normal. Furthermore, at doses adjusted to give an equal amount of cell killing in each strain, the frequency of UV-induced mutations per survivor was higher in the XP variant than in the normal cells (Figure 5). This suggests that XP-variant cells either use an abnormally "error-prone" process in dealing with unexcised lesion, or are defective in an "error-free" replication (or postreplication) process which is as yet unidentified.

Because caffeine has been demonstrated to interfere with one or more steps in "post replication repair" in certain mammalian cells, we examined its effect on UV-irradiated, XP-variant cells and normal, human cells. Caffeine (0.75 mM) given from immediately after irradiation until the end of the period required for expression of mutations to azaguanine resistance, dramatically increased the cytotoxic and mutagenic effect of UV in the XP-variant cells[109,110] (Figure 6). It had no effect on the normal human cells. A similar synergistic increase in the cytotoxic and mutagenic effect of UV or of MNU has been reported for Chinese hamster cells.[111-115] One interpretation offered to explain this increase is that of Chang et al.[115] They suggest that caffeine blocks or interferes with some "error-free" process which the cells use during replication to handle unexcised lesions, and allows an "error-prone" process to produce mutations. This interference leads to greater lethality, and to higher mutation frequencies. However, the same result could be obtained, even if the replication processes which caffeine interfered with were "error-prone" in the absence of caffeine, and introduced small-deletions, frame shifts, base-pair changes, etc. If caffeine caused a significant increase in large-sized deletions (loss of genetic information), this would increase both

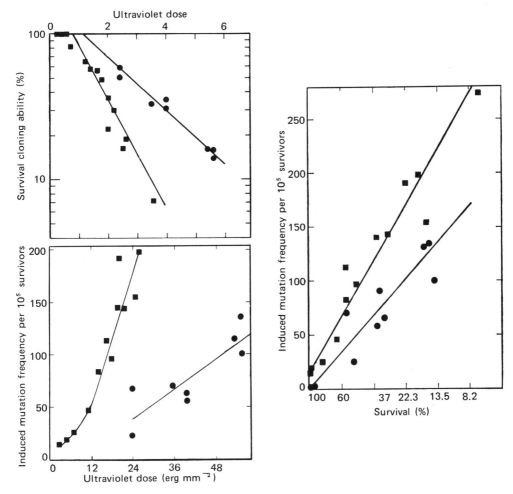

FIGURE 5. Cytotoxicity and mutagenicity of UV radiation in normal cells (●) and in an XP variant strain, XP4BE (■) as a function of dose (left two charts), and a comparison of the frequency of mutations to 8-azaguanine resistance induced in these strains as a function of the cytotoxic effect of the radiation (right chart). The procedures used for these experiments have been described.[108] The genetic marker is resistance to 8-azaguanine. (This figure combines three figures from Maher, V. M., Ouellette, L. M., Curren, R. D., and McCormick, J. J., *Nature*(London), 201, 593, 1976. With permission.)

the cytotoxicity and the frequency of mutations to 6-thioguanine or 8-azaguanine resistance. Roberts and co-workers[111,112] and Maher et al.[110] have put forward this latter explanation, which is supported by cytological evidence of shattered chromosomes.[111]

Such an explanation predicts however, that one should not observe a synergistic increase in the frequency of mutations if ouabain resistance were chosen as the genetic marker, since cells carrying deletions of the Na + /K + ATPase gene would not survive. We are presently investigating this question. If posttreatment with caffeine results in loss of chromosome material, the population of 8-azaguanine- or 6-thioguanine-resistant mutants generated in the presence of caffeine can be expected to include more cells with chromosome aberrations than are found in the absence of caffeine. Such defective cells could be expected to multiply at a slower rate than less damaged cells. If this is so, then if one replates the population at the beginning of selection instead of allowing the mutant population to form resistant colonies *in situ,* the increase in mutant frequency could be obscured. This may explain why Fox and collaborators report that caffeine results in an increased frequency in UV-induced, 6-thioguanine-resistant, mu-

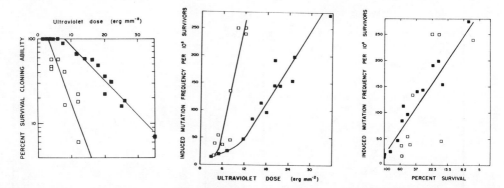

FIGURE 6.   Synergistic increase in the cytotoxic and mutagenic effect of UV radiation in an XP variant (XP4BE) caused by 0.75 m*M* caffeine given from immediately after irradiation until the beginning of selection of mutants with resistance to 8-azaguanine. No caffeine (■); caffeine present during expression period (□). Procedures used for these experiments have been described.[110] (This figure combines two figures taken from Maher, V. M., Ouellette, L. M., Curren, R. D., and McCormick, J. J., *Biochem. Biophys. Res. Commun.*, 71, 228, 1976. With permission.)

tant-V79 cells with the latter technique,[114] but not with the former.[116] Further investigation into the mechanism of caffeine's interference with DNA replication following exposure to various agents is clearly called for. Nevertheless, it has proved useful for demonstrating that "postreplication repair" processes are involved in at least some mammalian-cell mutagenesis as well as in the formation of sister-chromatid exchanges.[117,118]

IV. EVIDENCE THAT DNA REPAIR CAN ALTER THE FREQUENCY OF ONCOGENIC TRANSFORMATION OF CELLS IN CULTURE

It is important to develop quantitative transformation systems for diploid, human cells in culture, because the availability of repair-deficient strains in that species enables one to determine directly the effect of DNA repair on the frequency of oncogenic transformation. Efforts in this direction are underway in several laboratories, and Kakunaga has reported successful transformation of skin fibroblasts from normal donors using 4NQO and MNNG as carcinogens.[119] In his experiments, transformation was characterized by foci formation and the cells in the foci proved able to cause large tumors in nude mice.

In earlier studies, Kakunaga developed a quantitative in vitro transformation system involving a selected subclone of mouse 3T3 cells.[120] With this system he showed that if 4NQO or 3-methylcholanthrene-treated cells are prevented from undergoing a single cell division by maintaining them in a confluent state (to allow time for excision repair before releasing them and plating them for foci formation), induction of cell transformation is prevented.[121,122] In contrast, if he designed the experiment to allow a single, population doubling before confluency was reached, this was sufficient to "fix" the transforming event in the cells, since maintaining them in a nondividing state for a week before replating them at a lower cell density did not alter the frequency of transformed foci which ultimately developed. Similarly, if he held the carcinogen-treated cultures at confluency so that they could not divide, and released them from this block after 24, 72, or 120 hr, the frequency of transformation decreased dramatically with time held at confluency. Ikenaga and Kakunaga have recently determined the rate of loss of 4NQO-DNA adducts from carcinogen treated 3T3 cells.[123] They find that the decrease in transformation frequency is directly correlated with the enzymatic removal of adducts. These data provide evidence that excision repair which takes place in the absence of cell division can lower the frequency of carcinogen-induced, cell transformation.

Terzaghi and Little[124] confirmed the loss of transformation of X-irradiated 10T½ C3H mouse cells held in the confluent state. However, when they assayed for transformation frequency after much shorter intervals (2 hr, 4 hr, etc.) they observed a slight but significant dose-dependent increase in transformation frequency, which they attributed to errors introduced during prereplication repair of the X-ray-induced damage. When they maintained cells at confluency for 6 hr or longer postirradiation, the results were similar to Kakunaga's. They suggest that lesions which were introduced during the first few hours after irradiation were removed by the cell during the next couple of hours, before replication of the DNA was allowed to take place.

Donovan and DiPaolo showed that low doses of caffeine given to N-AcO-AAF-treated, Syrian hamster cells during the posttreatment expression period increased the frequency of morphological transformation.[125] Since low doses of caffeine also increase the mutation frequency in carcinogen-treated rodent cells,[111] and interfere with "postreplication repair" in Chinese hamster cells after N-AcO-AAF treatment,[126] the results with the Syrian hamster cells support the hypothesis that mutations are involved in bringing about cell transformation. Kakunaga found that if higher doses of caffeine are present during the expression time, the frequency of cell transformation decreases.[127] Mutation frequency is also observed to decrease if caffeine is present throughout the whole time that carcinogen-treated cells are kept in culture for selection of azaguanine-resistant mutants.[114]

V. EVIDENCE THAT DNA REPAIR CAN ALTER THE FREQUENCY OF TUMORS INDUCED IN ANIMALS OR HUMANS BY CARCINOGEN TREATMENT

A. Photoreactivation Can Prevent Tumors

Hart and Setlow reported[128] that if they exposed portions of cell suspensions of tissue from various organs of a nonsexually reproducing fish to 20 J/m² of UV radiation (254 nm), and then injected the cells into isogenic recipient fish, 10% of the fish developed granulomas and 100% developed thyroid carcinomas. However, if the UV-irradiated, cell suspenion was illuminated with photoreactivatng wavelengths of light before injection, the yields of both kinds of tumors were reduced ten fold. They conclude that pyrimidine dimers were ultimately responsible for the production of the tumors, and that photoreactivation can protect irradiated cells from becoming tumorigenic. Here, again, however, the cautionary note of Witkin referred to earlier in the section on photoreactivation must be kept in mind.

B. Excision Repair Can Reduce the Frequency of Tumors

1. Excision of UV-Induced Damage

Sunlight has been shown to introduce pyrimidine dimers into the DNA of cells in culture,[129] and pyrimidine dimers have been linked to tumor formation in fish.[128] XP patients from complementary-group A have been shown to be the most deficient of all XPs in carrying out excision repair of such pyrimidine dimers. Recently Takebe et al.[130] showed that Japanese patients from this group exhibited the earliest onset of skin tumors. Of a group of 50 patients studied, they found that all who had developed symptoms of XP disease early in life, i.e., from age 0 to 8 years, were from the group with the very lowest, or undetectable, levels of excision repair, and the most extreme sensitivity to the killing action of UV light (complementation group A). Malignant skin tumors were identified at the earliest age (5 years) in this group. Of patients with intermediate rates of excision repair (10 to 60% of normal), the earliest age of onset of skin tumors was 9 years, but the majority developed tumors only after age 17, and two, aged 28 and 42, had not developed any tumors as yet. In contrast, only one group-A patient, from among eight who were 12 years old or older, had attained age 12 without developing malignant skin tumors. A conclusion which follows from these data is that the efficient rate of excision found in normal persons protects them significantly from the possibility of developing skin tumors from normal amounts of exposure to radiation from the sun. Abundant epidemiological data[131] indicates, however, that individuals with normal rates of excision repair do develop skin tumors following many years of exposure to sunlight, e.g., ranchers, sailors. The fact that normal cells also become cancerous after such exposure to sunlight correlates with our data. These show that, at high doses of UV radiation, mutations are induced in normal cells with the same high frequencies as are found in XP cells exposed to much lower doses[23,24] (Figure 3).

2. Excision of Chemically Induced DNA Damage

Another example of how efficient excision repair can lower the possibility of developing tumors in animal organs exposed to a carcinogen comes from DNA repair studies in rodents exposed to directly acting, alkylating agents. Goth and Rajewsky[132] observed that, although there was an approximately equal molar amount of ethyl groups initially bound to purine bases in the liver and in the brain following a single pulse of N-ethyl-N-nitrosourea (ENU) given to BDIX rats during the perinatal period, only neuroectodermal neoplasms in the central and peripheral nervous system developed. They showed that N-7-ethylguanine and N-3-ethyladenine were lost at about the same rate from "high risk" and "low risk" organs, but that O^6-ethylguanine was removed from the brain DNA at a very much slower rate than from other tissues. They concluded that this slow rate of excision combined with the relatively high rate of DNA replication which takes place in the developing brain could account for the increased probability of neoplastic conversion. The O^6-ethylation of guanine has been shown to be the most likely alkyl lesion to cause miscoding and anomalous base-pairing during DNA replication.[133]

A similar conclusion, i.e., that the slow rate of excision was ultimately responsible for the production of tumors, was reached by Kleihues and Margison.[134] They found that exposure of rats to N-methyl-N-nitrosourea (MNU) over a period of 35 days resulted in selective persistance of O^6-methylguanine (O^6-MeG) in the brain, but not in the liver, and resulted in an increased frequency of brain tumors over liver tumors. More recently, Buechler and Kleihues reported[135] that the relationship between slow rate of excision of O^6-MeG and tumor susceptibility was not as straightforward as originally believed. They found essentially the same rate of loss of O^6-MeG from the brain of two strains of mice, although these strains differ significantly in their susceptibility to the neuro-oncogenic effect of MNU and related carcinogens. Furthermore, levels of O^6-MeG were highest in the brain and lung seven days after injection of ^{3}H-MNU, but the lung is the principal target organ for MNU-induced tumors in mice, and brain tumors are far less frequent. Noting that Rajewsky et al.[136] also have found that the rate of excision of O^6-ethylguanine was not measurably different in two strains of rats with widely different susceptibilities to brain tumors, these investigators conclude that, although rapid excision repair protects organs from tumor induction, the presence of unexcised O^6-alkylations is not the sole factor determining the preferential location of tumors.

Magee and co-workers have shown that the organ specificity of carcinogenic nitrosamines which require metabolic activation can be explained on the basis of differential rates of excision of O^6-methylated bases. Dimethylnitrosamine (DMN), administered as a series of low doses, causes tumors in the liver, but not in the kidney. After a single, high dose (approaching the lethal level), about 20% of the surviving animals have renal tumors,[137] and the incidence can approach 100% if preceded by a protein-deficient diet, which increases the proportion of DMN metabolized in the kidney.[138] After a very high dose, the extent of methylation in the liver is much higher than in the kidney, but only kidney tumors develop. This result has recently been explained by the finding that after the large dose the rate of loss of O^6-MeG from the liver was the same as after the low dose, but loss from the kidney was dramatically slower after the high dose.[139] No difference in the slow loss of N^7-MeG by chemical depurination was observed for the two organs.[140]

Additional evidence that excision may protect from DMN-induced carcinogenesis comes from Magee's observation[141] that if the administration of two doses is separated by only a few days, the incidence of kidney tumors is significantly higher than if they are separated by 8 or more days — sufficient time to permit removal of the DNA damage.

C. "Tolerance Repair" Mechanisms Can Increase the Frequency of Tumors in Animals

Evidence that replication of DNA templates containing unexcised lesions increases the possibility of tumorigenesis comes from many sources. We cite here only a few to indicate the kinds of studies undertaken. In mice there is a much higher incidence of thymic lymphomata caused by exposure to a single dose of MNU than there is to a dose of MMS, even though equal extents of alkylation of bone marrow DNA takes place. Frei and Venitt[142] explain this difference by demonstrating that the former agent causes greater chromosome damage and toxicity because of the increased levels of O^6-methylation of guanine and phosphotriesters it produces. They suggest that the much higher level of necrosis which occurs with MNU leads to enhanced stem-cell replication (reparative hyperplasia), and this is correlated with the induction of this particular form of cancer.

A somewhat similar conclusion has been reached by Craddock from her observation that the highest incidence of liver tumors is obtained when DMN is given to rats at the time of maximum DNA synthesis (produced by partial hepatectomy).[143] No measurable difference in the nature, extent, or persistence of DNA damage caused by alkylation was observed between the regenerating and the intact organ, but the rate of DNA replication was significantly higher in the former organ even after exposure to DMN.

Caffeine has also been used to investigate the role of "postreplication repair" processes in tumor induction. For example, Zajdela and Laterjet painted one of each pair of mouse ears with caffeine and exposed the animals to UV radiation. The incidence of tumors was lower in the caffeine-painted ears.[144] Nomura reported[145] that the average number of tumor nodules per lung in female mice treated with a single injection of 4NQO was decreased approximately 70% by caffeine (5 injections of 100 μg/g at 6- to 12-hr intervals) administered immediately, or 5 days after, the 4NQO treatment. Caffeine also increased the toxicity of 4NQO in this system. Kondo has interpreted these results as providing evidence that caffeine inhibits an "error-prone" mechanism which ordinarily leads ultimately to tumor production.[146] However, much more research on the mechanisms involved in DNA replication on damaged templates in vivo, as well as the role of such processes on the induction of mutations and tumors in vivo, is required before firm conclusions can be drawn.

VI. CONCLUSION

Although it has not been established with absolute certainty that the interaction of carcinogenic agents with DNA is causally related to the induction of cancer, there is now substantial evidence in support of this concept. Convincing evidence that DNA is the critical target comes from the studies on XP patients who are extraordinarily susceptible to sunlight-induced cancer, whose cells exhibit abnormally high frequencies of mutations induced by UV, and by metabolites of carcinogenic polycyclic aromatic hydrocarbons,[47] and who are deficient in the rate of DNA excision repair,[37] or "post-replication repair,"[38] as well as in other forms of DNA repair.[147,148] Studies comparing cells of normal persons with those of XP patients have broadened our understanding of the important protective effect of efficient, "error-free", excision repair found in the cells of normal persons, and suggest that "error-prone" mechanisms of replication (or "postreplication repair") are responsible for causing mutations, and that mutations are ultimately responsible for the induction of skin cancer. Additional evidence that carcinogen interaction with DNA plays a central role in the induction of cancer comes from the finding that several other genetic diseases characterized by a greatly increased frequency of cancer are also characterized by greatly increased rates of spontaneous and/or carcinogen-induced chromosome breakage (which can result in deletion mutations through loss of genetic material). They are also deficient in one or more DNA repair or replication processes.[149,150] The present review of the role of these cellular repair processes in altering the frequency of mutations induced in mammalian cells, of oncogenic transformation of cells in culture, and of tumor induction in animals and man, highlights recent discoveries in these areas. It underscores the need for further investigation into the role of DNA repair and mutagenesis in the mechanism of carcinogenesis.

ACKNOWLEDGMENTS

The work reported from the authors' laboratory was supported by National Cancer Institute Grants CA 21247 and CA 21253. We wish to acknowledge the supporting help of A. Aust, N. Birch, R. D. Curren, D. J. Dorney, R. H. Heflich, B. Konze-Thomas, J. W. Levinson, A. Mendrala, J. R. Otto, L. M. Ouellette, and M. Zakem who are past or present members of our research group.

REFERENCES

1. Boveri, T., *The Origin of Malignant Tumors,* Williams & Wilkins, Baltimore, 1929.
2. Burdette, W. J., The significance of mutation in relation to the origin of tumours. A review, *Cancer Res.,* 15, 201, 1955.
3. Kaplan, S. H., Some implications of indirect induction mechanisms in carcinogenesis: a review, *Cancer Res.,* 19, 791, 1959.
4. Miller, J. A. and Miller, E. C., Metabolic activation of carcinogenic aromatic amines and amides via N-hydroxylation and N-hydroxyesterification and its relationship to ultimate carcinogens as electrophilic reactants, in *The Jerusalem Symposia on Quantum Chemistry and Biochemistry. Physico-Chemical Mechanisms of Carcinogenesis,* Vol. 1, Bergmann, E. D. and Pullman, B., Eds., Israel Academy of Science and Humanities, Jerusalem, 1969, 237.
5. Hollender, A., Ed., *Chemical Mutagens, Principles and Methods for their Detection,* Vol. 1 and 2, Plenum Press, New York, 1971.
6. Ames, B. N., Lee, F. D., and Durston, W. E., An improved bacterial test system for the detection and classification of mutagens and carcinogens, *Proc. Natl. Acad. Sci.* U.S.A., 70, 782, 1973.

7. Chu, E. H. Y., Introduction and analysis of gene mutations in mammalian cells in culture, in *Chemical Mutagens, Principles and Methods for their Detection*, Vol. 2., Hollender, A., Ed., Plenum Press, New York, 1971, 411.

8. DeMars, R., Resistance of cultured human fibroblasts and other cells to purine and pyrimidine analogues in relation to mutagenesis detection, *Mutat. Res.*, 24, 335, 1974.

9. Thilly, W. G., De Luca, J. G., Hoppe, H., IV, and Penman, B. W., Mutation of human lymphoblasts by methylnitrosourea, *Chem. Biol. Interact.*, 15, 33, 1976.

10. Hill, R. F., A radiation-sensitive mutant of *Escherichia coli.*, *Biochim. Biophys. Acta*, 30, 636, 1958.

11. Hanawalt, P. C. and Setlow, R. B., Eds., *Molecular Mechanisms for Repair of DNA*, Parts A and B, Plenum Press, New York, 1975.

12. Grossman, L., Braun, A., Feldberg, R., and Mahler, I., Enzymatic repair of DNA, *Annu. Rev. Biochem.*, 44, 19, 1975.

13. Witkin, E. M., Ultraviolet mutagenesis and inducible DNA repair in *Escherichia coli*, *Bacteriol. Rev.*, 40, 869, 1976.

14. Cleaver, J. E., Repair processes for photochemical damage in mammalian cells, *Adv. Radiat. Biol.*, 4, 1, 1974.

15. Hanawalt, P. C., Friedberg, E. C., and Fox, C. F., Eds., *DNA Repair Mechanisms*, Academic Press, New York, 1978.

16. Cook, J. S., Photoenzymatic repair in animal cells, in *Molecular and Cellular Repair Processes*, Beers, R. F., Herriott, R. M., and Tilghman, R. C., Eds., Johns Hopkins University Press, Baltimore, 1972, 79.

17. Rupert, C. S., Photoenzymatic repair of ultraviolet damage in DNA. II. Formation of an enzyme-substrate complex, *J. Gen. Physiol.*, 45, 724, 1962.

18. Rupert, C. S., Enzymatic photoreactivation: overview, in *Molecular Mechanisms for Repair of DNA*, Part A, Hanawalt, P. and Setlow, R. B., Eds., Plenum Press, New York, 1975, 73.

19. Sutherland, B. M., Runge, P., and Sutherland, J. C., DNA photoreactivating enzyme from placental mammals. Origin and characteristics, *Biochemistry*, 13, 4710, 1974.

20. Sutherland, B. M., Photoreactivating enzymes from human leukocytes, *Nature* (London), 248, 109, 1974.

21. Mortelmans, K., Cleaver, J. E., Friedberg, E. C., Paterson, M. C., Smith, B. P., and Thomas, G. H., Photoreactivation of thymine dimers in UV-irradiated human cells: unique dependence on culture conditions, *Mutat. Res.*, 44, 433, 1977.

22. Witkin, E. M., Mutation-proof and mutation-prone modes of survival in derivatives of *Escherichia coli* B differing in sensitivity to ultraviolet light, *Brookhaven Symp. Biol.*, 20, 17, 1967.

23. Maher, V. M., Curren, R. D., Ouellette, L. M., and McCormick, J. J., Effect of DNA repair on the frequency of mutations induced in human cells by ultraviolet irradiation and by chemical carcinogens, in *Fundamentals in Cancer Prevention*, Magee, P. N., Takayama, S., Sugimura, T., and Matsushima, T., Eds., University of Tokyo Press, Tokyo, 1976, 363.

24. Maher, V. M., Curren, R. D., Ouellette, L. M., and McCormick, J. J., Role of DNA repair in the cytotoxic and mutagenic action of physical and chemical carcinogens, in *In Vitro Metabolic Activation in Mutagenesis Testing*, de Serres, F. J., Fouts, J. R., Bend, J. R., and Philpot, R. M., Eds., North-Holland, Amsterdam, 1976, 313.

25. Setlow, R. B. and Carrier, W. L., The disappearance of thymine dimers from DNA: an error-correcting mechanism, *Proc. Natl. Acad. Sci. U.S.A.*, 51, 226, 1964.

26. Lieberman, M. W. and Dipple, A., Removal of bound carcinogen during DNA repair in nondividing human lymphocytes, *Cancer Res.*, 32, 1855, 1972.

27. Amacher, D. E., Elliott, J. A., and Lieberman, M. W., Differences in removal of acetylaminofluorene and pyrimidine dimers from the DNA of cultured mammalian cells, *Proc. Natl. Acad. Sci. U.S.A.*, 74, 1553, 1977.

28. Ikenaga, M., Takebe, H., and Ishii, Y., Excision repair of DNA base damage in human cells treated with the chemical carcinogen 4-nitroquinoline-1-oxide, *Mutat. Res.*, 43, 415, 1977.

29. Paterson, M. C., Lohman, P. H. M., and Sluyter, M. L., Use of a UV endonuclease from *Micrococcus luteus* to monitor the progress of DNA repair in UV-irradiated human cells, *Mutat. Res.*, 19, 245, 1973.

30. Stich, H. F. and San, R. H., DNA repair synthesis and survival of repair deficient human cells exposed to the K-region epoxide of benz[a]anthracene, *Proc. Soc. Exp. Biol. Med.*, 142, 155, 1973.

31. Stich, H. F., San, R. H., Miller, J. A., and Miller, E. C., Various levels of DNA repair synthesis in xeroderma pigmentosum cells exposed to the carcinogens, N-hydroxy and N-acetoxy-2-acetylaminofluorene, *Nature (London) New Biol.*, 238, 9, 1972.

32. McCormick, J. J., Marks, C., and Rusch, H. P., DNA repair after ultraviolet irradiation in synchronous plasmodium of *Physarum polycephalum*, *Biochim. Biophys. Acta*, 287, 246, 1972.

33. Regan, J. D., Setlow, R. B., and Ley, R. D., Normal and defective repair of damaged DNA in human cells: a sensitive assay utilizing the photolysis of bromodeoxyuridine, *Proc. Natl. Acad. Sci. U.S.A.*, 68, 708, 1971.

34. **Cleaver, J. E.**, Repair replication of mammalian cell DNA: effects of compounds that inhibit DNA synthesis or dark repair, *Radiat. Res., 37*, 334, 1969.
35. **Poirier, M. C., De Cicco, B. T., and Lieberman, M. W.**, Nonspecific inhibition of DNA repair synthesis by tumor promoters in human diploid fibroblasts damaged with N-acetoxy-2-acetylamino-fluorene, *Cancer Res., 35*, 1392, 1975.
36. **Cleaver, J. E. and Painter, R. B.**, Absence of specificity in inhibition of DNA repair replication by DNA-binding agents, cocarcinogens, and steroids in human cells, *Cancer Res., 35*, 1773, 1975.
37. **Cleaver, J. E.**, Xeroderma pigmentosum: a human disease in which an initial stage of DNA repair is defective, *Proc. Natl. Acad. Sci. U.S.A., 63*, 428, 1969.
38. **Lehmann, A. R., Kirk-Bell, S., Arlett, C. F., Paterson, M. C., Lohmann, P. H. M., De Weerd-Kastelein, E. A., and Bootsma, D.**, Xeroderma pigmentosum cells with normal levels of excision repair have a defect in DNA synthesis after UV-irradiation, *Proc. Natl. Acad. Sci. U.S.A., 72*, 219, 1975.
39. **Taylor, A. M. R., Harnden, D. G., Arlett, C. F., Harcourt, S. A., Lehmann, A. R., Stevens, S., and Bridges, B. A.**, Ataxia telangiectasia: a human mutation with abnormal radiation sensitivity, *Nature* (London), *258*, 427, 1975.
40. **Paterson, M. C., Smith, B. P., Lohmann, P. H., Anderson, A. K., and Fishman, L.**, Defective excision repair of γ-ray-damaged DNA in human (ataxia telangiectasia) fibroblasts, *Nature* (London), *260*, 444, 1976.
41. **Poon, P. K., Parker, J. W., and O'Brien, R. L.**, Faulty DNA repair following ultraviolet irradiation in Fanconi's anemia, in *Molecular Mechanisms for Repair of DNA*, Part B, Hanawalt, P. C. and Setlow, R. B., Eds., Plenum Press, New York, 1975, 821.
42. **Fujiwara, Y., Tatsumi, M., and Sasaki, M. S.**, Cross-link repair in human cells and its possible defect in Fanconi's anemia cells, *J. Mol. Biol., 113*, 635, 1977.
43. **Remson, J. F. and Cerutti, P. A.**, Deficiency of gamma-ray excision repair in skin fibroblasts from patients with Fanconi's anemia, *Proc. Natl. Acad. Sci. U.S.A., 73*, 2419, 1976.
44. **Stich, H. F., San, R. H., and Kawazoe, Y.**, Increased sensitivity of xeroderma pigmentosum cells to some chemical carcinogens and mutagens, *Mutat. Res., 17*, 127, 1973.
45. **Regan, J. D. and Setlow, R. B.**, Two forms of repair in the DNA of human cells damaged by chemical carcinogens and mutagens, *Cancer Res., 34*, 3318, 1974.
46. **Maher, V. M., Birch, N., Otto, J. R., and McCormick, J. J.**, Cytotoxicity of carcinogenic aromatic amides in normal and xeroderma pigmentosum fibroblasts with different DNA repair capabilities, *J. Natl. Cancer Inst., 54*, 1287, 1975.
47. **Maher, V. M., McCormick, J. J., Grover, P. L., and Sims, P.**, Effect of DNA repair on the cytotoxicity and mutagenicity of polycyclic hydrocarbon derivatives in normal and xeroderma pigmentosum fibroblasts, *Mutat. Res., 43*, 117, 1977.
48. **Heflich, R. H., Dorney, D. J., Maher, V. M., and McCormick, J. J.**, Reactive derivatives of benzo[a]pyrene and 7,12-dimethylbenz[a]anthracene cause S_1 nuclease sensitive sites in DNA and "UV-like" repair, *Biochem. Biophys. Res. Commun., 77*, 634, 1977.
49. **Lindahl, T.**, New class of enzymes acting on damaged DNA, *Nature* (London), *259*, 64, 1976.
50. **Ljunquist, S. and Lindahl, T.**, A mammalian endonuclease specific for apurinic sites in double-stranded DNA. I. Purification and general properties, *J. Biol. Chem., 249*, 1530, 1974.
51. **Verly, W. G., Paquette, Y., and Thibodeau, L.**, Nuclease for DNA apurinic sites may be involved in the maintenance of DNA in normal cells, *Nature* (London) *New Biol., 244*, 67, 1973.
52. **Strauss, B., Karran, P., Bose, K., and Higgins, P.**, *Abstr. 2nd Int. conference on environmental mutagens, Mutat. Res., 53*, 268, 1978.
53. **Rupp, W. D. and Howard-Flanders, P.**, Discontinuities in the DNA synthesized in an excision-defective strain of *Escherichia coli* following ultraviolet irradiation, *J. Mol. Biol., 31*, 291, 1968.
54. **Iyer, V. N. and Rupp, W. D.**, Usefulness of benzoylated napthoylated DEAE-cellulose to distinguish and fractionate double-stranded DNA bearing different extents of single-stranded regions, *Biochim. Biophys. Acta, 228*, 117, 1971.
55. **Ganeson, A. R.**, Persistance of pyrimidene dimers during post-replication repair in ultraviolet light-irradiated *Escherichia coli* K12., *J. Mol. Biol., 87*, 102, 1974.
56. **Lin, P-F., Bardwell, E. and Howard-Flanders, P.**, Initiation of genetic exchanges in λ phage-pro-phage crosses, *Proc. Natl. Acad. Sci. U.S.A., 74*, 291, 1977.
57. **Witkin, E. M. and George, D. L.**, Ultraviolet mutagenesis in *polA* and *uvrA polA* derivatives of *Escherichia coli* B/r: evidence for an inducible error-prone repair system, *Genetics* Suppl., *73*, 91, 1973.
58. **Witkin, E. M.**, Thermal enhancement of ultraviolet mutability in a *tif*-1 *uvrA* derivative of *Escherichia coli* B/r: evidence that ultraviolet mutagenesis depends upon an inducible function, *Proc. Natl. Acad. Sci. U.S.A., 71*, 1930, 1974.

59. Radman, M., Phenomenology of an inducible mutagenic DNA repair pathway in *Escherichia coli*: SOS repair hypothesis, in *Molecular and Environmental Aspects of Mutagenesis,* Prokash, L., Sherman, F., Miller, M., Lawrence, C., and Tabor, H. W., Eds., Charles C Thomas, Springfield, Ill., 1974, 128.

60. Witkin, E. M., Persistence and decay of thermo-inducible error-prone repair activity in nonfilamentous derivatives of *tif-1 Escherichia coli* B/r: the timing of some critical events in ultraviolet mutagenesis, *Mol. Gen. Genet.,* 142, 87, 1975.

61. Radman, M., SOS repair hypothesis: phenomenology of an inducible DNA repair which is accompanied by mutagenesis, in *Molecular Mechanisms for Repair of DNA,* Part A, Hanawalt, P. and Setlow, R. B., Eds., Plenum Press, New York, 1975, 355.

62. Witkin, E. M., Elevated mutability of *polA* and *uvrA polA* derivatives of *Escherichia coli* B/r at sublethal doses of ultraviolet light: evidence for an inducible error-prone repair system ("SOS repair") and its anomalous expression in these strains, *Genetics* Suppl., 79, 199, 1975.

63. Sedgwick, S. G., Inducible error-prone repair in *Escherichia coli, Proc. Natl. Acad. Sci. U.S.A.,* 72, 2753, 1975.

64. Sedgwick, S. G., Misrepair of overlapping daughter-strand gaps as a possible mechanism for UV induced mutagenesis in *uvr* strains of *Escherichia coli*: a general model for induced mutagenesis by misrepair (SOS repair) of closely spaced DNA lesions, *Mutat. Res.,* 41, 185, 1976.

65. Defais, M., Caillet-Fauquet, P., Fox, M. S., and Radman, M., Induction kinetics of mutagenic DNA activity in *E. coli* following ultraviolet irradiation, *Mol. Gen. Genet.,* 148, 125, 1976.

66. Sedgwick, S. G., Inducible error-prone repair in *Escherichia coli, Proc. Natl. Acad. Sci. U.S.A.,* 72, 2753, 1975.

67. Youngs, D. A. and Smith, K. C., Genetic control of multiple pathways of post-replicational repair in uvrB strains of *Escherichia coli* K-12, *J. Bacteriol.,* 125, 102, 1976.

68. Bridges, B. A., Recent advances in basic mutation research, *Mutat. Res.,* 44, 149, 1977.

69. McCann, J., Springarn, N. E., Kobori, J., and Ames, B., Detection of carcinogens as mutagens: bacterial tester strains with R factor plasmids, *Proc. Natl. Acad. Sci. U.S.A.,* 72, 979, 1975.

70. Kimball, R. F., Boling, M. E., and Perdue, S. W., Evidence that UV-inducible error-prone repair is absent in *Haemophilus influenzae* Rd, with a discussion of the relation to error-prone repair of alkylating-agent damage., *Mutat. Res.,* 44, 183, 1977.

71. Kondo, S., Ichikawa, H., Iwo, K., and Kato, T., Base-change mutagenesis and prophage induction in strains of *E. coli* with different DNA repair capacities, *Genetics,* 66, 187, 1970.

72. Lehmann, A. R., Postreplication repair of DNA in ultraviolet-irradiated mammalian cells, *J. Mol. Biol.,* 66, 319, 1972.

73. Buhl, S. N., Setlow, R. B., and Regan, J. D., Steps in DNA chain elongation and joining after ultraviolet irradiation of human cells, *Int. J. Radiat. Biol.,* 22, 417, 1972.

74. Fujiwara, Y., Postreplication repair of alkylation damage to DNA of mammalian cells in culture, *Cancer Res.,* 35, 2780, 1975.

75. Koerner, I., Malz, W., and Pitra, C., Dark repair processes in mammalian cells, *Biol. Zentralbl.,* 95, 561, 1976.

76. Cleaver, J. E., Xeroderma pigmentosum: variants with normal DNA repair and normal sensitivity to ultraviolet light, *J. Invest. Dermatol.,* 58, 124, 1972.

77. Koerner, I. J. and Malz, W., Postreplication gap filling in the DNA of X-ray damaged Chinese hamster cells, *Stud. Biophys.,* 51, 115, 1975.

78. Meyn, R. E. and Humphrey, R. M., Deoxyribonucleic acid synthesis in ultraviolet-light-irradiated Chinese hamster cells, *Biophys. J.,* 11, 295, 1971.

79. Lehmann, A. R. and Kirk-Bell, S., Postreplication repair of DNA in ultraviolet-irradiated mammalian cells: no gaps in DNA synthesized late after ultraviolet irradiation, *Eur. J. Biochem.,* 31, 438, 1972.

80. Hewitt, R. R. and Meyn, R. E., Concerning pyrimidine dimers as "blocks" to DNA replication in bacteria and mammalian cells, in *Molecular Mechanisms for Repair of DNA,* Part B, Hanawalt, P. and Setlow, R. B., Eds., Plenum Press, New York, 1975, 635.

81. Buhl, S. N., Setlow, R. B., and Regan, J. D., Recovery of the ability to synthesize DNA in segments of normal size at long times after ultraviolet irradiation of human cells, *Biophys. J.,* 13, 1265, 1973.

82. Maher, V. M., Dorney, D. J., Mendrala, A., Konze-Thomas, B., and McCormick, J. J., Biological relevance in diploid human cells of excision repair of lesions in DNA caused by ultraviolet light or *N*-AcO-AAF, *Proc. Am. Assoc. Cancer Res.,* 19, 70, 1978.

83. Buhl, S. N. and Regan, J. D., Repair endonuclease-sensitive sites in daughter DNA of ultraviolet irradiated human cells, *Nature* (London), 246, 484, 1973.

84. Meneghini, R. and Hanawalt, P. C., T4-endonuclease V-sensitive sites in DNA from ultraviolet irradiated human cells, *Biochim. Biophys. Acta.,* 425, 428, 1976.

85. Fujiwara Y. and Tatsumi, M., Low-level DNA exchanges in normal human and xeroderma pigmentosum cells after UV radiation, *Mutat. Res.,* 43, 279, 1977.

86. **Higgins, N. P., Kato, K., and Strauss, B.,** A model for replication repair in mammalian cells, *J. Mol. Biol.,* 101, 417, 1976.
87. **Fujiwara, Y. and Tatsumi, M.,** Replicative by-pass repair of ultraviolet damage to DNA of mammalian cells: caffeine sensitive and caffeine resistant mechanisms, *Mutat. Res.,* 37, 91, 1976.
88. **D'Ambrosio, S. M. and Setlow, R. B.,** Enhancement of postreplicative repair in Chinese hamster cells, *Proc. Natl. Acad. Sci. U.S.A.,* 73, 2396, 1976.
89. **Chang, C. C., d'Ambrosio, S. M., Schultz, R., Trosko, J. E., and Setlow, R. B.,** Modification of UV-induced mutation frequencies in Chinese hamster cells by dose fractionation, cycloheximide and caffeine treatments, *Mutat. Res.,* 52, 231, 1978.
90. **Cole, R. S.,** Inactivation of *Escherichia coli* F′episomes at transfer and bacteriophage lambda by psoralen plus 360-nm light: significance of deoxyribonucleic acid cross-links, *J. Bacteriol.,* 107, 846, 1971.
91. **Hariharan, P. V. and Cerutti, P. A.,** Excision of ultraviolet and gamma ray products of the 5,6-dihydroxy-dihydrothymine type by nuclear preparations of xeroderma cells, *Biochim. Biophys. Acta,* 447, 375, 1976.
92. **Remsen, J. F., Cerutti, P. A.,** Excision of gamma ray-induced thymine lesions by preparations from ataxia telangiectasia fibroblasts, *Mutat. Res.,* 43, 139, 1977.
93. **Feldman, R. S. and Grossman, L.,** A DNA binding protein from human placenta specific for ultraviolet damaged DNA, *Biochemistry,* 15, 2402, 1976.
94. **Dean, C. J.,** DNA strand breakage in cells irradiated with X-rays, *Nature* (London), 222, 1042, 1969.
95. **Sawada, S. and Okada, S.,** Rejoining of single-strand breaks of DNA in cultured mammalian cells, *Radiat. Res.,* 41, 145, 1970.
96. **Epstein, J., Williams, J. R., and Little, J. B.,** Rate of DNA repair in progeric and normal human fibroblasts, *Biochem. Biophys. Res. Commun.,* 59, 850, 1974.
97. **Regan, J. D. and Setlow, R. B.,** DNA repair in human progeroid cells, *Biochem. Biophys. Res. Commun.,* 59, 858, 1974.
98. **Bradley, M. O., Erickson, L. C., and Kohn, K. W.,** Normal DNA strand rejoining and absence of DNA cross-linking in progeroid and aging human cells, *Mutat. Res.,* 37, 279, 1977.
99. **Carry, P. M. and Cole, A.,** Double-strand joining in mammalian DNA, *Nature,* (London) *New Biol.,* 245, 100, 1973.
100. **Harm, H.,** Repair of UV-irradiated biological systems: photoreactivation, in *Photochemistry and Photobiology of Nucleic Acids,* Vol. 2, Wang, S. Y. Ed., Academic Press, New York, 1966, 219.
101. **Witkin, E. M.,** Radiation induced mutations and their repair, *Science,* 152, 1345, 1966.
102. **Bridges, B. A. and Munson, R. J.,** Excision repair of DNA damage in an auxotrophic strain of E. coli., *Biochem. Biophys. Res. Commun.,* 22, 268, 1966.
103. **Hill, R. F.,** Ultraviolet-induced lethality and reversion to prototrophy in *Escherichia coli* strains with normal and reduced dark repair ability, *Photochem. Photobiol.,* 4, 563, 1965.
104. **Maher, V. M. and McCormick, J. J.,** Effect of DNA repair on the cytotoxicity and mutagenicity of UV irradiation and of chemical carcinogens in normal and xeroderma pigmentosum cells, in *Biology of Radiation Carcinogenesis,* Yuhas, J. M., Tennant, R. W., and Regan, J. B., Eds., Raven Press, New York, 1976, 129.
105. **Robbins, J. H., Kraemer, K. H., Lutzner, M. A., Festoff, B. W., and Coon, H. G.,** Xeroderma pigmentosum — an inherited disease with sun sensitivity, multiple cutaneous neoplasms and abnormal DNA repair, *Ann. Intern. Med.,* 80, 221, 1974.
106. **Maher, V. M., Dorney, D. J., Mendrala, A. L., Konze-Thomas, B., and McCormick, J. J.,** DNA excision repair processes in human cells can eliminate the cytotoxic and mutagenic consequences of ultraviolet irradiation, *Mutat. Res.,* in press.
107. Effects of liquid holding on cell killing, and mutation induction in normal and repair-deficient human cell strains, in *DNA Repair Mechanisms,* Hanawalt, P. C., Friedberg, E. C., and Fox, C. F., Eds., Academic Press, New York, 1978, 729.
108. **Maher, V. M., Ouellette, L. M., Curren, R. D., and McCormick, J. J.,** Frequency of ultraviolet light-induced mutations is higher in xeroderma pigmentosum variant cells than in normal human cells, *Nature* (London), 201, 593, 1976.
109. **Maher, V. M., Ouellette, L. M., Mittlestat, M., and McCormick, J. J.,** Synergistic effect of caffeine on the cytotoxicity of ultraviolet irradiation and of hydrocarbon epoxides in strains of xeroderma pigmentosum, *Nature* (London), 258, 760, 1975.
110. **Maher, V. M., Ouellette, L. M., Curren, R. D., and McCormick, J. J.,** Caffeine enhancement of the cytotoxic and mutagenic effect of ultraviolet irradiation in a xeroderma pigmentosum variant strain of human cells, *Biochem. Biophys. Res. Commun.,* 71, 228, 1976.
111. **Roberts, J. J. and Sturrock, J. E.,** Enhancement by caffeine of N-methyl-N-nitrosourea induced mutations and chromosome aberrations in Chinese hamster cells, *Mutat. Res.,* 20, 243, 1973.
112. **Roberts, J. J., Sturrock, J. E., and Ward, K. N.,** The enhancement by caffeine of alkylation induced cell death, mutations and chromosomal aberrations in Chinese hamster cells, as a result of inhibition of postreplication DNA repair, *Mutat. Res.,* 26, 129, 1974.

113. **Arlett, C. F. and Harcourt, S. A.,** Expression time and spontaneous mutability in the estimation of induced mutation frequency following treatment of Chinese hamster cells by ultraviolet light, *Mutat. Res.,* 16, 301, 1972.

114. **Fox, M.,** Factors affecting the quantitation of dose response curves for mutation induction in V79 Chinese hamster cells after exposure to chemical and physical mutagens, *Mutat. Res.,* 29, 449, 1975.

115. **Chang, C. C., Philipps, C., Trosko, J. E., and Hart, R. W.,** Mutagenic and epigenetic influence of caffeine on the frequencies of UV-induced ouabain-resistant Chinese hamster cells, *Mutat. Res.,* 45, 125, 1977.

116. **Fox, M. and McMillan, S.,** Relationship between caffeine sensitive and resistant DNA repair, cell lethality and mutagenesis in mammalian cell after X-rays and alkylating agents, *Stud. Biophys.,* 61, 71, 1977.

117. **Kato, H.,** Induction of sister chromatid exchanges by UV light and its inhibition by caffeine, *Exp. Cell Res.,* 82, 383, 1973.

118. **Sasaki, M. S.,** Sister chromatid exchange and chromatid interchange as possible manifestations of different DNA repair processes, *Nature* (London), 269, 623, 1977.

119. **Kakunaga, T.,** Neoplastic transformation of human diploid fibroblast cells by chemical carcinogens, *Proc. Natl., Acad. Sci. U.S.A.,* 75, 1334, 1978.

120. **Kakunaga, T.,** A quantitative system for assay of malignant transformation by chemical carcinogens using a clone derived from BALB/3T, *Int. J. Cancer,* 12, 463, 1973.

121. **Kakunaga, T.,** Requirement for cell replication in the fixation and expression of the transformed state in mouse cells treated with 4-nitro-quinoline-1-oxide, *Int. J. Cancer,* 14, 736, 1974.

122. **Kakunaga, T.,** The role of cell division in the malignant transformation of mouse cells treated with 3-methylcholanthrene, *Cancer Res.* 35, 1637, 1975.

123. **Ikenaga, M. and Kakunaga, T.,** Excision of 4-nitroquinoline-1-oxide damage and transformation in mouse cells, *Cancer Res.,* 37, 3672, 1977.

124. **Terzaghi, M. and Little, J. H. B.,** Repair of potentially lethal radiation damage in mammalian cells is associated with enhancement of malignant transformation, *Nature* (London) 253, 548, 1975.

125. **Donovan, P. J. and Di Paolo, J. A.,** Caffeine enhancement of chemical carcinogen-induced transformation of culture Syrian hamster cells, *Cancer Res.,* 34, 2720, 1974.

126. **Trosko, J. E., Frank, P., Chu, E. H. Y., and Becker, J. E.,** Caffeine inhibition of postreplication repair of N-acetoxy-2-acetylaminofluorene-damaged DNA in Chinese hamster cells, *Cancer Res.,* 33, 2444, 1973.

127. **Kakunaga, T.,** Caffeine inhibits cell transformation by 4-nitroquinoline-1-oxide, *Nature* (London), 258, 248, 1975.

128. **Hart, R. W., Setlow, R. B., and Woodhead, A. D.,** Evidence that pyrimidine dimers in DNA can give rise to tumors, *Proc. Natl. Acad. Sci. U.S.A.,* 74, 5574, 1977.

129. **Trosko, J. E., Krause, D., and Isoun, M.,** Sunlight-induced pyrimidine dimers in human cells *in vitro, Nature* (London), 228, 358, 1970.

130. **Takebe, H., Miki, Y., Kozuka, T., Furuyama, J., Tanaka, K., Sasaki, M., Fujiwara, Y., and Akiba, H.,** DNA repair characteristics and skin cancers of xeroderma pigmentosum patients in Japan, *Cancer Res.,* 37, 490, 1977.

131. **Urbach, F., Ross, D. B., and Bonnem, M.,** Genetic and environmental interactions in skin carcinogenesis, in *Environment and Cancer: A Collection of Papers,* 24th Symp. on Fundamental Cancer Res., M. D. Anderson Hospital and Tumor Institute, Williams & Wilkins, Baltimore, 1971, 355.

132. **Goth, R. and Rajewsky, M. F.,** Persistence of O^6-ethylguanine in rat brain DNA: correlation with nervous system specific carcinogenesis by ethylnitrosourea, *Proc. Natl. Acad. Sci. U.S.A.,* 71, 639, 1974.

133. **Loveless, A.,** Possible relevance of O-6 alkylation of deoxyguanosone to the mutagenicity and carcinogenicity of nitrosamines and nitrosamides, *Nature* (London), 223, 206, 1969.

134. **Kleihues, P. and Margison, G. P.,** Carcinogenicity of N-methyl-N-nitrosourea: possible role of repair excision of O^6-methylguanine from DNA, *J. Nat. Cancer Inst.,* 53, 1839, 1974.

135. **Buechler, J. and Kleihues, P.,** Excision of O^6-methylguanine from DNA of various mouse tissues following a single injection of N-methyl-N-nitrosourea, *Chem. Biol. Interact.* 16, 325, 1977.

136. **Rajewsky, M. F., Augenlicht, L. H., Biessman, H., Goth, R., Husler, D. F., Laerum, O. D., and Lomakina, L. Y.,** Nervous system-specific carcinogenesis by ethylnitrosourea in the rat: molecular and cellular aspects, in *Cold Spring Harbor Conferences on Cell Proliferation,* in press.

137. **Magee, P. N. and Barnes, J. M.,** Induction of kidney tumours in the rat with dimethylnitrosamine (N-nitroso-dimethylamine), *J. Pathol. Bacteriol.,* 84, 19, 1962.

138. **Swann, P. F. and McLean, A. E. M.,** Cellular injury and carcinogenesis. The effect of a protein-free, high-carbohydrate diet on the metabolism of dimethylnitrosamine in the rat, *Biochem. J.,* 124, 283, 1971.

139. **Nicoll, J. W., Swann, P. F., and Pegg, A.,** Effect of dimethylnitrosamine on persistence of methylated guanines in rat liver and kidney DNA, *Nature* (London), 254, 261, 1975.

140. **Craddock, V. M.**, Stability of deoxyribonucleic acid methylated in the intact animal by administration of dimethylnitrosamine, *Biochem. J.*, 111, 497, 1967.

141. **Magee, P. N., Swann, P. F., Mohr, U., Resnik, G., and Green, U.**, Possible repair of carcinogenesis by nitroso compounds, in *Fundamentals in Cancer Prevention*, Magee, P. N., Takayama, S., Sugimura, T., and Matsushima, T., Eds., University of Tokyo Press, Tokyo, 1976, 281.

142. **Frei, J. V. and Venitt, S.**, Chromosome damage in the bone marrow of mice treated with the methylating agents methyl methanesulfonate and N-methyl-N-nitrosourea in the presence or absence of caffeine and its relationship with thymoma induction, *Mutat. Res.*, 29, 89, 1975.

143. **Craddock, V. M.**, Replication and repair of DNA in livers of rats treated with dimethylnitrosamine and with methyl methanesulfonate, in *Fundamentals in Cancer Prevention*, Magee, P. N., Takayama, S., Sugimura, T., and Matsushima, T., Eds., University of Tokyo Press, Tokyo, 1976, 293.

144. **Zajdela, F. and Latarjet, R.**, Effet inhibiteur de la cafeine sur l'induction de cancers cutanes par les rayons ultraviolets chez la souris, *C. R. Acad. Sci.*, 277, 1073, 1973.

145. **Nomura, T.**, Diminution of tumorigenesis initiated by 4-nitroquinoline-1-oxide by post-treatment with caffeine in mice., *Nature (London)*, 260, 547, 1976.

146. **Kondo, S.**, A test for mutation theory of cancer: carcinogenesis by misrepair of DNA damaged by 4-nitroquinoline-1-oxide, *Br. J. Cancer*, 35, 595, 1977.

147. **Sutherland, B. M., Rice, M., and Wagner, E. K.**, Xeroderma pigmentosum cells contain low levels of photoreactivating enzyme, *Proc. Natl. Acad. Sci. U.S.A.*, 72, 103, 1975.

148. **Kuhnlein, U., Penhoet, E. E., and Linn, S.**, An altered apurinic DNA endonuclease activity in group A and group D xeroderma pigmentosum fibroblasts, *Proc. Natl. Acad. Sci. U.S.A.*, 73, 1169, 1976.

149. **Knudsen, A. G., Jr.**, Mutation and human cancer, *Adv. Cancer Res.*, 17, 317, 1973.

150. **German, J.**, Genes which increase chromosomal instability in somatic cells and predispose to cancer, in *Progress in Medical Genetics*, Vol. 8, Grune & Stratton, New York, 1972, 61.

151. **Howard-Flanders, P.**, personal communication, 1977.

152. **Arlett, C. F., Cox, R., and Simons, J. W. I. M.**, personal communication, 1977.

153. **Kato, T., Rothman, R. H., and Clark, A. J.**, Analysis of the role of recombination and repair in mutagenesis of *Escherichia coli* UV irradiation, *Genetics*, 87, 1, 1977.

Chapter 6

DNA — THE CRITICAL CELLULAR TARGET IN CHEMICAL CARCINOGENESIS?

Hans Marquardt

TABLE OF CONTENTS

I. INTRODUCTION

A tumor cell is a persistently altered cell against the growth of which there is no adequate control mechanism in the host. Thus, during the transition from a normal to a tumor cell, there occurs a profound and permanent change that is transmitted from cell to cell for many generations, allowing the tumor cell to be autonomous, i.e., to determine its own activities irrespective of the laws that so precisely govern the growth of normal cells.[1] Therefore, it seems inescapable that the carcinogen must alter the expression of the genome and thus the phenotype. The question that needs to be answered is whether this alteration of expression of the genome results from a somatic mutation or from epigenetic alterations or from a combination of both mechanisms.

II. CARCINOGENESIS — INITIATION BY SOMATIC MUTATION

The thesis that a single chromosomal or mutational event in somatic cells is the specific change reponsible for tumorigenesis has become known as the "somatic mutation theory". This theory was put forward by Boveri[2] and by Bauer[3] long before there was knowledge either of the molecular structure of the genetic material or of the chemical nature of carcinogens and has been sustained ever since, but with fluctuating levels of support. It accounts for the monoclonal character of cancer as well as for the inheritability and the permanence of the malignant change. DNA alterations, as an efficient means for preserving and perpetuating new information, remain the most logical mechanism for the initiation of cancer. The genetic susceptibility to certain forms of cancer and the occurrence of some familial cancers are also consistent with the hypothesis that the initiation process proceeds via a genetic change.[4] From analyses of such disorders, Knudson has suggested that the initiation of carcinogenesis results from at least two mutational events, the first of which may or may not be inherited.[4] Similarly, experimental carcinogenesis studies have led to the suggestion that two mutations are required for initiation and five to six mutations for further development of carcinogenesis.[5,6] In addition, fibroblasts derived from patients suffering from genetic disorders such as von Recklinghausen's disease,[7] Down's syndrome,[8] Fanconi's anemia,[9] and familial polyposis[10] appear to be more easily transformed by viruses or by chemicals than fibroblasts from normal individuals.

A. Carcinogens and Mutation

Carcinogenesis and mutagenesis are complex cellular processes which are superficially similar in that each produces heritable changes. Chemical carcinogens and mutagens also have much in common and the active forms of both are frequently electrophilic reactants which are often generated through metabolism.[11] Such reactants produce various forms of DNA damage, such as chromosomal aberrations (it should be noted that carcinogen-specific chromosomal changes have been observed[12]), frameshift mutations, and missense mutations.[13] Such studies are just beginning, and it is not yet possible to find any correlation between the induction of these varied types of genetic damage and neoplastic transformation by chemicals. Prior to 1960, the correlation between the carcinogenic and mutagenic properties of chemicals was poor, but the situation changed dramatically following the discovery that many such chemicals require metabolic activation by microsomal and other enzymes before they become biologically active.[11] This has led to the development of appropriate mutagenesis tests using microbial and mammalian cell systems that incorporate a metabolic activation step and to results that suggest that many, and perhaps all, chemical carcinogens are mutagens in their ultimate reactive forms, and that many but not all chemical mutagens are potential carcinogens.[14] At present, the exceptions among the mutagens include some base analogs, nitrous acid and acridine dyes,[14] and some diol-epoxides of benzo[a]pyrene.[15] Parenthetically, it should be noted that virus-induced oncogenesis also involves a change in host cell DNA,[16] and that viruses can induce mutations, too.[16-18] However, while this general qualitative correlation exists, quantitatively, a strong mutagen is not necessarily also a strong carcinogen. For instance, the strong skin carcinogen, benzo[a]pyrene-7,8-oxide, is a weak mutagen, while the weak carcinogen, benzo[a]pyrene-4,5-oxide, is a potent mutagen.[19,20] However, it should also be noted that, at present, attempts to correlate mutagenic and oncogenic potencies of chemicals are beset by practical difficulties. No test system exists in which both processes can be studied simultaneously in one cloned cell line (see below), and no one single optimal mutation assay is available. Thus, some compounds are mutagenic in one test, but not in another assay: (a) in the Ames test with *Salmonella typhimurium*, as many as 31% of the carcinogens tested, such as urethan, ethionine, and dimethylhydrazine, give "false negative" results;[21-23] (b) the potent mutagen and carcinogen, *N*-methyl-*N*'-nitro-*N*-nitrosoguanidine, is barely mutagenic in a host-mediated assay using *Neurospora conidia;*[13] (c) *N*-hydroxy-1-naphthylamine is mutagenic in *Escherichia coli* but nonmutagenic in bacteriophage T4;[24] and (d) the anthracycline antitumor antibiotic, 4-demethoxydaunomycin, is strongly mutagenic in *S. typhimurium* but nonmutagenic in an assay employing mammalian cells in vitro.[25] Perhaps even more disturbing (at least from the standpoint of drug development) are the 17% "false-positive results" with noncarcinogens found when the Ames test is used.[21] Therefore, at present, mutagenesis testing requires the use of a battery of different test assays. The difficulties one encounters in correlating the mutagenic and oncogenic potential of chemicals, which mostly require microsomal activation, are further exacerbated by the great individual- and species-related variations in the activity of microsomal metabolism.[26] Nevertheless, the correlation so far observed between both processes appears convincing. However, the interpretation of this correlation in terms of mechanisms of action of chemical carcinogenesis remains a difficult problem. While even a one-to-one correlation cannot be taken as proof that carcinogenesis is a mutational event, this concept is an attractive one and is supported by the following further evidence.

B. Carcinogen Interactions with DNA

1. Covalent Interaction of Carcinogens with Nuclear DNA and Its Repair

In 1947 the Millers made the important discovery that hepatocarcinogenic aminoazo dyes become covalently bound to cellular proteins,[27] and in 1961 Heidelberger and Davenport reported for the first time that carcinogenic hydrocarbons also become bound covalently to mouse skin DNA following local application.[28] Since then, it has become axiomatic that most chemical carcinogens in their ultimate form, i.e., after metabolic activation, are electrophilic and react covalently with negatively charged regions in host cell DNA[11,29] and often interfere with its synthesis.[30] The nature of the reactions of various chemical carcinogens with DNA has been described in detail in other chapters in this volume. Many types of DNA damage have thus been produced by physical or by chemical agents. However, attempts to correlate certain types of damage with carcinogenicity have not yet been successful. While, qualitatively, ultimate carcinogens do react with DNA, quantitatively, the capacity of carcinogens to react with DNA does not correlate well with their carcinogenic potency. Magee and Barnes, for instance, had found no correlation between the extent of in vitro methylation of the N^7 of guanine and the biological activities of carcinogenic and noncarcinogenic methylating agents.[31] It was subsequently suggested that O^6-alkylguanine may be among those derivatives most likely to be involved in the initiation of malignant transformation, since it leads to mispairing and thus can be considered promutagenic.[32] However, the formation and persistence of O^6-alkylguanines after chemical treatment does not correlate well with the carcinogenic activity of these chemicals, as will also be discussed later. With polycyclic hydrocarbons, the noncarcinogenic dibenz[a,c]anthracene and the carcinogenic dibenz[a,h]anthracene interact equally well with DNA[33] and the nontransforming K-region phenol of dibenz[a,h]anthracene showed a greater capacity to interact with DNA than the transforming K-region epoxide.[34] Similarly, a comparison between DNA binding and induction of malignant transformation by 7,12-dimethylbenz[a]anthracene and its K-region oxide at 4 hr after treatment showed no correlation at all. At that time after treatment, when the binding of the parent hydrocarbon to DNA is minimal and that of its K-region oxide maximal (Figure 1), we observed transformation almost exclusively with the parent hydrocarbon.[35] While the initiation of malignant transformation by the K-region oxide of 7,12-dimethylbenz[a]anthracene is cell-cycle dependent (see below), the binding to DNA of this agent does not show cell-cycle-dependent variations (Figure 2). In the case of aflatoxins, too, binding capacity and oncogenicity are poorly correlated.[36] Thus, while total binding of carcinogens to DNA does not correlate well quantitatively with their carcinogenic potency and though covalent binding of carcinogens to macromolecules can often be detected in tissues apart from those in which tumors are induced, the fact that covalent binding to cellular DNA has been found for almost all carcinogens with their enormous variation in chemical structure is, nevertheless, in itself evidence that

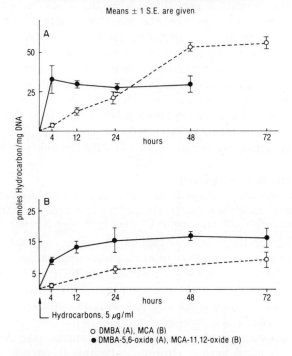

TIME COURSE OF THE BINDING OF DMBA AND MCA AND
THEIR RESPECTIVE K-REGION EPOXIDES TO DNA OF M2 CELLS

Means ± 1 S.E. are given

o DMBA (A), MCA (B)
● DMBA-5,6-oxide (A), MCA-11,12-oxide (B)

FIGURE 1.   Time course of the binding of tritiated 7,12-
dimethylbenz[*a*]anthracene (DMBA), methylcholanthrene
(MCA), and their respective K-region epoxides to the DNA
of logarithmically growing cultures of M2 mouse fibroblasts. Means ± standard error are given. (From Marquardt, H., *Screening Tests in Chemical Carcinogenesis*,
IARC Publ. No. 12, Montesano, R., Bartsch, H., and Tomatis, L. Eds., International Agency for Research on Cancer, Lyon, 1976, 389. With permission).

this binding may be necessary for tumor induction. It seems likely that very specific
binding sites on DNA, which have not yet been elucidated, play an important role.[37,38]

Repair of carcinogen-induced DNA damage may be as important for tumor development as the production of the initial DNA damage, i.e., as the ability of chemicals
to covalently react with DNA. Since one can assume that no species or individual
organisms have DNA molecules that are refractory to deleterious environmental
agents, one or more DNA repair systems must be available for the maintenance of
genetic integrity. Indeed, several forms of DNA repair mechanisms have been extensively characterized in microorganisms and to a lesser extent in mammalian cells,[6] and
these are discussed in detail in Volume II, Chapters 4 and 5. Circumstantial evidence
links such mechanisms to mutagenesis and carcinogenesis. In man, for instance, xeroderma pigmentosum, a syndrome which is clinically characterized by hypersensitivity
of the skin to solar radiation and a high incidence of multiple skin carcinomas, is
biochemically characterized by various DNA repair deficiencies.[6] Fibroblasts from patients with this[39,40] and similar diseases, such as Fanconi's anemia[6] or ataxia telangiectasia,[41] are more susceptible than normal human fibroblasts to mutagenesis induced
by irradiation or some chemical agents. Likewise, the high incidence of malignanacies
in xeroderma pigmentosum patients may be a consequence of DNA repair deficiencies.
DNA repair has been shown to affect oncogenesis. Thus, Setlow and co-workers were

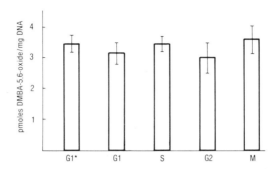

BINDING OF DMBA-5,6-OXIDE TO DNA OF M2 CELLS AT DIFFERENT TIMES AFTER RELEASE OF DOUBLE-THYMIDINE-BLOCK

DMBA-5,6-oxide, 5 μg/ml for 30 min; means ± 1 S.E. are given.

FIGURE 2.   The binding of tritiated 7,12-dimethylbenz[-a]anthracene 5,6-oxide to the DNA of synchronized M2 mouse fibroblasts. Cells were synchronized by the double-thymidine block and treated, for 30 min, with 5 μg/ml of the epoxide; means ± standard error are given. (From Marquardt, H., *Screening Tests in Chemical Carcinogenesis*, IARC Publ. No. 12, Montesano, R., Bartsch, H., and Tomatis, L., Eds., International Agency for Research on Cancer, Lyon, 1976, 389. With permission.)

able to prevent vent UV-irradiation-induced malignant transformation in vitro of fish thyroid cells by activating the photoreactivation repair process.[42] The possibility that DNA repair processes may affect oncogenesis is further demonstrated by the biological activities of caffeine. Caffeine, which also inhibits error-prone "postreplication repair" in mammalian cells,[6] was shown to inhibit malignant transformation in vitro[43] and lung tumorigenesis in vivo[44] induced by 4-nitroquinoline-1-oxide. In other experiments, however caffeine enhanced malignant transformation induced by a variety of chemical carcinogens,[45] and Heidelberger and co-workers were unable to find a correlation between the production and repair of single-stranded breaks in the DNA and malignant transformation in vitro produced by N-methyl-N-nitro-N-nitrosoguanidine in asynchronous and in synchronized mouse fibroblasts.[46].

Recently, much attention has been given to the suggestion that the persistence, i.e., lack of repair, of the promutagenic miscoding bases,[47] O^6-methylguanine or O^6-ethylguanine,[32] in target tissues for particular chemical carcinogens may be important in oncogenesis.[48-50] Thus, Craddock initially found that O^6-methylguanine is present in liver DNA following in vivo administration of the carcinogenic dimethylnitrosamine, but not following the noncarcinogenic methyl methanesulfonate.[51] However, in her more recent studies, she has been unable to find differences in extent and duration of O^6-methylguanine formation in rat liver between dimethylnitrosamine treatment at 6 hr after partial hepatectomy, which gives a low hepatoma incidence, and at 24 hr after partial hepatectomy, which gives high hepatoma incidence.[52] This and other recent studies[53-56] argue against the attractive hypothesis that O^6-alkylation of guanine and its persistence is responsible for the carcinogenic action of alkylating agents.

Finally, a good correlation has been found between the extent of repair synthesis provoked by, and the carcinogenic activity of, a variety of chemicals,[57] and in addition, sensitivity to chemical transformation has been related to inability to repair carcinogen-induced DNA lesions.[58] It appears, therefore, that this is similar to the situation that exists with the ability of chemical carcinogens to covalently interact with DNA in that this apparently good correlation between the carcinogenic activities of chemicals and the repair that they induce provides evidence that DNA repair may be involved in chemical carcinogenesis and, consequently, that DNA may be the primary macromolecular target of chemical carcinogens.

2. Noncovalent Interactions of Carcinogens with Nuclear DNA

It is conceivable that chemical carcinogenesis may also result from a noncovalent interaction between chemical carcinogens and DNA. There is extensive literature on the noncovalent binding to DNA of compounds possessing biological activity.[29] Such noncovalent interactions may take the form of intercalation or of external binding of the carcinogen. In this context, it must also be remembered that it has not yet been possible to demonstrate covalent linkage to DNA for chemical carcinogens like tricycloquinazoline,[59] purine-N-oxides,[60] and anthracycline antibiotics.[61] The role of noncovalent interaction in chemical carcinogenesis, however, is in dispute. There is no strong relationship between the carcinogenicity of various polycyclic hydrocarbons and their ability to intercalate into DNA in vitro,[29] and compounds such as the acridine dyes and ethidium bromide, which bind firmly but noncovalently to macromolecules, are not carcinogens.[62] On the other hand, our own most recent results indicate that the intercalation of the antitumor antibiotic, adriamycin, into DNA without covalent interaction may initiate oncogenesis.[61] We had reported that adriamycin is a strong oncogen, inducing mammary tumors in rats as well as in vitro mutagenesis and malignant transformation in mammalian cells.[25,30] Adriamycin binds to DNA, most probably by intercalation,[63] and it can be removed from DNA by extraction of the complex with water-saturated phenol.[64] We now find that, in a test tube assay, addition of a rat liver microsomal or a rat liver postmitochondrial preparation will not facilitate DNA binding that is resistant to extraction with water-saturated phenol, but does reduce the noncovalent interaction between the agent and DNA[61] (Tables 1 and 2). In accordance with these findings, addition of rat liver postmitochondrial preparations

TABLE 1

Effect of a Rat Liver Postmitochondrial Preparation
on Adriamycin-DNA Interactions

Adriamycin (μg/ml)	Addition	nmoles [a] ^{3}H-adriamycin per mg DNA after incubation[b] (min)			
		5	15	30	60
50	—	29	35	—	49
100	—	51	64	—	81
200	—	88	108	123	155
200	heat-inactivated S9[c]	—	112	121	151
200	active S9	—	117	94	26

[a] ^{3}H-adriamycin (sp.act., 13.8 μCi/μmole). Gift of Dr. F. Arcamone, Farmitalia, Italy.

[b] Four milligrams calf thymus DNA per 6 ml incubation mixture.

[c] S9, postmitochondrial preparation, prepared according to McCann et al.[22] from rat liver and added so as to give 5 mg protein per ml incubation mixture.

TABLE 2

Effect of Purified Rat Liver Microsomes on Adriamycin-DNA Interactions

Adriamycin (μg/ml)	Addition	nmoles ^{3}H-adriamycin[a] per mg DNA after incubation[b] (min)		
		5	60	300
100	Heat-inactivated microsomes	44, 46, 65	59, 59, 77	50, 54, 81
100	Microsomes without cofactors	42, 52	49, 66	58
100	Microsomes and cofactors			
	0.6 mg protein/ml	53, 55	31, 33	19, 21
	1.2 mg protein/ml	48, 52, 66	21, 23, 33	1, 4, 17
	2.4 mg protein/ml	49	25	16

[a] ^{3}H-adriamycin (specific activity, 13.8 μCi/μmole). Gift of Dr. F. Arcamone, Farmitalia, Italy.

[b] Four milligrams calf thymus DNA per 6 ml incubation mixture.

to a bacterial mutagenesis assay (Table 3) and induction of microsomal enzyme activity in mouse M2 fibroblasts (Table 4) decreases the ability of adriamycin to induce mutagenesis and malignant transformation, respectively.[61] Conversely, inhibition of microsomal enzyme activity in mouse cells increases the yield of drug-induced transformants[61] (Table 4). These data indicate that adriamycin is detoxified, not activated, by microsomal metabolism and permit, for the first time, the suggestion that a noncovalent DNA interaction may also be responsible for initiation of chemical carcinogenesis. These studies are being continued in our laboratory in collaboration with Dr. A. Feinberg.

3. Interactions of Carcinogens with Replicating Nuclear DNA

The somatic mutation theory of chemical carcinogenesis is further supported by observations indicating that proliferating cells, possibly even replicating DNA, may be the initial site of attack by chemical carcinogens.[65-68] Haddow et al. were the first to observe the inhibitory effect of polycyclic hydrocarbons on body growth.[69] Later, the selective cytotoxic effect of 7,12-dimethylbenz[a]anthracene[70] as well as of antitumor agents[71] on cell renewal systems was observed by various groups. Indeed, induction of inhibition of DNA synthesis in such a cell renewal system, i.e., in mouse testis, has been suggested as a simple mammalian assay for chemical carcinogens and mutagens,[72,73] and this author certainly agrees that this merits further investigation. Cytotoxic effects of chemicals in cell renewal systems, which often indicate an early interference with DNA synthesis, frequently suggest the possibility that a mutagenic/ carcinogenic hazard exists.

Thus, there is evidence, though still indirect and incomplete, which suggests that DNA replication and cell division may play an important role in the process of malignant transformation.[74,75] Clinical and experimental experience indicates that malignant growth in vivo does not occur in cell systems normally lacking proliferating cells or cells which can be triggered back into cycle from a nonproliferative state. The tumorigenicity of many oncogenic agents appears to be more pronounced in embryonic or neonatal tissues with a high rate of cell proliferation,[76] in some adult tissues with a higher proliferation rate such as bone marrow, Zymbal's gland, ovary, mammary gland, and skin during wound healing,[65] and in adult tissues which have been stimu-

TABLE 3

Effect of Rat Liver Postmitochondrial Preparations on Adriamycin-Induced Bacterial Mutagenesis

Adriamycin (μg/plate)	His+ Revertants per 10⁶ Survivors	
	Without S9	With S9
0	1.6	0.5
0.2	1.6	1.4
2	5.7	1.3
10	24.2	5.3
20	65.4	14.9
30	122.5	26.7
40	272.3	119.0

Note: Procedures were carried out as described by McCann et al.[22] using *Salmonella typhimurium*, strain TA98.

TABLE 4

Effect of Inducers and Inhibitors of Microsomal Enzyme Activity on Adriamycin-Induced Cytotoxicity and Malignant Transformation in Mouse M2 Fibroblasts

	Plating Efficiency (%) after Adriamycin (μg/mℓ)				Transformed Foci/No. of Treated Dishes after Adriamycin (μg/mℓ)			
Pretreatment	0	0.001	0.005	0.01	0	0.001	0.005	0.01
None	23	18	14	8	0/12	6/12	12/12	8/12
PPO (2.5 μg/mℓ)	22	23	21	19	0/12	0/12	3/12	1/12
ANF (1.5 μg/mℓ)	23	12	9	1	0/12	21/12	17/12	—
SKF-525A (10 μg/mℓ)	19	18	4	0	0/12	11/12	26/12	—

Note: Inducer, PPO (2,5-diphenyloxazole), was present in cultures only during the 24 hr preceding adriamycin treatment. Inhibitors, SKF-525A and ANF (α-naphthoflavone), were present during that time and during the 24-hr period of adriamycin treatment. For methods, see Marquardt.[30]

lated to divide[68,74,77-99] (Table 5). It must also be pointed out that a property common to many chemical carcinogens applied in vivo or in vitro is the causation of an elevated level of DNA synthesis and cell proliferation in the respective target cell systems.[75,100] Our own in vivo results with 7,12-dimethylbenz[a]anthracene in regenerating rat liver have demonstrated an increased ability of the carcinogen to bind to replicating DNA, leading to the suggestion that replicating DNA may be the primary target of chemical carcinogens.[65-67] It should also be mentioned, however, that there are some studies reporting an equal[101,102] or even a decreased[103] tumor yield in tissues which were treated with carcinogens during regeneration.

From tissue culture studies, it is well known that both mutagenesis and oncogenesis require DNA replication for initiation and expression. Expression of chemical mutagenesis depends on the elapse of an optimal expression time during which the treated

TABLE 5

Examples of Increases in Carcinogenesis in Tissues Stimulated to Divide

Tissue	Stimulus	Carcinogen	Ref.
Liver	Regeneration	Urethan	74, 77—80
		Ethyl methanesulfonate	78, 81, 83
		Dimethylnitrosamine	82, 85
		Diethylnitrosamine	85
		Nitrosoguanidine	85
		Methylnitrosourea	86
		Dimethylaminoazobenzene	87
		Dimethylbenz[a]anthracene	68, 80
	Schistoma infection	Hycanthone	88
Lung	Butylated hydroxytoluene	Urethan	89
Intestine	Wound	Dimethylhydrazine	90
Kidney	Unilateral nephrectomy	Dimethylnitrosamine	91—93
Urinary bladder	Glass bead implantation	Bracken fern	94
	Stone formation	Ethylsulphonyl naphthalenesulfonamide	95, 96
		Saccharine	97
Gall bladder	Cholesterol pellet implantation	Dimethylnitrosamine	98
Bone marrow	Erythropoietin	Dimethylbenz[a]anthracene	99

cells can divide.[104] Similarly, in cultures in which DNA synthesis is inhibited, malignant transformation by viruses,[105,106] X-rays,[107] and chemicals[108-110] does not occur. Apparently, some temporary change is converted into a stable change in either genetic information or in its expression by the replication of some cellular constituent, presumably DNA. This conclusion may possibly explain the higher susceptibility (discussed above) of S-phase cells to the neoplastic change: alterations of the DNA occurring while the DNA is replicating are more likely to become fixed in the genome before they can be repaired.[110] This high susceptibility of S-phase cells to initiation of oncogenesis by chemicals, which is suggested by results summarized above, is clearly documented by observations in tissue culture. We were able to demonstrate in mitotically synchronized cultures of M2 mouse fibroblasts that the initiation of malignant transformation occurs only during the S-phase of the cell cycle[110] (Figure 3), and a similar cell-cycle dependence of transformation was observed with cytosine arabinoside[111] and 5-fluorodeoxyuridine.[112] Similarly, the initiation of chemical mutagenesis in yeast[113] and in mammalian cells[114] (Table 6) occurs preferentially in S-phase cells.

4. Interactions of Carcinogens with Cytoplasmic DNA

It has also been suggested that mitochondria, especially mitochondrial DNA, may play a role in oncogenesis: (a) damage to the mitochondria may lead to the release of its genome, enabling mitochondrial DNA, like viral DNA, to "infect" the nucleus,[115] and carcinogens are known to damage mitochondria,[116] and (b) mitochondrial genes, altered by mutation, may lead to aberrant cell membranes and thus to malignant transformation.[117] In support of this theory that cytoplasmic mutations are involved in carcinogenesis, preferential methylation of mitochondrial DNA by N-methyl-N-nitrosourea[118] and dimethylnitrosamine[119] has been observed.

C. Malignant Transformation Caused by Tumor Cell DNA

The chemical nature of genetic determinants was elucidated in 1944 by Avery et al. in their classic findings of DNA-mediated transformation of pneumococcal types.[120] The transfer of heritable characteristics mediated by preparations of DNA has now

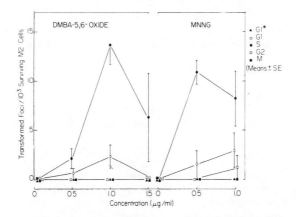

FIGURE 3.   Cell-cycle dependence of malignant transformation induced by 7,12-dimethylbenz[a]anthracene 5,6-oxide (DMBA 5,6-oxide) and N-methyl-N'-nitro-N-nitrosoguanidine (MNNG) (From Marquardt, H., *Cancer Res.*, 34, 1612, 1974. With permission.)

TABLE 6

Cell Cycle Dependence of Chemical Mutagenesis in V79 Chinese
Hamster Cells

	8-Azaguanine-resistant colonies per 10^5 survivors after treatment with MNNG ($\mu g/m\ell$)		
Treatment during	0.25	0.5	1.0
G1	31	85	136
S	141	246	406
G2	39	86	114
M	65	121	142

Note: Cells were synchronized by double-thymidine block; treatment
time, 30 min. MNNG, N-methyl-N'-nitro-N-nitrosoguanidine.
For methods, see Marquardt et al.[14]

been authenticated in a variety of microbial systems.[121] Convincing examples for mammalian cells, however, are rare, although suggestions for a "gene therapy" of human genetic diseases have been made.[122] Roosa and Bailey[121] and McBride and Ozer[123] were able to demonstrate the development of resistance to 8-azaguanine in mouse cells by treatment with DNA or with chromosomes from resistant cells, i.e., from cells lacking the X-chromosome-linked gene for hypoxanthine-guanine-phosphoribosyltransferase. This provides evidence that transfer and expression of genetic information by uptake of genetic material is also possible in mammalian cells.[124] If malignant transformation by chemicals were due to a gene mutation, it should, therefore, be possible to transform cells by exposing them to DNA isolated from cells which had been transformed in vitro by chemical carcinogens, and experiments of this type are at present underway in our laboratory. Borenfreund et al.[125] have already succeeded in demonstrating this type of phenomenon. They treated Chinese hamster cells with DNA isolated from mouse Ehrlich ascites tumor cells and found that the treated hamster cells had acquired oncogenic potential and also the ability to express mouse cell antigens. Of course, viral transformation of cells also involves the incorporation of viral genetic information into host cell DNA,[16,126] and it is worth noting in this context that in cell hybrids between malignant and normal cells, malignancy is sometimes expressed, and in other experiments it is suppressed.[127]

D. Carcinogen Interactions with RNA

Chemical carcinogens interact with RNA as well as with DNA, and another theory of oncogenesis, involving RNA and linking mutagenesis and oncogenesis and differentiation, has been presented by Temin.[128] The relatively recent phenomenon of reverse transcription provides a mechanism by which an initial RNA alteration can be fixed in the genome. Temin speculates that RNA from one cell may be transported to others where it would undergo reverse transcription, thus bringing about a progressive change in the genetic properties of the cell. Indeed, the amplification of genes coding for ribosomal RNA, which normally takes place in differentiating oocytes of the frog *Xenopus*, is blocked by an inhibitor of reverse transcriptase.[129] Thus, Temin visualizes reverse transcriptase as playing a role not only in transformation by oncogenic RNA viruses but also during normal development and in differentiation as well as in chemical carcinogenesis.[128] It was, therefore, of interest to study the effect of inhibitors of reverse transcription on chemically induced malignant transformation in vitro. In our experiments[130] (Table 7), we used polyriboinosinic-polyribocytidylic acid and polyribocytidylic-oligodeoxyriboguanylic acid which, like other polynucleotides,[131] inhibit reverse transcription.[166] Both polymers markedly inhibit malignant transformation by *N*-methyl-*N'*-nitro-*N*-nitrosoguanidine, while mutagenesis is unaffected. It must be pointed out in this context that (a) like others with similar mouse cell lines,[132] we were unable to detect the expression of oncornaviruses in our M2 cell line; and (b) an antiviral mouse interferon preparation did not affect chemical transformation.[130] Further studies in this area are at present underway in our laboratory.

III. CARCINOGENESIS — A PROBLEM IN DEVELOPMENT

The high degree of correlation between mutagenesis and carcinogenesis by chemicals might well be circumstantial and cannot prove a causal relationship between these two biological processes. Both processes, however, apparently require the initiating action of highly reactive chemicals. Indeed, the relatively high yields of transformants (over 10%; see Table 8) sometimes obtained with chemical carcinogens[133-135] when compared to the very low frequencies of induced mutation in mammalian cell cultures (10^{-6} per gene per cell division)[136] speak strongly against conventional random mutations as the basis of chemical carcinogenesis. In an effort to overcome one argument against such comparisons, namely, that these two biological effects were studied in different cells (see above), we are currently attempting to determine the mutation rates resulting from treatment with chemicals in our cloned, transformable M2 mouse cell line. In accordance with the results in Table 8, our preliminary results also indicate that malignant transformation is an event that is much more frequent than mutagenesis (Table 9). It should be noted, however, that with mouse myeloma cells in which the spontaneous mutation frequency (to variants producing an altered immunoglobulin) is unusually high (10^{-3} per cell generation), treatment with chemical mutagens results in the induction of an even higher yield of variants that are probably mutants.[137] As far as the high transformation frequency is concerned, the results of some experiments by Di-Paolo and co-workers[167] argue against the somatic mutation theory. They found that, while pretreatment of Syrian hamster embryo cells with the alkylating agent methyl methanesulfonate did enhance malignant transformation by *N*-acetoxy-2-acetylaminofluorene, such pretreatment did not affect mutagenesis induced in V79 Chinese hamster cells with *N*-acetoxy-2-acetylaminofluorene.

TABLE 7

Effect of Polynucleotides on Chemically Induced Malignant Transformation
and Mutagenesis in Mammalian Cell Cultures

Treatment		Malignant transformation (mouse M2 cells: transformed foci per no. of dishes treated)	Mutagenesis (V79 Chinese hamster cells: 8-azaguanine-resistant colonies per 10^5 survivors)
Polynuc-leotide[a] (10μg/mℓ)	MNNG (0.2μg/mℓ)		
none	none	0/30	3
P(I:C)	none	0/20	2
P(C):O(dG)	none	0/12	4
none	+	76/30	83
P(I:C)	+	0/21	86
P(C):O(dG)	+	4/8	79

[a] P(I:C) = Polyriboinosinic-polyribocytidylic acid; P(C):O(dG) = Polyribocytidylic-oligodeoxyriboguanylic acid. For methods, see Marquardt et al.[14] and
Marquardt.[130]

TABLE 8

Frequencies of Malignant Transformation in Mammalian Cell
Cultures

Compound	Concentration (μg/mℓ)	% Transfor-mants	Ref.
Syrian hamster embryo cells			
Aflatoxin B₁	0.5	7.0	133
N-Acetoxy-2-acetyl-aminofluorene	5.0	15.4	133
N-Methyl-N′-nitro-N-nitrosoguanidine	0.5	6.9	133
3-Methylcholanthrene	7.5	4.3	134
3-Methylcholanthrene 11,12-oxide	7.0	16.5	134
7,12-Dimethylbenz-[a]anthracene	5.0	3.0	134
Mouse cell lines			
Aflatoxin B₁	1.0	1.2	135
N-Acetoxy-2-acetyl-aminofluorene	1.0	1.5	135
N-Methyl-N′-nitro-N-nitrosoguanidine	0.2	1.7	35
	0.5	1.3	135
3-Methylcholanthrene	10.0	0.2	35
3-Methylcholanthrene 11,12-oxide	1.5	2.1	35
7,12-Dimethylbenz-[a]anthracene	0.1	3.7	135
	10.0	11.0	35

TABLE 9

Malignant Transformation and Mutagenesis by Chemicals in M2 Mouse Fibroblasts

Compound	$\mu g/ml$	Plating efficiency (%)	Transformed foci/10^6 survivors	Ouabain resistant colonies/10^6 survivors	Ratio transformants: ouabain resistant colonies
Acetone	0.5%	50	0	0.7	
MNNG	0.25	41	2,700	90	30
	0.5	32	5,000	211	24
	1.0	21	19,760	618	32
7MBA-3,	1.0	39	3,800	3.4	1118
4-diol	5.0	15	14,000	17	859

Note: Transformation and mutagenesis were determined under optimal conditions. Details of the transformation assay are given in Reference 30. For determination of mutagenesis, 1.5×10^6 cells were treated in a plastic petri dish (10 ml) for 24 hr. After an optimal expression time (48 hr), the cells were trypsinized and replated, 10^5 cells per dish (5 ml). Selection media contained ouabain, 2 mM. MNNG, N-methyl-N'-nitro-N-nitrosoguanidine; 7MBA-3,4-diol, 3,4-dihydro-3,4-dihydroxy-7-methylbenz[a]anthracene.

Thus, an alternative to the somatic mutation theory can be proposed: perhaps every nucleated cell in a multicellular organism has the potential for malignant expression, and neoplasia may therefore be one of the diseases of cell differentiation.[138] Like normal cellular differentiation, cancer may arise by the action of epigenetic, cytoplasmic mechanisms[139] leading to a persistent change in the expression of information. Since differentiation is potentially reversible, then carcinogenesis, too, should be potentially reversible. Nuclear transplantation experiments, in which nuclei from Lucké frog tumor cells were implanted into enucleated normal frog eggs and gave rise to fully functional tadpoles,[140] provide experimental evidence that such epigenetic mechanisms may also govern oncogenesis. This view is supported by the numerous observations that reversion of malignancy can occur in plants,[1] in animals,[1,141-143] and in humans[1,144,145] as well as in cells in culture.[146-155] Especially noteworthy in this context are the reversion results obtained by treatment with nonlethal concentrations of 5-bromodeoxyuridine[150,151] that exclude selection as a possible mechanism of action (Table 10). This compound has also been shown to affect differentiation in many cell types.[156-158] At present, we are investigating whether such revertant cells are more easily transformed by chemical carcinogens. It is conceivable that a kind of dynamic biological equilibrium between a cancer cell and its normal progenitor may exist which also would indicate the noninvolvement of irreversible genetic (karyotypic) alterations in the causation of transformation.[24] The present biochemical and molecular biological knowledge of differentiation is clearly insufficient to permit speculations about mechanisms, but the similarities between differentiation and carcinogenesis such as the influence of cytoplasmic factors and reversibility suggest that the mechanisms involved in both processes may be similar if they are not actually identical.[159] Transformation, like differentiation, may represent heritable changes that are phenotypic rather than genotypic.[160] The possible role of chromosomal proteins in this regard has been discussed,[24,161] and it should also be noted that the state of differentiation can affect DNA repair.[6] It has also been proposed that development may depend on enzymic modifications of DNA bases[162,163] or, alternatively, on RNA stability and membrane-RNA interaction.[164]

TABLE 10

Reversion of Malignancy by BUdR Treatment in Chemically Transformed Mouse M2 Fibroblasts

Cell	Saturation density (cells/cm²)	Tumors after s.c. injection of		
		10^4 cells	10^5 cells	10^6 cells
M2	47,500	0/7	0/7	0/7
M2, MCA-transformed	133,500	1/7	6/7	7/7
M2, MCA-transformed after 3 weeks of BUdR-treatment[a]	52,500	0/7	0/7	0/7
M2, MCA-transformed, 3 weeks of BUdR treatment, followed by 3 weeks in normal medium	47,500	0/7	0/7	0/7

Note: BUdR, 5-bromodeoxyuridine; MCA, 3-methylcholan-
threne.

[a] 0.1 µg/ml of medium.

IV. CONCLUSIONS

The high degree of correlation between mutagenic and carcinogenic agents and the rapidity and simplicity of short-term mutagenesis tests has made the use of a combination of such mutation assays valuable for prescreening our environment for hazardous chemicals, mutagens, and carcinogens. Such tests will certainly be of help in guiding the selection of high-priority compounds for long-term in vivo carcinogenesis testing. With a world capacity for in vivo carcinogenesis testing of about 400 compounds per year,[165] it is impossible to test, in animals, the enormous number of new chemicals entering our environment. It must be emphasized that up to 90% of human cancer may be caused by exposure to such environmental chemicals.[5] As regards the cellular mechanisms that may be involved in carcinogenesis, one may speculate that in some situations carcinogens cause mutational changes while in others they may cause changes in, for example, gene expression without inducing mutation or, alternatively, they may sometimes cause a mixture of the two types of effect.

This review has attempted to summarize the existing evidence for and against DNA as the critical cellular target in chemical carcinogenesis. Chemical mutagenesis and oncogenesis appear to be well correlated and both are certainly induced by reactive chemicals; however, at this stage it is by no means certain that they are causally related.

"Oh, if only it were possible to find understanding!" Joseph Knecht exclaimed. "If only there were a dogma to believe in. Everything is contradictory, everything is tangential, there are no certainties anywhere. Everything can be interpreted one way and then again interpreted in the opposite sense ..... Isn't there any truth? Is there no real and valid dogma?"

Herman Hesse,
The Glass Bead Game

Acknowledgments

I gratefully acknowledge the help and encouragement I received from discussions with Dr. Hildegard Marquardt, American Health Foundation, Valhalla, N.Y. and Dr. Morris S. Zedeck, Sloan-Kettering Institute. The superb assistance of Ms. Stephanie Baker in my experimental work and of Ms. Susan London in the preparation of this manuscript has been invaluable. My research is supported by USPHS Grants CA-15205 and CA-08748. I am the recipient of Research Career Development Award 1K04-CA-00127 from the National Institutes of Health, U.S. Public Health Service.

REFERENCES

1. **Braun, A. C.**, *The Biology of Cancer,* Addison-Wesley, London, 1974.
2. **Boveri, T.**, *The Origin of Malignant Tumors,* Fischer Verlag, Jena (reprinted by Williams & Wilkins, Baltimore, 1929).
3. **Bauer, K. H.**, *Das Kresbsproblem,* Springer-Verlag, Berlin, 1963.
4. **Knudson, A. G., Jr.**, Mutation and human cancer, *Adv. Cancer Res.,* 17, 317, 1973.
5. **Cairns, J.**, The cancer problem, *Sci. Am.,* 233, 64, 1975.
6. **Trosko, J. E. and Chu, E. H. Y.**, The role of DNA repair and somatic mutation in carcinogenesis, *Adv. Cancer Res.,* 21, 391, 1975.
7. **Igel, H. J., Freeman, A. E., Spiewak, J. E., and Kleinfeld, K. L.**, Chemical transformation of diploid human cells: a rare event, *In Vitro,* 11, 117, 1975.
8. **Todaro, G. and Martin, G.**, Increased susceptibility of Down's syndrome fibroblasts to transformation by SV40, *Proc. Soc. Exp. Biol. Med.,* 124, 1232, 1967.
9. **Miller, R. W. and Todaro, G. J.**, Viral transformation of cells from persons at high risk of cancer, *Lancet,* 1, 81, 1969.
10. **Pfeffer, L. M. and Kopelovich, L.**, Differential genetic susceptibility of cultured human skin fibroblasts to transformation by murine sarcoma virus, *Cell,* 10, 313, 1977.
11. **Miller, J. A.**, Carcinogenesis by chemicals: an overview — G. H. A. Clowes Memorial Lecture, *Cancer Res.,* 30, 559, 1970.
12. **Sugiyama, T.**, Specific vulnerability of the largest telocentric chromosome of rat bone marrow cells to 7,12-dimethylbenz[a]anthracene, *J. Natl. Cancer Inst.,* 47, 1267, 1971.
13. **Malling, H. V. and Chu, E. H. Y.**, Development of mutational model systems for study of carcinogenesis, in *Chemical Carcinogenesis, Part B,* Ts'o, P. O. P. and DiPaolo, J. A., Eds., Marcel Dekker, New York, 1974, 545.
14. **Miller, J. A. and Miller, E. C.**, Chemical carcinogenesis: mechanisms and approaches to its control, *J. Natl. Cancer Inst.,* 47, V, 1971.
15. **Marquardt, H., Baker, S., Grover, P. L., and Sims, P.**, Malignant transformation and mutagenesis in mammalian cells induced by vicinal diol epoxides derived from benzo[a]pyrene, *Cancer Lett.,* 3, 31, 1977.
16. **Dulbecco, R.**, From the molecular biology of oncogenic viruses to cancer, *Science,* 192, 437, 1976.
17. **Marshak, M. I., Varshaver, N. B., and Shapiro, N. I.**, Induction of gene mutations and chromosomal aberrations by Symian virus 40 in cultured mammalian cells, *Mutat. Res.,* 30, 383, 1975 .
18. **Nichols, W. W.**, Viruses and chromsomes, in *The Cell Nucleus,* Busch, H., Ed., Academic Press, New York, 1974, 437.
19. **Wood, A. W., Goode, R. L., Chang, R. L., Levin, W., Conney, A. H., Yagi, H., Dansette, P. M., and Jerina, D. M.**, Mutagenic and cytotoxic activity of benzo[a]pyrene 4,5-, 7,8- and 9,10-oxides and the six corresponding phenols, *Proc. Natl. Acad. Sci. U.S.A.,* 72, 3176, 1975.
20. **Levin, W., Wood, A. W., Yagi, H., Dansette, P. M., Jerina, D. M., and Conney, A. H.**, Carcinogenicity of benzo[a]pyrene 4,5-, 7,8- and 9,10-oxide on mouse skin, *Proc. Natl. Acad. Sci. U.S.A.,* 73, 243, 1975.
21. **Brookes, P. and DeSerres, F. J.**, Report of the workshop on mutagenicity of chemical carcinogens, *Mutat. Res.,* 38, 155, 1976.
22. **McCann, J., Choi, E., Yamasaki, E., and Ames, B.**, Detection of carcinogens as mutagens in the Salmonella/microsome test: assay of 300 chemicals, *Proc. Natl. Acad. Sci. U.S.A.,* 72, 5135, 1975.

23. McCann, J. and Ames, B., Detection of carcinogens as mutagens in the Salmonella/microsome test: assay of 300 chemicals: discussion, *Proc. Natl. Acad. Sci. U.S.A.,* 73, 950, 1976.

24. Nery, R., Carcinogenic mechanisms: a critical review and a suggestion that oncogenesis may be adaptive ontogenesis, *Chem. Biol. Interact.,* 12, 145, 1976.

25. Marquardt, H. and Marquardt, H., Induction of malignant transformation and mutagenesis in cell culture by cancer chemotherapeutic agents, *Cancer,* 40, 1930, 1977.

26. Marquardt, H., Microsomal metabolism of chemical carcinogens in animals and man, in *Air Pollution and Cancer in Man,* Mohr, U., Schmähl, D., and Tomatis, L., Eds., IARC Publ. No. 16, International Agency for Research on Cancer, Lyon, 1977, 309.

27. Miller, E. C. and Miller, J. A., The presence and significance of bound amino azo dyes in the livers of rats fed p-dimethylaminoazobenzene, *Cancer Res.,* 7, 468, 1947.

28. Heidelberger, C. and Davenport, G. R., Local functional components of carcinogenesis, *Acta Unio Int. Contra Cancrum,* 17, 55, 1961.

29. Irving, C. C., Interaction of chemical carcinogens with DNA, in *Methods in Cancer Research,* Vol. 7, Busch, H., Ed., Academic Press, New York, 1973, 189.

30. Marquardt, H., Malignant transformation in vitro: a model system to study mechanisms of action of chemical carcinogens and to evaluate the oncogenic potential of environmental chemicals, in *Screening Tests in Chemical Carcinogenesis,* Montesano, R., Bartsch, H., and Tomatis, L., Eds. IARC Publ. No. 12 International Agency for Research on Cancer, Lyon, 1976, 389.

31. Magee, P. N. and Barnes, J. M., Carcinogenic nitroso compounds, *Adv. Cancer Res.,* 10, 163, 1967.

32. Loveless, A., Possible relevance of O-6-alkylation of deoxyguanosine to the mutagenicity and carcinogenicity of nitrosamines and nitrosamides, *Nature (London),* 223, 206, 1969.

33. Jerina, D. M. and Daly, J. W., Arene oxides: a new aspect of drug metabolism, *Science,* 185, 573, 1974.

34. Kuroki, T., Huberman, E., Marquardt, H., Selkirk, J. E., Heidelberger, C., Grover, P. L., and Sims, P., Binding of K-region epoxides and other derivatives of benz[a]anthracene and dibenz[a,h]anthracene to DNA, RNA, and proteins of transformable cells, *Chem. Biol. Interact.,* 4, 389, 1971—1972.

35. Marquardt, H., Sodergren, J. E., Grover, P. L., and Sims, P., Malignant transformation *in vitro* of mouse fibroblasts by 7,12-dimethylbenz[a]anthracene and 7-hydroxymethylbenz[a]anthracene and by their K-region derivatives, *Int. J. Cancer,* 13, 304, 1974.

36. Lijinsky, W., Lee, K. Y., and Gallagher, C. H., Interaction of aflatoxin B_1 and G_1 with tissues of the rat, *Cancer Res.,* 30, 2280, 1970.

37. Singer, B., All oxygens in nucleic acids react with carcinogenic ethylating agents, *Nature (London),* 264, 333, 1976.

38. Swenson, D. H., Farmer, P. B., and Lawley, P. D., Identification of the methylphosphotriester of thymidylyl(3'-5')thymidine as a product from reaction of DNA with the carcinogen N-methyl-N-nitrosourea, *Chem. Biol. Interact.,* 15, 91, 1976.

39. Maher, V. M., Birch, N., Otto, J. R., and McCormick, J. J., Cytotoxicity of carcinogenic aromatic amides in normal and xeroderma pigmentosum fibroblasts with different DNA repair capabilities, *J. Natl. Cancer Inst.,* 54, 1287, 1975.

40. Maher, V. M., Oulette, L. M., Mittlestat, M., and McCormick, J. J., Synergistic effect of caffeine on the cytotoxicity of ultraviolet irradiation and of hydrocarbon epoxides in strains of xeroderma pigmentosum, *Nature (London)* 258, 760, 1975.

41. Taylor, A. M. R., Metcalf, J. A., Oxford, J. M., and Harnden, D. G., Is chromatide-type damage in ataxia telangiectasia after irradiation at G_o a consequence of defective repair?, *Nature (London),* 260, 441, 1976.

42. Weinstein, I. B., Molecular events in chemical carcinogenesis, in *Cancer Biology II, Etiology and Therapy,* Fenoglio, C. M. and King, D. W., Eds., Stratton Intercontinental Medical Book Corp., New York, 1976, 106.

43. Kakunaga, T., Caffeine inhibits cell transformation by 4-nitroquinoline-1-oxide, *Nature (London),* 258, 248, 1975.

44. Nomura, T., Diminution of tumorigenesis by 4-nitroquinoline-1-oxide by post-treatment with caffeine in mice, *Nature (London),* 260, 547, 1976.

45. DiPaolo, J. A. and Casto, B. C., In vitro transformation: interaction of chemical carcinogens with viruses and physical agents, in *Screening Tests in Chemical Carcinogenesis,* Montesano, R., Bartsch, H., and Tomatis, L., Eds., IARC Publ. No. 12, International Agency for Research on Cancer, Lyon, 1976, 415.

46. Heidelberger, C., Chemically and metabolically induced DNA adducts: relationship to chemical carcinogenesis, in *Aging, Carcinogenesis and Radiation Biology,* Smith, K. C., Ed., Press, New York, 1976, 341.

47. Frei, J. V. and Lawley, P. D., Methylation of DNA in various organs of C57B1 mice by a carcinogenic dose of N-methyl-N-nitrosourea and stability of some methylation products up to 18 hr, *Chem. Biol. Interact.,* 10, 413, 1975.

48. Goth, R. and Rajewsky, M. F., Persistence of O⁶-ethylguanine in rat brain DNA: correlation with nervous system-specific carcinogenesis by ethylnitrosourea, *Proc. Natl. Acad. Sci. U.S.A.*, 71, 639, 1974.

49. Kleihues, P. and Margison, G. P., Carcinogenicity of N-methyl-N-nitrosourea: possible role of excision repair of O⁶-methylguanine from DNA, *J. Natl. Cancer Inst.*, 53, 1839, 1974.

50. Nicoll, J. W., Swann, P. F., and Pegg, A. E., Effect of dimethylnitrosamine on persistence of methylated guanines in rat liver and kidney DNA, *Nature (London)*, 254, 261, 1975.

51. Craddock, V. M., The pattern of methylated purines formed in DNA of intact and regenerating livers of rats treated with the carcinogen dimethylnitrosamine, *Biochim. Biophys. Acta*, 312, 202, 1973.

52. Craddock, V. M., Effect of a single treatment with the alkylating carcinogens dimethylnitrosamine, diethylnitrosamine and methyl methanesulphonate on liver regeneration after partial hepatectomy, *Chem. Biol. Interact.*, 10, 323, 1975.

53. Nicoll, J. W., Swann, P. F., and Pegg, A. E., The accumulation of O⁶-methylguanine in the liver and kidney DNA of rats treated with dimethylnitrosamine for a short or a long period, *Chem. Biol. Interact.*, 16, 301, 1977.

54. Buecheler, J. and Kleihues, P., Excision of O⁶-methylguanine from DNA of various mouse tissues following a single injection of N-methyl-N-nitrosourea, *Chem. Biol. Interact.*, 16, 325, 1977.

55. Rogers, K. J. and Pegg, A. E., Formation of O⁶-methylguanine by alkylation of rat liver, colon, and kidney DNA following administration of 1,2-dimethylhydrazine, *Cancer Res.*, 37, 4082, 1977.

56. Margison, G. P., Margison, J. M., and Montesano, R., Accumulation of O⁶-methylguanine in nontarget-tissue deoxyribonucleic acid during chronic administration of dimethylnitrosamine, *Biochem. J.*, 165, 463, 1977.

57. Stich, H. F., San, R. H. C., Lam, P. P. S., Koropatnik, D. J., Lo, L. W., and Laishes, B. A., DNA fragmentation and DNA repair as an *in vitro* and *in vivo* assay for chemical precarcinogens, carcinogens, and carcinogenic nitrosation products, in *Screening Tests in Chemical Carcinogenesis*, Montesano, R., Bartsch, H., and Tomatis, L., Eds., IARC Publ. No. 12, International Agency for Research on Cancer, Lyon, 1976, 617.

58. Waters, R., Mishra, N., Bouck, N., DiMayorca, G., and Regan, J. D., Partial inhibition of postreplication repair and enhanced frequency of chemical transformation in rat cells injected with leukemia virus, *Proc. Natl. Acad. Sci. U.S.A.*, 74, 238, 1977.

59. Baldwin, R. W., Palmer, H. C., and Partridge, M. W., Studies on tricycloquinazoline carcinogenesis: interaction of carcinogen with skin components, *Br. J. Cancer*, 16, 740, 1962.

60. McCuen, R. W., Stöhrer, G., and Sirotnak, F. M., Mutagenicity of derivatives of oncogenic purine-N-oxides, *Cancer Res.*, 34, 378, 1974.

61. Marquardt, H., Baker, S., Grab, D., and Marquardt, H., Oncogenic and mutagenic activity of adriamycin decreased by microsomal metabolism, *Proc. Am. Assoc. Cancer Res.*, 18, 13, 1977.

62. Brookes, P., Role of covalent binding in carcinogenicity, in *Biological Reactive Intermediates*, Jollow, D. J., Kocsis, J. J., Snyder, R., and Vainio, H., Eds., Plenum Press, New York, 1977, 470.

63. DiMarco, A. and Arcamone, F., DNA-complexing antibiotics: daunomycin, adriamycin and their derivatives, *Arzneim. Forsch.*, 25, 368, 1975.

64. DiMarco, A., Zunino, F., Orezzi, P., and Gambetta, R. A., Interaction of daunomycin with nucleic acids: effect of photoirradiation of the complex, *Experientia*, 28, 327, 1972.

65. Marquardt, H. and Philips, F. S., The effect of 7,12-dimethylbenz[a]anthracene on the synthesis after nucleic acids in rapidly dividing hepatic cells in rats, *Cancer Res.*, 30, 2000, 1970.

66. Marquardt, H., Bendich, A., Philips, F. S., and Hoffmann, D., Binding of (G-³H)-7,12-dimethylbenz[a]anthracene to DNA of normal and of rapidly dividing hepatic cells of rats, *Chem. Biol. Interact.*, 3, 1, 1971.

67. Marquardt, H., Philips, F. S., and Bendich, A., DNA binding and inhibition of DNA synthesis of 7,12-dimethylbenz[a]anthracene administered during the early prereplicative phase in regenerating rat liver, *Cancer Res.*, 32, 1810, 1972.

68. Marquardt, H., Sternberg, S. S., and Philips, F. S., 7,12-Dimethylbenz[a]anthracene and hepatic neoplasia in regenerating rat liver, *Chem. Biol. Interact.*, 2, 401, 1970.

69. Haddow, A., Scott, C. M., and Scott, J. D., The influence of certain carcinogenic and other hydrocarbons on body growth in the rat, *Proc. Roy. Soc., (B)*, 122, 477, 1937.

70. Philips, F. S., Sternberg, S. S., and Marquardt, H., *In vivo* cytotoxicity of polycyclic hydrocarbons, in *Pharmacology and the Future of Man*, Proc. 5th Int. Cong. Pharmacol., Loomis, T. A., Ed., S. Karger Publ., Basel, 1973, 75.

71. Philips, F. S. and Sternberg, S. S., The lethal action of antitumor agents in proliferating cell systems *in vivo*, *Am. J. Pathol.*, 81, 205, 1975.

72. Friedman, M. A. and Staub, J., Inhibition of mouse testicular DNA synthesis by mutagens and carcinogens as a potential simple mammalian assay for mutagenesis, *Mutat. Res.*, 37, 67, 1976.

73. Seiler, J. P., Inhibition of testicular DNA synthesis by chemical mutagens and carcinogens. Preliminary results in the validation of a novel short term test, *Mutat. Res.,* 46, 305, 1977.
74. Warwick, G. P., Effect of the cell cycle on carcinogenesis, *Fed. Proc. Fed. Am. Soc. Exp. Biol.,* 30, 1760, 1971.
75. Rajewsky, M. F., Proliferative parameters of mammalian cell systems and their role in tumor growth and carcinogenesis, *Z. Krebsforsch.,* 78, 12, 1972.
76. Druckrey, H., Preussmann, R., Ivancovic, S., and Schmähl, D., Organotrope carcinogene Wirkung bei 65 verschiedenen N-Nitroso-Verbindungen an BD-Rattens, *Z. Krebsforsch.,* 69, 103, 1967.
77. Lane, M., Liebelt, M., and Calvert, J., Effect of partial hepatectomy on tumor incidence in BALB mice treated with urethane, *Cancer Res.,* 30, 1812, 1970.
78. Hollander, C. F. and Bentvelzen, P., Enhancement of urethan induction of hepatoma in mice by prior partial hepatectomy, *J. Natl. Cancer Inst.,* 41, 1303, 1968.
79. Pound, A. W. and Lawson, T. A., Effects of partial hepatectomy on carcinogenicity, metabolism and binding to DNA of ethyl carbamate, *J. Natl. Cancer Inst.,* 53, 423, 1974.
80. Pound, A. W., Carcinogenesis and cell proliferation, *N.Z. Med. J.,* 67, 88, 1968.
81. Craddock, V. M. and Frei, J. V., Induction of tumors in intact and partially hepatectomized rats with ethyl methane sulphonate, *Br. J. Cancer,* 34, 207, 1977.
82. Pound, A. W. and Lawson, T. A., Partial hepatectomy and toxicity of dimethylnitrosamine and carbon tetrachloride in relation to the carcinogenic action of dimethylnitrosamine, *Br. J. Cancer,* 32, 596, 1975.
83. Craddock, V. M., Effect of a single treatment with the alkylating carcinogens, dimethylnitrosamine, diethylnitrosamine and methyl methanesulphonate on liver regeneration after partial hepatectomy, *Chem. Biol. Interact.,* 10, 313, 1975.
84. Craddock, V. M., Liver carcinogenesis induced by single administration of dimethylnitrosamine after partial hepatectomy, *J. Natl. Cancer Inst.,* 47, 889, 1971.
85. Craddock, V. M., Induction of liver tumors in rats by a single treatment with nitroso compounds given after partial hepatectomy, *Nature (London),* 245, 386, 1973.
86. Craddock, V. M. and Frei, J. V., Induction of liver cell adenomata in the rat by a single treatment with N-methyl-N-nitrosourea given at various times after partial hepatectomy, *Br. J. Cancer,* 30, 503, 1974.
87. Glinos, A. D., Bucher, N. L. R., and Aub, J. C., The effect of liver regeneration on tumor formation in rats fed 4-dimethylaminoazobenzene, *J. Exp. Med.,* 93, 313, 1951.
88. Haese, W. H. and Bueding, E., Long-term hepatocellular effect of hycanthone and of two other antischistosomal drugs in mice injected with *Schistosoma mansoni, J. Pharmacol. Exp. Ther.,* 197, 703, 1976.
89. Witschi, H., Williamson, D., and Lock, S., Enhancement of urethan-tumorigenesis in mouse lung by butylated hydroxytoluene, *J. Natl. Cancer Inst.,* 58, 301, 1977.
90. Pozharisski, K. M., The significance of unspecific injury for colon carcinogenesis in rats, *Cancer Res.,* 35, 3824, 1975.
91. Ito, N., Hiasha, Y., Tamai, A., Kamamoto, Y., Makiura, Y., and Kondo, Y., The Influence of Unilateral Nephectomy on the Development of Renal Tumor in Rats Treated with Dimethylnitrosamine and Basic Lead Acetate, *Proc. 10th Int. Cancer Congr., Houston,* 1970, 12.
92. Ito, N., Hiasha, Y., Tamai, A., and Yoshida, K., Effect of unilateral nephectomy on the development of kidney tumors in rats treated with N-nitrosodimethylamine, *Gann,* 60, 319, 1969.
93. Terracini, B., Palestro, G., Rua, S., and Trevisio, A., A study on the role of compensatory hyperplasia in renal carcinogenesis with dimethylnitrosamine in the rat, *Tumori,* 55, 357, 1970.
94. Miyakawa, M. and Yoshida, O., Induction of tumors of the urinary bladder in female mice following surgical implantation of glass beads and feeding of bracken fern, *Gann,* 66, 437, 1975.
95. Lawson, T. A., Dzhioev, F. K., Lewis, F. A., and Clayson, D. B., Acute changes in nucleic acid synthesis induced by carcinogens in the mouse bladder, *Biochem. J.,* 111, 12, 1968.
96. Dzioev, F. K., Wood, M., Cowens, M., Campbasso, O., and Clayson, D. B., Further investigation on the proliferative response of mouse bladder epithelium to 4-ethylsulphonylnaphthalene-1-sulphonamide, *Br. J. Cancer,* 23, 772, 1969.
97. Bryan, G. T., Ertürk, E., and Yoshida, O., Production of urinary bladder carcinomas in mice by sodium saccharine, *Science,* 168, 1238, 1970.
98. Kowalewski, K. and Todd, E. F., Carcinoma of the gall bladder induced in hamsters by insertion of cholesterol pellets and feeding dimethylnitrosamine, *Proc. Soc. Exp. Biol. Med.,* 136, 482, 1971.
99. Sugiyama, T., Role of erythropoietin in 7,12-dimethylbenz[a]anthracene induction of acute chromosome aberrations and leukemia in the rat, *Proc. Natl. Acad. Sci. U.S.A.,* 68, 2761, 1971.
100. Marquardt, H. and Heidelberger, C., Stimulation of DNA synthesis in hydrocarbon-transformable hamster embryo cells by the K-region epoxide of benz[a]anthracene, *Chem. Biol. Interact.,* 5, 69, 1972.

101. Zedeck, M. S. and Sternberg, S. S., Tumor induction in intact and regenerating liver of adult rats by a single treatment with methylazoxymethanol, *Chem. Biol. Interact.*, 17, 291, 1977.

102. Rogers, A. E., Kula, N. S., and Newberne, P. M., Absence of an effect of partial hepatectomy on aflatoxin B₁ carcinogenesis, *Cancer Res.*, 31, 491, 1971.

103. Outzen, H. C., Custer, R. P., and Prehn, R. T., Demonstration of an inverse relationship between regenerative capacity and oncogenesis in the adult frog, *Rana pipiens*, in *Advances in Experimental Biology and Medicine*, Hildemann, H. H. and Benedict, A. A., Eds., Plenum Press, New York, in press.

104. Arlett, C. F., Turnbull, D., Harcourt, S. A., Lehmann, A. R., and Corella, C. M., A comparison of the 8-azaguanine and ouabain-resistance systems for the selection of induced mutant Chinese hamster cells, *Mutat. Res.*, 33, 261, 1975.

105. Todaro, G. J. and Green, H., Cell growth and the initiation of transformation by SV40, *Proc. Natl. Acad. Sci. U.S.A.*, 55, 302, 1966.

106. Scher, L. D., SV40-induced DNA synthesis and the fixation of the transformed state, *Virology*, 46, 956, 1971.

107. Borek, C. and Sachs, L., Cell susceptibility to transformation by x-irradiation and fixation of the transformed state, *Proc. Natl. Acad. Sci. U.S.A.*, 57, 1522, 1967.

108. Chen, T. T. and Heidelberger, C., Quantitative studies on the malignant transformation of mouse prostate cells by carcinogenic hydrocarbons in vitro, *Int. J. Cancer*, 4, 166, 1969.

109. Kakunaga, T., Requirement for cell replication in the fixation and expression of the transformed state in mouse cells treated with 4-nitroquinoline-1-oxide, *Int. J. Cancer*, 14, 736, 1974.

110. Marquardt, H., Cell cycle dependence of chemically induced malignant transformation in vitro, *Cancer Res.*, 34, 1612, 1974.

111. Benedict, W. F., Rucker, N., Faust, J., and Louri, R. E., Malignant transformation with ara-C, FUdR, MTX, and bleomycin in 10T 1/2 C1.8 cells, *Proc. Am. Assoc. Cancer Res.*, 16, 40, 1975.

112. Jones, P. A., Benedict, W. F., Baker, M. S., Mondal, S., Rapp, U., and Heidelberger, C., Oncogenic transformation of C3H/10T 1/2 clone 8 mouse embryo cells by halogenated pyrimidine nucleosides, *Cancer Res.*, 36, 101, 1976.

113. Kee, S. G. and Haber, J. E., Cell-cycle-dependent induction of mutations along a yeast chromosome, *Proc. Natl. Acad. Sci. U.S.A.*, 72, 1179, 1975.

114. Berman, J. J. and Williams, G. M., Enhanced susceptibility of cultured rat liver cells to mutagenesis during DNA synthesis, *Proc. Am. Assoc. Cancer Res.*, 17, 158, 1976.

115. Hadler, H. I., Daniel, B. G., and Pratt, R. D., The induction of ATP energized mitochondrial volume changes by carcinogenic N-hydroxy-N-acetyl-aminofluorenes when combined with showdomycin. A unitary hypothesis for carcinogenesis, *J. Antibiot.*, 24, 405, 1971.

116. Hadler, H. I. and Daniel, B. G., A correlation between the carcinogenicity of isomeric N-hydroxy-N-acetylaminofluorenes and their *in vitro* effect on mitochondria, *Cancer Res.*, 33, 117, 1973.

117. Wilkie, D., Egilsson, V., and Evans, I. H., Mitochondria in oncogenesis. *Lancet*, 1, 697, 1975.

118. Wunderlich, V., Schütt, M., Böttger, M., and Graffi, A., Preferential alkylation of mitochondrial deoxyribonucleic acid by N-methyl-N-nitrosourea, *Biochem. J.*, 118, 99, 1970.

119. Wunderlich, V., Tetzlaff, I., and Graffi, A., Studies on nitrosodimethylamine: preferential methylation of mitochondrial DNA in rats and hamsters, *Chem. Biol. Interact.*, 4, 81, 1971/72.

120. Avery, O. T., MacLeod, C. M., and McCarty, M., Studies of the chemical nature of the substance inducing transformation of pneumococcal type, *J. Exp. Med.*, 79, 137, 1944.

121. Roosa, R. A. and Bailey, E., DNA-mediated transformation of mammalian cells in culture. Increased transforming efficiency following sonication, *J. Cell. Physiol.*, 75, 137, 1970.

122. Friedmann, T. and Roblin, R., Gene therapy for human genetic disease?, *Science*, 175, 949, 1972.

123. McBride, O. W. and Ozer, H. L., Transfer of genetic information by purified metaphase chromosomes, *Proc. Natl. Acad. Sci., U.S.A.*, 70, 1258, 1973.

124. Ottolenghi-Nightingale, E., DNA-mediated transformation in mammalian cells, in *Cell Communications*, Cox, R. P., Ed., John Wiley & Sons, New York, 1974, 233.

125. Borenfreund, E., Honda, Y., Steinglass, M., and Bendich, A., Studies of DNA-induced heritable alterations of mammalian cells, *J. Exp. Med.*, 132, 1071, 1970.

126. Dulbecco, R., Cell transformation by virus, *Science*, 166, 962, 1969.

127. Stanbridge, E. J., Suppression of malignancy in human cells, *Nature (London)*, 260, 17, 1976.

128. Temin, H., The protovirus hypothesis: speculations on the significance of RNA-directed DNA synthesis for normal development and carcinogenesis, *J. Natl. Cancer Inst.*, 46, III, 1971.

129. Tocchini-Valentini, G. P. and Crippa, M., On the mechanisms of gene amplification, in *The Biology of Oncogenic Viruses*, Silvestri, L. G., Ed., North-Holland, Amsterdam, 1971, 237.

130. Marquardt, H., Polyriboinosinic-polyribocytidylic acid prevents chemically-induced malignant transformation in vitro, *Nature (London) New Biol.*, 246, 228, 1973.

131. Tuominen, F. W. and Kenney, F. T., Inhibition of the DNA polymerase of Rauscher leukemia virus by single-stranded polyribonucleotides, *Proc. Natl. Acad. Sci. U.S.A.*, 68, 2198, 1971.

132. Rapp, U. R., Nowinski, R. C., Reznikoff, C. A., and Heidelberger, C., Endogenous oncornaviruses in chemically induced transformation, *Virology,* 65, 392, 1975.

133. DiPaolo, J. A., Nelson, R. L., and Donovan, P. J., In vitro transformation of Syrian hamster embryo cells by diverse chemical carcinogens, *Nature (London),* 235, 278, 1972.

134. Huberman, E., Kuroki, T., Marquardt, H., Selkirk, J. K., Heidelberger, C., Grover, P. L., and Sims, P., Transformation of hamster embryo cells by epoxides and other derivatives of polycyclic hydrocarbons, *Cancer Res.,* 32, 1391, 1972.

135. DiPaolo, J. A., Takano, T., and Popescu, N. C., Quantitation of chemically induced neoplastic transformation of BALB/3T3 cloned cell lines, *Cancer Res.,* 32, 2686, 1972.

136. Cairns, J., Mutation selection and the natural history of cancer, *Nature (London),* 255, 197, 1975.

137. Birschtein, B. K., Pseud'homme, J. L., and Scharff, M. D., Variants of mouse myeloma cells that produce short immunoglobulin heavy chains, *Proc. Natl. Acad. Sci. U.S.A.,* 71, 3478, 1974.

138. Markert, C. L., Neoplasia: a disease of cell differentiation, *Cancer Res.,* 28, 1908, 1968.

139. Pitot, H. C. and Heidelberger, C., Metabolic regulatory circuits and carcinogenesis, *Cancer Res.,* 23, 1694, 1963.

140. McKinnell, R. G., Deggins, B. A., and Labat, D. D., Transplantation of pluripotential nuclei from triploid frog tumors, *Science,* 165, 394, 1969.

141. Pierce, G. B., Teratocarcinoma: model for a developmental concept of cancer, in *Current Topics in Developmental Biology,* Vol. 3, Monroy, A. and Moscona, A. A., Eds., Academic Press, New York, 1967, 223.

142. Mintz, B. and Illmensee, K., Normal genetically mosaic mice produced from malignant teratocarcinoma cells, *Proc. Natl. Acad. Sci. U.S.A.,* 72, 3585, 1975.

143. Pierce, G. B. and Wallace, C., Differentiation of malignant to benign cells, *Cancer Res.,* 31, 127, 1971.

144. Everson, T. C. and Cole, W. H., *Spontaneous Regression of Cancer,* W. B. Saunders, Philadelphia, 1966.

145. Fibach, E., Landau, T., and Sachs, L., Normal differentiation of myeloid leukemia cells induced by a differentiation-inducing protein, *Nature (London) New Biol.,* 237, 276, 1972.

146. Rabinowitz, Z. and Sachs, L., Reversion of properties in cells transformed by polyoma virus, *Nature (London),* 220, 1203, 1968.

147. Rabinowitz, Z. and Sachs, L., Control of reversion of properties in transformed cells, *Nature (London),* 225, 136, 1970.

148. Pollack, R. E., Green, H., and Todaro, G. J., Growth control in cultured cells: selection of sublines with increased sensitivity to contact inhibition and decreased tumor-producing activity, *Proc. Natl. Acad. Sci. U.S.A.,* 60, 126, 1968.

149. Pollack, R. E., Cellular and viral contributions to maintenance of the SV40-transformed state, *In Vitro,* 6, 58, 1970.

150. Silagi, S. and Bruce, S. A., Suppression of malignancy and differentiation in melanotic melanoma cells, *Proc. Natl. Acad. Sci. U.S.A.,* 66, 72, 1970.

151. Marquardt, H., Treatment in tissue culture: loss of malignancy in a methylcholanthrene-transformed cell clone, *Naunyn Schmiedebergs Arch. Pharm.,* 227, R45, 1973.

152. Hsie, A. W. and Puck, T. T., Morphological transformation of Chinese hamster cells by dibutyryl adenosine cyclic 3′:5′-monophosphate and testosterone, *Proc. Natl. Acad. Sci. U.S.A.,* 68, 358, 1971.

153. Johnson, G. S., Friedman, R. M., and Pastan, J., Restoration of several morphological characteristics of normal fibroblasts in sarcoma cells treated with adenosine-3′:5′-cyclic monophosphate and its derivatives, *Proc. Natl. Acad. Sci. U.S.A.,* 68, 425, 1971.

154. Prasad, K. N. and Sinha, P. K., Effect of sodium butyrate on mammalian cells in culture. A review, *In Vitro,* 12, 125, 1976.

155. Leder, A. and Leder, P., Butyric acid, a potent inducer of erythroid differentiation in cultured erythroleukemic cells, *Cell,* 5, 319, 1975.

156. Schubert, S. and Jacob, F., 5-Bromodeoxyuridine-induced differentiation of a neuroblastoma, *Proc. Natl. Acad. Sci. U.S.A.,* 67, 247, 1970.

157. Strom, C. M. and Dorfman, A., Distribution of 5-bromodeoxyuridine and thymidine in the DNA of developing chick cartilage, *Proc. Natl. Acad. Sci. U.S.A.,* 73, 1019, 1976.

158. Braun, A. C., Differentiation and dedifferentiation, in *Cancer,* Vol. 3, Becker, F. F., Ed., Plenum Press, London, 1975, 3.

159. Dustin, P., Jr., Cell differentiation and carcinogenesis: a critical review, *Cell Tissue Kinet.,* 5, 519, 1972.

160. Finckh, E. S., The genesis of tumours — mutation or abnormal differentiation?, *Med. J. Aust.,* 61, 438, 1974.

161. Bonner, J., Molecular events in differentiation and dedifferentiation, in *Chemical Carcinogenesis, Part B.,* Ts'o, P. O. P. and DiPaolo, J. A., Eds., Marcel Dekker, New York, 1974, 531.

162. Holliday, R. and Pugh, J. E., DNA modification mechanisms and genetic activity during development, *Science,* 187, 226, 1975.
163. Scarano, E., The control of gene function in cell differentiation and in embryogenesis, in *Advances in Cytopharmacology,* Vol. 1, Clementi, F. and Ceccarelli, B., Eds., Raven Press, New York, 1971, 13.
164. Pitot, H. C., Neoplasia: a somatic mutation or a heritable change in cytoplasmic membranes?, *J. Natl. Cancer Inst.,* 53, 905, 1974.
165. Bartsch, H., Predictive value of mutagenesis tests in chemical carcinogenesis, *Mutat. Res.,* 38, 177, 1976.
166. Cavalieri, L., personal communication.
167. DiPaolo, J. A. et al., personal communication.

Chapter 7

CHEMICAL CARCINOGENESIS AS A CONSEQUENCE OF ALTERATIONS IN THE STRUCTURE AND FUNCTION OF DNA

J. E. Trosko and C. C. Chang

TABLE OF CONTENTS

> ..., cancer is a problem in regulatory dysfunction,
> which in this case results in a failure to
> orchestrate the available repertory of gene
> capabilities in a manner appropriate to the
> whole organism at any given time.
> Van R. Potter[1]

I. INTRODUCTION

Cancer is a word (symbol) used to encompass a wide variety of observations related to one of the major diseases known to mankind. Disease, itself, is a concept whose meaning is heavily influenced by cultural philosophy.[2] The ultimate understanding of cancer as a disease[3,4] and as a biological phenomenon[1,5] will depend, in part, on a concise definition. Without a universally agreed upon concept of this major and complex disease, rapid progress in its control will be difficult. If the quotation used above is correct, then the fundamental problem is to determine in what way(s) chemicals that influence carcinogenesis can disrupt the ability of a cell to "orchestrate" its genes in order to stay integrated within an organism. Although the state of knowledge related to carcinogenesis is by no means complete, it is our contention that sufficient information exists which allows one to speculate about broad concepts of carcinogenesis. Our main objective, therefore, is to provide a theoretical framework that will attempt to unify a plethora of observations bearing on carcinogenesis, such as those discussed in the preceding chapters.

II. GENERAL CONCEPTS OF CARCINOGENESIS

A. Cancer as a Phenotype

Although at present no universally accepted theory exists for the mechanism of carcinogenesis, Temin[6] critically reviewed five major theories of carcinogenesis (i.e., mutation, differentiation, oncogene, protovirus, and provirus). In the context of this review, we will limit our analysis to how chemicals, which interact with DNA, might relate to the mutation and epigenetic (differentiation) theories of carcinogenesis. This is in no way meant to imply that chemical carcinogens and viruses, which might induce cancers, are not causally related.[7] In general, the five theories of carcinogenesis can be classified either as mutation or epigenetic theories. Moreover, if one accepts the concept that every phenotype is the consequence of the interaction between the genotype and environmental factors,[8,9] then cancer, as an "abnormal" phenotype, is not the result only of inherited genes or environmental exposure, but of the interaction of particular genetic backgrounds with particular environmental agents at particular developmental periods. An excellent example of the identification of genetic and environmental factors and of the subsequent use of that knowledge for cancer prevention is provided by Lynch,[10] who demonstrated that avoidance of exposure to UV light was sufficient to prevent skin cancer in pairs of xeroderma pigmentosum twins.

In principle, at least, any phenotype, including cancer, could be the result of either a mutation or modulation (repression or derepression) in genes which are responsible for an "orchestrated" integration of a cell with the whole organism. Therefore, the specific question of mechanism now becomes, "How can carcinogenesis be triggered by chemical reactions with DNA (or DNA-protein complexes) which might lead to either a mutation or an epigenetic change in a gene?"

B. Two-Stage Theory of Carcinogenesis

Another major observation which must be considered in the analysis of how chemical reactions with DNA influence carcinogenesis is that of the two-stage phenomenon of carcinogenesis. The concepts of tumor *initiation* and *promotion* have been generated to explain the observation that, months or years after the exposure of mouse skin to a carcinogen, tumors would appear (which would not otherwise appear) when a particular noncarcinogenic promoter, such as croton oil, was applied.[11-13] Although not all cancers appear to involve these two stages, some carcinogenic processes have been conceptualized as a two-stage process, involving the initiation of normal cells to a potential cancer state and the subsequent promotion of these precancerous cells.[12] Chemicals that interact with DNA in such a way as to induce an irreversible (but latent) process would be considered as initiators. Other chemicals, such as the phorbol esters, which are constituents of croton oil, would be considered as promoters if, when administered to an animal after the initiating agent, they in some manner* enhance the process of tumor formation.

Since it is important to recognize that tumor cells go through a "staged" evolution during their natural history of development,[14-17] it should be obvious that the promotion phase is not a simple or uniform process. The natural history of many tumors seems to include a period in which (1) a tumor that is growth-factor or promoter dependent becomes autonomous, and (2) in the case of an euploid cell-derived tumor, some initiated cells give rise to aneuploid tumor cells. In this case, it might then be more appropriate to refer to this complex process of tumorigenesis as a multistage phenomenon.

The two-stage phenomenon related to carcinogenesis has been demonstrated in several in vitro[18-23] and in vivo[11-13,24-26] model systems, as well as in human carcinogenesis. A recent hypothesis has been advanced which assigned, on the biological level, *mutagenesis* to be responsible for initiation and epigenetic mechanisms to be responsible for promotion.[22] Moreover, on the molecular level, we have postulated that an "error-prone" DNA repair/replication mechanism is responsible for the major cause of mutagenesis, and perturbation in cyclic nucleotide pools triggers the modulation of gene expression.[27]

It must also be noted that the concept of "cocarcinogenesis" might be expected, theoretically, to be an important explanation for several chemicals, which by themselves are poor or noninitiators or promoters, but which in combination interact synergistically to trigger the carcinogenic process. Recent work by Van Duuren and Goldschmidt[28] indicates this phenomenon is experimentally demonstrable.

In addition, we do not believe, on the basis of the theory to be presented, that all carcinogenic events need both the initiation and promotion phases. There might be some which require only initiation; some which require both initiation and promotion; while others would require only promotion.** A summary of the two-stage concept of carcinogenesis is presented with the following definitions.

1. Carcinogenesis = initiation and/or promotion.
2. a. Initiation = DNA damage + "mutation fixation".
   b. Anti-initiation = prevention of DNA damage and its repair by "error-prone" mechanisms.
3. a. Promotion = gene modulation (gene repression or derepression).
   b. Antipromotion = negation of tumor promoter functions.

C. Role of Genes in Carcinogenesis

The role of heredity and genes in the etiology of some cancers has been recognized and accepted by investigators for some time. Specific genes and chromosomal anomalies have been clearly associated with a predisposition to various types of cancers.[29,30] Recessive and dominant mutations in human beings have given rise to cancer-prone syndromes such as xeroderma pigmentosum, ataxia telangiectasia, retinoblastoma, and familial polyposis. Chromosomal aberrations, such as those found in Downs syndrome and the various sex chromosome syndromes[31] (i.e., Klinefelter's syndrome) predispose these individuals to various types of tumors. Moreover, the involvement of specific human chromosomes has been implicated with SV_{40} transformation of human cells,[32] with chronic myeloid leukemia, which is associated with a chromosome 22 translocation,[33] with meningiomas, associated with a deletion of chromosome 22,[34] with Burk-

---

* See later section.
** See later discussion on the "integrated theory".

itt's lymphoma, associated with an additional terminal fluorescent band on chromosome 14,[35] and with retinoblastoma, having a deletion in chromosome 13.[36]

Since mutations can and do occur in both the somatic and germ cells of mammalian organisms after exposure to chemicals inducing DNA damage, and since these mutations, which can be of the "gene-type" (i.e., deletions, structural, and regulatory) or of the "chromosomal-type", can have their expression influenced by many factors (i.e., recessive, dominant or codominant nature of the gene, diploid state, "penetrance", differentiation, period of development when mutation occurred, and exposure to particular environmental agents), clear patterns of genetic influence in carcinogenesis are often not seen. On another conceptual level, genes have been postulated to play an important role in chemical carcinogenesis. Based on the two-stage theory of carcinogenesis, Trosko and Chu[9] postulated the existence of three functional classes of genes which related either to the initiation (induction of DNA damage) or to the promotion (derepression of genes which cause the proliferation of quiescent, but initiated, cells) phases of carcinogenesis. Within this model, these three functional classes of genetic and environmental factors predisposing to cancer (representing large numbers of specific genes or environmental chemicals) were postulated in addition to the regulatory and "transforming" genes, which were postulated to be directly involved in controlling the neoplastic phenotype:[37] genes and environmental chemicals involved

1. In carcinogenic initiation (anti or super initiation)
2. In the replication and repair of damaged DNA
3. In tumor promotion (or antipromotion)

To illustrate this concept, genetic variability in drug-metabolizing enzymes, which might convert noncarcinogenic chemicals to chemicals that interact with DNA to induce damage, are, theoretically, distributed among individuals. Genetically-controlled pigmentation seems to influence the amount of UV light-induced DNA damage and the amount of sunlight-induced skin cancer.[38] Although contradictory experimental evidence exists with regard to the demonstration of a correlation between aryl hydrocarbon hydroxylase activity and lung cancer[39,40] in human beings, in principle, genes, which influence the ability of a chemical to interact with DNA, probably exist. However, there is clearly a strong correlation of a specific gene controlling polycyclic hydrocarbon metabolism with an increased risk for tumorigenesis, mutagenesis, toxicity, and teratogenesis in mice.[41]

Genes responsible for the repair of the DNA after it has been damaged by various physical and chemical carcinogens are known through a variety of human syndromes which predispose the individuals to cancer or to premature aging after exposure to specific environmental agents. For example, xeroderma pigmentosum,[42] Fanconi's anemia,[43,44] ataxia telangiectasia,[45] Hutchinson-Gilford (progeria),[46,47] and possibly Cockayne's syndrome[48] and retinoblastoma[49] seem to be genetically deficient in specific DNA repair functions for coping with particular environmentally-induced DNA damage.

In the case of xeroderma pigmentosum, the genetic imbalance seems to contribute to what Burnet[50] calls "intrinsic" mutagenesis, possibly by affecting the mutation process in the cells of these individuals.[51] It is not yet known if other DNA-repair-deficient syndromes, as well as other genetic deficiencies that lead to chromosomal aberrations (i.e., Bloom's syndrome), contribute to "intrinsic" mutagenesis on the structural gene or on the chromosomal level. On the other hand, genetic influence on cancer predisposition, which does not contribute to "intrinsic" mutagenesis by altering either the amount or rate of DNA damage or repair (i.e., initiation), might be conceptualized as "extrinsic" mutagenesis (i.e., altering the expression of genes or promotion).

Finally, genetic deficiencies in the immunological mechanism[52] or hormone balance[53,54] seem to predispose individuals to cancer, possibly by altering the influence of these vital functions on the antipromotion of cells initiated by various physical or chemical carcinogens.

Obviously, within a "nature and nurture" concept of carcinogenesis, environmental chemicals, which either alter (1) the expression of normal genes in these three functional classes or (2) the function of the normal enzymes coded for by these genes, can mimic the effect of genetic alterations of these three classes of genes. Chemical modification of initiation (DNA damage and repair) and of promotion (growth of initiated cells) will be illustrated in the next section.

Recapitulating then, when a tumor finally appears in an individual, many defense barriers on several biological levels (cellular, physiological, and biochemical) have been overcome. Within this view, a chemical initiator has overcome a genetic barrier which protects the DNA molecule (i.e., drug-metabolizing enzymes, transport or receptor proteins). Overcoming this first barrier, the chemical could interact with other chemicals ("comutagenesis")[55] or with DNA in such a way so as to alter the DNA structure and function ("irreversible" mutation or reversible gene modulation). If the DNA is damaged, genetic variation or environmental-modification of DNA repair enzymes could influence "error-free" vs. "error-prone" repair. If the repair is less than 100% accurate, a mutation could be expected. If the mutation occurs in a gene which is repressed in a viable cell, the biological consequence of such a mutation is not detected at this point. (Figure 1) If the carcinogen does not damage DNA (i.e., hormones), but causes an unscheduled modulation (gene repression or derepression) of genes, then the developmental pattern of the cell is sequentially altered.

Finally, if these genetically-altered, "nontumor" (initiated) cells are exposed to a promoter, these cells must overcome the third protective defense of the body, namely the immunological and hormonal influences (antipromoter genes). Variation in the genetic control of these systems, as well as environmental stimulation or repression of the immune or hormone control of cell proliferation, would determine if the initiated and promoted cell will eventually develop into a tumor.

III. MUTATION THEORY OF CARCINOGENESIS

The mutation theory of cancer was postulated by Boveri[56] long before the molecular structure of the genetic material, the nature of carcinogenesis, or the nature of the interaction between DNA and carcinogenic chemicals were known. The mutation theory was put forward to explain the observations that the daughter cells of a cancer maintain their neoplastic properties in spite of a progressive series of changes and that there is a seemingly unlimited variety of tumor types. Several predictions of the mutation theory, which are listed below, have been reviewed by Trosko and Chang.[5,37,57] An expanded discussion will be made of only one of the predictions.

A. Predictions and Evidence in Support of Theory
1. Alteration in Genes or Gene Products That Control Cell Proliferation and Integration Within Organisms

If a cancer cell differs from a normal cell by a mutation, then one would expect to find an alteration in the regulatory DNA sequences or in the polypeptide constituents of gene products controlling cell division and differentiation: no direct evidence bearing on this prediction exists to date.

2. Mutagenicity of Carcinogens
If cancers arise via mutagenic events, then carcinogens must be shown to be muta-

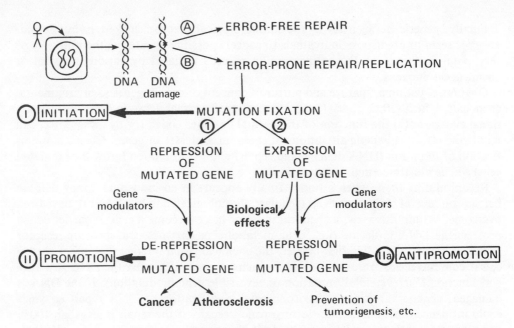

FIGURE 1.   This diagram aims to conceptualize the two-stage theory of carcinogenesis (initiation and promotion) in terms of the molecular and biological basis of each phase. Initiation is that process which includes the induction of molecular damage to DNA molecules and the error-prone repair and/or replication of that DNA molecule which leads to mutation fixation. Treatment of cells prior to the exposure to an initiating agent can enhance the amount of DNA damage. DNA repair, either error-free excision and post-replication repair or error-prone postreplication repair, occurs after DNA damage. Mutations are fixed during this repair period (first S-phase) and either expressed or repressed. The expressed mutations manifest themselves after dilution or decay of the product of the original gene. Repressed, but mutated, genes can be derepressed by agents that modulate gene activity. Promotion would be the process of modulating (depressing) gene expression, whereas antipromotion would repress the expression of mutated genes. In brief, initiation is a mutagenic event, depending on DNA damage and error-prone repair and/or replication, and promotion is an epigenetic event that derepresses mutated genes.

gens: approximately 90% of the chemical carcinogens tested have been shown to be mutagens.[58]

3. Clonal Nature of Tumors

If the cells of a tumor arose via a mutation, then all cells of the tumor must have a common ("clonal") origin: most, if not all, malignant tumors have indicated a clonal origin.[14,16,17,29] It must be noted that a stable epigenetic change, such as that which occurs during normal differentiation, could also explain the clonal nature of tumors.[59]

4. Certain Human Syndromes, Genetically Predisposed to Cancer, Have High Mutation Frequencies

If certain genetic syndromes predispose individuals to cancer, then cells from some of these cancer-prone individuals would be expected to have higher mutation frequencies induced in their cells than in cells from nonsusceptible human beings: xeroderma pigmentosum cells have higher gene and chromosomal mutation frequencies than "normal" human cells.[51,60]*

5. Age of Onset of "Hereditary" Tumors

If certain genetic syndromes predispose individuals to cancer because they inherit at least one mutated allele in a gene which is necessary for normal cell division and dif-

* See Chapter 5 in this volume by Maher and McCormick.

ferentiation, then random mutations leading to cancer would be expected to trigger carcinogenesis earlier in these syndromes than in normal individuals, who would require two independent mutations in both alleles of a gene in a single cell: hereditary Wilms' and retinoblastoma tumors appear earlier than nonhereditary tumors of the same tissue.[61]

6. Correlation Between Photoreactivation of DNA Damage and Biological Amelioration of UV Light-Induced Neoplasms

If carcinogen-induced molecular lesions in the DNA molecule that lead to mutations are eliminated in an "error-free" manner, then one would expect an amelioration of the induced tumors: photoreactivation of UV-induced pyrimidine dimers and a reduction of tumors in fish has been accomplished.[12]

7. Correlation of In Vitro DNA Damage with In Vitro Mutagenesis, In Vitro Transformation, and In Vivo Carcinogenesis

If DNA damage, its error-prone repair, in vitro mutagenesis, in vitro transformation, and in vivo tumorigenesis are causally related, then modifications in the frequency of one ought to be correlated with similar modifications in the others; evidence related to this prediction will be discussed at length.[27] Obviously, if mutagenesis is an important biological process leading to carcinogenesis, one would predict from the two-stage theory of carcinogenesis that those chemicals which influence the two-stage process of tumorigenesis (e.g., phorbol esters, caffeine, and hormones) also will influence the frequencies of mutations. As mentioned previously, the two-stage phenomenon has been demonstrated in several in vivo model systems.[11-13,24-26] Several chemicals that indirectly or directly affect gene expression, such as cyclic AMP, steroid hormones, caffeine, phorbol esters, protease inhibitors, retinoic acid, and other compounds, reduce or enhance the frequency of tumors induced by various physical and chemical carcinogens. If we assume for the moment that mutations are responsible for these carcinogen-induced tumors and that error-prone DNA repair/replication is responsible for the mutations, one would predict that these chemicals that modify the frequency of tumors are able to do so, depending on how they are applied to cells, by either modifying (1) the initial DNA damage; (2) the repair of DNA (hence, the mutation production); or (3) the expression of the mutations.

Phorbol esters are powerful promoters for chemical or UV light-induced tumors.[63] If phorbol esters are given to cells in vitro, prior to a chemical carcinogen, it appears to decrease the amount of induced DNA damage.[64] If phorbol esters are given to cells immediately after carcinogen-induced DNA damage (during the DNA repair and mutation fixation period), there are no significant molecular or biological consequences.[22,64] However, if phorbol ester is given well after the DNA repair and mutation fixation period, it causes an increase in the recovery of induced mutation,[22] an increase of induced transformation of cells in vitro,[18,21] and an increase of induced tumors.[13,63]

Caffeine and its analogues seem to act in a manner exactly the opposite to phorbol esters. Huberman and Sachs[65] showed that aminophylline, given to cells in vitro prior to exposure to chemical carcinogens, will enhance the mutagenic and transformation potentials of chemical carcinogens. Although it is difficult to generalize from experiments performed on different cells under various conditions, it does appear that caffeine can enhance the frequency of induced chromosomal aberrations,[66] structural gene mutations,[67-70] and in vitro transformation,[71,72] if it is present only during the DNA repair and mutation fixation period. In this respect, caffeine is different from phorbol esters, in that it does inhibit a constitutive postreplication repair enzyme in several rodent cell lines, and therefore, one does observe that cell killing and mutation frequencies are affected since DNA repair mechanisms are necessary for survival and mutation fixation. Furthermore, if caffeine is given to carcinogen-treated cells after DNA has been repaired and after mutations have been fixed, then there is no effect on cell survival, but there seems to be a decrease in the frequency of structural gene mutations[73] and of in vitro cell transformation.[74] It has been repeatedly demonstrated that prolonged caffeine (or theophylline) posttreatment of carcinogen treated mice also reduces the appearance of skin tumors.[75-79]

Many hormones have been shown to modify tumor frequencies. Antiinflammatory agents such as dexamethasone and fluocinolone acetonide have been shown to be very potent inhibitors of the phorbol ester promotion of 7,12-dimethylbenz[a]anthracene-induced mouse skin tumorigenesis.[80-82] These hormones were also found to inhibit the production of plasminogen activator.[82,83] Moreover, we have recently observed a negation of TPA-enhanced recovery of UV-induced, ouabain-resistant mutations in Chinese hamster cells with dexamethasone and fluocinoline acetonide.[27] On the other hand, some sex steroid hormones increase tumor formation in vivo. 17-β estradiol increases the formation of tumors, while it is well documented that diethylstilbesterol (DES) induces vaginal carcinogenesis.[84] It has been shown that both 17-β estradiol and DES induce ornithine decarboxylase activity in the chick oviduct in vivo and in vitro.[85] Recently we have shown that 17-β estradiol modifies the recovery of UV-induced, ouabain-resistant mutations in Chinese hamster cells.[27]

Additional evidence relevant to the understanding of the basic mechanisms for initiation (anti-initiation) and promotion (anti-promotion) can be found in studies (1) on the prevention of chemical carcinogenesis;[86] (2) on the amelioration of the tumor-promoting activity of phorbol esters by vitamin A and its synthetic analogues;[87,88] and (c) on the biochemical action of known tumor promoters. It has been observed that tumor promoters induce plasminogen activator[89] and ornithine decarboxylase.[90-93] In addition, since neither promoters nor antitumor promoters act as mutagens,[27] it is only reasonable to attribute their phenotypic-modifying potential to their ability to act as gene modulators.[22] Further evidence for this explanation is provided by the postulated mechanism of hormone action[94] and by the studies of Verma and Boutwell,[87] who demonstrated that vitamin A inhibited a phorbol ester-induced ornithine decarboxylase activity in mouse epidermis, but did not inhibit the enzyme activity when added to soluble extracts under in vitro conditions. In addition, based on our working hypothesis that tumor promotion is due to the derepression of "transforming" genes in cells with a mutated regulatory gene, we have reasoned that all of the tumor and antitumor promoting chemicals could be acting through some common mechanism (i.e., the biochemical basis for gene expression). Our first guess was that cyclic nucleotides might be the critical molecules for the following reasons.

Phorbol esters have been shown, in some systems, to increase 3':5'-cyclic GMP[64,95,96] and to decrease 3':5'-cyclic AMP.[78] On the other hand, caffeine, an antitumor promoter, increases the concentration of cellular 3':5'-cyclic AMP by inhibiting phosphodiesterase.[97] We have recently demonstrated that both the TPA enhancement[22] and caffeine reduction[73] on UV-induced mutations were negated when both compounds were added together.[27]

Cyclic AMP has been postulated to mediate the activity of steroid hormones.[98] Dixon-Shanies and Knittle,[99] as well as Lee and Reed,[100] have shown that certain steroid hormones affect the regulation of the levels of cyclic AMP in human lymphocytes. As mentioned previously, steroidal agents are known to inhibit tumor promotion by phorbol esters,[80] as well as the production of plasminogen activator.[82] Theophylline and papaverine (cyclic AMP phosphodiesterase inhibitors) increase cyclic AMP levels and depress the production of plasminogen activator.[101] More direct evidence was provided by the report that the growth of two-hormone-dependent mammary tumors was inhibited by cyclic AMP.[102]

Other reports also support the hypothesis that tumor promoters (antipromoters) act by cyclic nucleotide-influenced modulation of genes. For example, Yasui and Takasugi,[103] and Chopra and Wilkoff[104] have shown that vitamin A prevented 17-β estradiol-induced vaginal epithelial proliferation and testosterone-induced hyperplastic lesions of the prostatic epithelium of mice, respectively. The major relevance of these observations is that these two nonmutagenic chemicals (vitamins, hormones), which are known to affect the expression of genes, negated each other. Cho-Chung and Redler[105] have shown that the growth of 7,12-dimethylbenz [a] anthracene-induced mammary tumors can be arrested by either ovariectomy or treatment with dibutyryl cyclic AMP and that 17β estradiol, or cessation of the dibutyryl cyclic AMP treatment, can reverse the regression of growth. Cotzias and Tang[106] have demonstrated a correlation between increased adenylate cyclase activity (increased cyclic AMP) in various strains of mice and a reduction in mammary cancers. Chang et al.[27] have also shown that dibutyryl cyclic AMP drastically reduced the recovery of UV-induced, ouabain-resistant mutation frequencies.

It must be noted, however, that Mufson et al.[93] seemed to have disassociated the induction of ornithine decarboxylase by TPA from detectable changes in cyclic nucleotide levels in mouse skin. It is conceivable that TPA, in some systems, acts to induce the expression[107] or activity of a specific gene or enzyme (i.e., ornithine decarboxylase), which, in turn, produces other chemicals (i.e., polyamines) that could modulate gene expression. Supporting that hypothesis is the observation that polyamines can alter growth, behavior, and morphological appearance of hamster cells.[108]

The observation that retinoic-acid amelioration of N-methyl-N-nitrosourea-induced bladder[86] and mammary cancers,[109] as well as the inhibition of TPA-induction ornithine decarboxylase activity in mouse epidermis,[87] leads to the prediction (based on the aforementioned two-stage theory of carcinogenesis) that retinoic acid acts as a gene modulator. Chang et al.[27] have shown that retinoic acid can reduce the recovery of UV-induced, ouabain-resistant mutations.

On a different level, several protease inhibitors have been shown to negate the promoting activity of TPA on 7,12-dimethylbenz [a] anthracene-induced tumorigenesis in mouse skin.[110] Unlike the chemicals mentioned above, these protease inhibitors seem to act as antiinitiators (i.e., reduce the mutation induction) rather than as antipromoters (i.e., repression of genes).

In summary, the literature does contain evidence which tends to support our hypothesis that mutagenesis plays an important role in the initiation phase of the two-stage hypothesis of carcinogenesis. Moreover, chemicals that modify the expression of genes (repression or derepression) can, again by inference, modify the promotion step of carcinogenesis. (Figure 1)

B. Criticisms of the Mutation Theory

In spite of the evidence supporting the mutation theory of carcinogenesis, critics point to at least three major observations which strain the mutation theory:

1. Not all known chemical carcinogens are mutagens (i.e., hormones).[53,54]
2. Some cancer cells do not lose their genetic "totipotency".[111,112]
3. The correlation between mutagenesis and in vitro transformation frequencies is not quantitatively strong.

Those in favor of the mutation theory try to argue away the observation that some chemical carcinogens do not seem to be mutagenic by explaining that either the in vivo cancer or in vitro mutation test systems are inadequate. However, experiments, using nuclei or cells from malignant tissue from frogs[111] or mice,[112] clearly indicate that in these specific types of tumors the malignant phenotype is completely reversible. For example, Mintz and Illmensee[112] showed that injection of a normal blastocyst cell into the testis capsule of an adult mouse led to the formation of malignant teratocarcinomas. By reimplanting single cells, which must be euploid, of the malignant teratocarcinoma back into a normal blastocyst, a normal mosaic mouse could develop, having tissues derived from both the malignant teratocarcinoma and its own genetic origin. These studies clearly demonstrate that in these kinds of tumors the genes of the tumor cells retained their genetic integrity, as shown by their ability to govern normal development when placed in a different environment (i.e., an enucleated egg or blastocyst). Obviously, in order to explain these observations, one has to postulate that the genes that were active (or inactive) in the tumor cells were repressed (or derepressed) when placed in these new environments. If these particular cells were mutated, it would be highly unlikely that they could have retained and regained their ability to govern normal development and differentiation. In fact, malignant cells which were mutated or which were aneuploid, cannot, when put through this type of regime, give rise to normal development.

If DNA damage, mutagenesis, and in vitro transformation are steps in carcinogenesis, then studies related to the correlation of mutation and in vitro transformation ought to be examined to test this hypothesis. In general, there is strong qualitative evidence that mutagenesis is correlated with in vitro cell transformation.[113,114] However, in all cases, the frequency of that which is arbitrarily measured as in vitro transformants is extremely high compared to the mutation frequency. If one assumes that mutagenesis can lead to transformation, one would have to postulate that (1) most transformation phenotypes in vitro would not lead to tumorigenesis in vivo, as has been shown,[115,116] and/or (2) that most in vitro transformants, by virtue of the technique used to measure them in vitro, are mainly due to epigenetic changes rather than mutations, and therefore, they would be reversible.

IV. INTEGRATIVE THEORY OF CARCINOGENESIS

Since there is strong compelling evidence for and against both the mutation and epigenetic theories of carcinogenesis, Trosko et al.[37,57] have postulated an "integrative" theory of carcinogenesis, rather than having to ignore either the observations that in some cases the neoplastic state can be reverted to the normal state or that mutations can influence carcinogenesis. This integrative theory is a synthesis of (1) the mutation and epigenetic theories of carcinogenesis, (2) the two-stage theory of carcinogenesis, and (3) Comings' general theory of cancer.[117] A general illustration of this integrative theory is seen in Figure 2.

The fundamental assumption of this integrative theory is that there are regulatory DNA sequences in each cell which control the expression of a series of genes ("transforming" genes) in these cells. These "transforming" genes are genes which allow a cell to proliferate within an organism, such as during embryogenesis and in the normal loss of cells due to use or injury. The term "transformation" gene is not meant, necessarily, to imply the existence of "cancer" genes. However, if exogenous genes are incorporated into the eukaryotic genome (i.e., viral insertion) which are not controlled by the host regulatory DNA sequences, or if the host regulatory DNA sequences are rendered inoperative (repression of the two alleles; two-recessive mutations of the alleles; or a deletion of one and a mutation or repression of the other), then those genes which foster cell division are no longer responsive to the signals of the whole body to stop cell division and to differentiate normally.

Another feature of this integrative theory is that carcinogenesis can induce tumorigenesis by mutational or epigenetic alteration in gene expression. In effect, carcinogens can be mutagens that induce irreversible changes in the regulatory gene(s) (structural

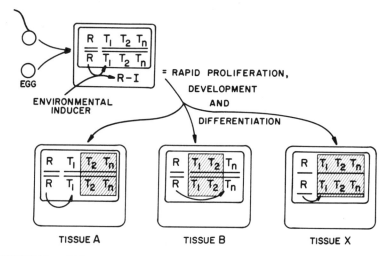

FIGURE 2. Using Comings' hypothesis[117] as the fundamental mode by which cells control their proliferative capacity, this diagram illustrates how simple environmental inducers divert products of gene regulators(R) from repressing (→) a series of genes that contribute to normal cell proliferation (T, "transforming" genes). It must be stressed that the symbol, "T", is meant to represent particular genes (normally present or inserted by viruses), which when unregulated, lead to uncontrolled cell division. Its use in these models does not imply the presence of "cancer" genes. The shaded areas of the genome represent heterochromatin or nucleoprotein-repressed areas of the chromosome. (Reproduced from Trosko, J. E., Chang, C. C., and Glover, T., *Colloq Int. C.N.R.S.*, 256, 353, 1977. With permission.)

gene mutations, as well as gene deletions), or gene modulators that induce stable, but reversible, repression or derepression of these regulatory or "transforming" genes.

This integrative theory is able to account for the two-stage phenomenon of carcinogenesis as well. For example, carcinogenesis is possible after the mutagenic (initiation) step if (1) both the alleles of the regulatory gene are inoperative (i.e., two-somatic-mutations, point and/or deletion; one germ and one somatic mutation), and (2) the "transforming" genes are in a transcribable condition (Figure 3). If they are not (as seems to be the case in most differentiated cells), then the transition of the transforming genes from a nontranscribable state to a transcribable state could be accomplished epigenetically (promotion) by differentiation with tissue-specific tumor promoters (e.g., hormones) or by the action of non-tissue-specific tumor promoters (e.g., phorbol esters).

Quite clearly, this integrative theory explains carcinogenic phenomenon that do not require the two phases (initiation and promotion). There are some circumstances that would require only initiation (if the "transforming" genes are already in a transcribable condition), while some cancers (such as the mouse teratocarcinoma example[112]) would only require the promotion step (repression of the regulatory DNA sequences) as seen in Figure 4. The Yasui and Takasugi,[103] as well as the Chopra and Wilkoff,[104] experiments would also be explained by this model.

Furthermore, this model explains the earlier onset of tumors, as well as the presence of bilateral-type tumors in individuals with hereditary predispositions to cancer (i.e., Wilms' kidney tumors and retinoblastoma). Knudson[61] and Bonaiti-Pellie et al.[118] postulated multimutation models to explain this phenomenon, in that, for hereditary tumors, one mutation is inherited via the germ line, and the second somatic mutation occurs after conception, relatively early in development.

A "deletion" mutation model has been proposed by Kondo[119] after he reviewed the work done on the oncogenic chemical, 4-nitroquinoline-1-oxide. This "deletion" mu-

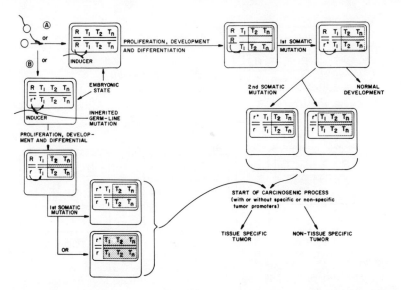

FIGURE 3.   This diagram integrates the Comings' hypothesis with the observations on, and interpretations of, heredity tumors made by Knudson.[61] In series A, the acquisition of two somatic mutations at the regulatory locus (R+) leads to the loss of control of genes that contribute to cell proliferation. If, during the course of differentiation and transformation, genes are put in a nontranscribable state (e.g., by histones), then another step is needed to activate these genes (promotion). If the promoter is tissue-specific (e.g., a hormone), then the tumor will originate only in the hormone-target tissue. If the promoter is nontissue-specific (e.g., phorbol ester), then the tumors could conceivably arise from any tissue having both dominant regulatory genes (R) mutated to the recessive state (r). Alternatively, an individual could inherit one or both mutated regulatory genes at conception. In the former case, the onset of tumors would be earlier, and in the latter, death of the fetus would probably occur. (Reproduced from Trosko, J. E., Chang, C. C., and Glover, T., *Colloq Int. C.N.R.S.*, 256, 353, 1977. With permission.)

tation model can be subsumed by this integrative theory because the deletion and inactivation of the regulatory alleles would have the same effect as mutating or repressing each of them. Moreover, it is noted that human, cancer-predisposing syndromes that have high chromosome aberration frequencies (i.e., Bloom's, Fanconi's) might be explained by this integrative model.

V. POTPOURRI: CHEMICALS, GENES, MUTATIONS, AND EVOLUTION

Any analysis of chemical carcinogenesis, particularly at the DNA level, must include an evolutionary perspective. Organisms have always been inexorably linked to environmental chemicals by mechanisms that controlled the expression of genes, in order to be adaptive and to allow normal development. Many adaptive somatic (short-term) and germ (long-term) line mechanisms have evolved which enabled the organism to cope with environmental chemical assaults. For example, there are genes that (1) protect or predispose DNA to various types of environmentally induced damage (i.e., drug metabolizing or transport enzymes); (2) repair DNA damage caused by physical and chemical agents; and (3) identify and control the proliferation and differentiation of cells (i.e., immune surveillance and hormone systems). If one accepts the conceptual view that mutagenesis is an adaptive feature for the survival of the species, and if certain mutations can lead to cancer, then it would seem that cancer is the price we, as individuals, must pay for the possession of this adaptive feature.[9,120]

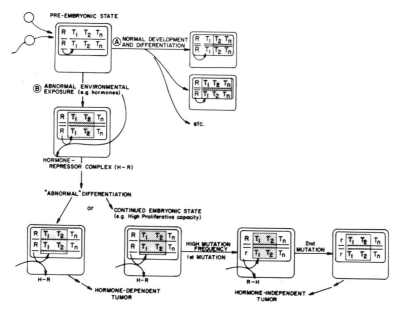

FIGURE 4. This diagram is a heuristic scheme to explain nonmutation-initiated tumors. It assumes that the regulatory gene of the Comings' hypothesis is rendered ineffective by an abnormal environmental inducer during a critical period of embryonic development (e.g., DES during development of vaginal tissue). This environmental agent removes the regulator product which allows the "transforming" genes to promote cell proliferation. However, because these cells are "out of place" with normal development, they do not respond to normal exogenous "signals" for the control of cell division. Moreover, some cells would at this stage be dependent on the continous presence of the agent (e.g., hormone), which would remove the regulatory product from potential control. Alternatively, the rapid proliferation of the cells, without concommitant increase in environmental mutagens or in the mutation rate, could have an increased spontaneous mutation frequency (gene or chromosome). This might explain observations relating to the loss of hormone dependency of some tumors with time and the increase of chromosomal aneuploidy in many tumors. (Reproduced from Trosko, J. E., Chang, C. C., and Glover, T., *Colloq Int. C.N.R.S.*, 256, 353, 1977. With permission.)

If one accepts the theory of evolution and assumes that (1) genes do exist that regulate normal cell division, differentiation, and integration within the whole organism, and (2) germ and somatic mutations can occur at random in any of these and all other genes, then it seems to us that it is no longer a question of whether mutagenesis can or cannot lead to carcinogenesis, but rather, "What is (or are) the gene(s), when inactivated by either mutations or epigenetic mechanisms, that can give rise to tumors?"

O'Brien et al.[90] and O'Brien and Diamond[91] have hypothesized that the gene(s) affecting the level of ornithine decarboxylase activity might be obligatory for tumor promotion. In effect, they have speculated that tumor promoters induce, transiently, the tumor phenotype in all cells (namely, the induction of ornithine decarboxylase enzyme and high proliferative activity). If a cell has had an initiator-caused error, it would be unable to reverse the induced-tumor phenotype back to the normal. They postulated that the initiator induces a deletion in some cellular component of the system controlling the level of ornithine decarboxylase. Prasad and Sinha have speculated that a defect in the regulation of cyclic AMP binding proteins may be one of the critical steps in the transformation of some cells.[121]

From our theoretical model, that initiator-caused error leading to a "deletion" in some cellular component controlling ornithine decarboxylase activity might well be a mutation in the regulatory DNA sequence negatively controlling ornithine decarboxylase (or other proliferation requiring enzymes). Since the neoplastic phenotype appears, genetically, to be recessive in character[122,123] and since there are data suggesting regulatory genes (DNA sequences) controlling several enzymes in mammalian cells,[124] it would not be unreasonable to assume two mutations (point and/or deletion type) in the postulated regulatory gene of the integrative model.

It has been postulated previously[125] that mutagenesis, as a fundamental biological process in both germ and somatic cells, could be responsible for the somatic diseases correlated with aging (i.e., degenerative diseases) as well as with cancer. Trosko and Chang[120] hypothesized that DNA damage of somatic cells, if mutationally fixed, would lead primarily to "aging" (i.e., most genes if mutated would lead to enzyme dysfunction and would not confer a selective advantage to a cell). On the other hand, mutations in a few particular genes (for example, the regulatory gene for ornithine decarboxylase or a cyclic AMP binding protein) would have the potential of conferring a selective advantage to that cell.

Two diverse observations, namely (1) higher ornithine decarboxylase activity in promoted cells than in nonpromoted cells and in malignant tumors than in benign tumors; (2) lower ornithine decarboxylase in senescent cells than in proliferating cells,[126] would be consistent with the hypothesis that mutations leading to regulatory dysfunction of the levels of structural genes could lead to cancer, whereas mutations in the structural genes themselves, leading to altered function of the enzyme, could lead to senescence. It would also be reasonable to assume that cellular dysfunction, in general, could in principle be the result of epigenetic changes affecting many other genes, similar to the model suggested by Holliday et al.[127]

Based on the assumption that (1) mutations can arise via error-prone DNA repair/replication, and (2) there are genes in all cells which regulate the levels of other genes needed for proliferation and integration into the whole body, one would assume that cancer, as well as other somatic diseases (i.e., atherosclerosis,[128,129] some teratogenic defects,[130] diabetes, and aging), would be a natural consequence of the evolutionary process, since DNA damage and repair leading to mutations occur in both somatic[131] and germ[132-134] cells. It has been suggested that with eradication of contagious disease-related deaths in modern technological societies,[5,135] human beings live longer only to suffer the consequence of somatic diseases caused by longer and more exposure to environmental initiators (mutagens) and promoters (gene modulators). The similarity of many of the same risk factors associated with cancer, atherosclerosis, diabetes, and teratogenic defects (namely, smoking, hormones, obesity, diet, genetic factors, and age) suggest to us a common underlying mechanism. That mechanism, in our view, might be mutagenesis.

The varied nature of the evidence compels us to believe that mutagenesis does play a major role in carcinogenesis. We do believe, however, that nonmutagenic alteration of genes by chemicals which interact with DNA (e.g., epigenetic modulation) can contribute to carcinogenesis in the repression or derepression of genes crucial to the regulation of cell division, or in the derepression of previously mutated genes (e.g., tumor promoters). Finally, recognizing that somatic mutations do occur in all cells and that there are several genes which could regulate the cells integration into the whole organism, it would be extremely difficult, if not impossible, to argue that mutations caused by chemical agents could not contribute to carcinogenesis.

VI. CONCLUSIONS

The roles of chemicals in the induction and modification of carcinogenesis is well documented. Furthermore, chemical-induced DNA damage appears to play a major role in mutation-fixation and carcinogenesis. Theoretically, many nonmutagenic chemicals, known to modify carcinogenesis, can modify (1) the amount of DNA damage,

(2) the repair of that molecular damage, and (3) the expression of the genetic consequences of the DNA damage.

Evidence was presented which seems to support the hypothesis that both mutations and epigenetic processes are components to chemical carcinogenesis. The clonal nature of tumors, the mutagenicity of many, but not all, carcinogens, the correlation of high mutation frequencies in cells of cancer-prone human fibroblasts lacking DNA repair enzymes, correlation of in vitro DNA damage, in vitro mutation and transformation frequencies with in vivo tumorigenesis, age related incidences of various hereditary tumors, and the correlation between photoreactivation of DNA damage and the biological amelioration of UV-induced neoplasms are all consistent with the mutation theory of cancer.

In order to reconcile the observations that both mutagens and gene modulators can be carcinogenic, we have made an analysis of how carcinogens could affect the genes which control cell division. We have attempted an integration of the mutation and epigenetic theories of cancer with the "two-stage" theory and Comings' general theory of carcinogenesis. The integrative theory postulates that chemical carcinogens can affect the regulatory genes (DNA sequences) which control a series of genes responsible for integrating the division and differentiation of the cell within an organism.

ACKNOWLEDGMENTS

The research reported from the authors' laboratory was supported by National Cancer Institute grants CA 13048-05 and CA 21107-01 to J.E.T. and a NIEHS Young Environmental Scientist Award (ES01809) to C.C.C. We wish to acknowledge the supporting help of J. Funston, L. P. Yotti, S. Warren, T. Glover, R. Schultz, and S. Austin.

REFERENCES

1. Potter, V. R., Hormonal induction of enzyme functions, cyclic AMP levels and AIB transport in Morris hepatomas and in normal liver systems, in *Morris Hepatomas: Mechanisms of Regulation*, Morris, H. P. and Criss, W. E., Eds., Plenum Press, New York, 1977, 87.
2. Copeland, D. D., Concepts of disease and diagnosis, *Perspect. Biol. Med.*, 20, 528, 1977.
3. Rabkin, J. G. and Struening, E. L., Life events, stress, and illness, *Science* 194, 1013, 1976.
4. Engel, G. L., The need for a new medical model: a challenge for biomedicine, *Science,* 196, 129, 1977.
5. Trosko, J. E. and Chang, C. C., Genes and environmental factors in carcinogenesis: an integrative theory, *Q. Rev. Biol.,* 53, 115, 1978.
6. Temin, H. M., On the origin of the genes for neoplasia: G. H. A. Clowes Memorial Lecture, *Cancer Res.,* 34, 2835, 1974.
7. Casto, B. C., Enhancement of adenovirus transformation by treatment of hamster cells with ultraviolet irradiation, DNA base analogs, and dibenz [a,h]anthracene., *Cancer Res.,* 33, 402, 1973.
8. Lynch, H. T. and Kaplan, A. R., Cancer genetic problems: host-environmental considerations., *Immunol. Cancer Prog. Exp. Tumor Res.,* 19, 332, 1974.
9. Trosko, J. E. and Chu, E. H. Y., The role of DNA repair and somatic mutation in carcinogenesis, in *Adv. Cancer Res.,* 21, 391, 1975.
10. Lynch, H. T., Cancer control in xeroderma pigmentosum, *Arch. Dermatol.,* 113, 193, 1977.
11. Berenblum, I., A speculative review: the probable nature of promoting action and its significance in the understanding of the mechanism of carcinogenesis, *Cancer Res.,* 14, 471, 1954.
12. Boutwell, R. K., Some biological aspects of skin carcinogenesis, *Prog. Exp. Tumor Res.,* 4, 207, 1964.
13. Boutwell, R. K., The function and mechanism of promoters of carcinogenesis, *CRC Crit. Rev. Toxicol.,* 3, 419, 1974.

14. Burnet, F. M., The biology of cancer, in *Chromosomes and Cancer*, German, J., Ed., John Wiley & Sons, New York, 1974, 21.
15. Cairns, J., Mutation, selection and the natural history of cancer, *Nature (London)*, 255, 197, 1975.
16. Nowell, P. C., The clonal evolution of tumor cell populations, *Science*, 194, 23, 1976.
17. Fialkow, P. J., Clonal origin and stem cell evolution of human tumors, in *Genetics of Human Cancer*, Mulvihill, J. J., Miller, R. W., and Fraumeni, J. F., Eds., Raven Press, New York, 1977, 439.
18. Lasne, C., Gentil, A., and Chouroulinkov, I., Two stage malignant transformation of rat fibroblasts in tissue culture, *Nature (London)*, 247, 490, 1974.
19. Mondal, S., Brankow, D. W., and Heidelberger, C., Two-stage chemical oncogenesis in cultures of C3H/10T½ cells, *Cancer Res.*, 36, 2254, 1976.
20. Mondal, S. and Heidelberger, C., Transformation of C3H/10T½ CL8 mouse embryo fibroblasts by ultraviolet irradiation and a phorbol ester, *Nature (London)*, 260, 710, 1976.
21. Kennedy, A. R., Mondal, S., Heidelberger, C., and Little, J. B., Enhancement of X-radiation transformation by a phorbol ester using C3H/10T½CL8 mouse embryo fibroblast, *Cancer Res.*, 38, 439, 1978.
22. Trosko, J. E., Chang, C. C., Yotti, L. P., and Chu, E. H. Y., Effect of phorbol myristate acetate on the recovery of spontaneous and ultraviolet light-induced 6-thioguanine and ouabain-resistant Chinese hamster cells, *Cancer Res.*, 37, 188, 1977.
23. Lankas, G. R., Baxter, C. S., and Christian, R. T., Effect of tumor-promoting agents on chemically-induced mutagenesis in cultured V79 Chinese hamster cells, *Mutat. Res.*, 45, 153, 1977.
24. Periano, C., Fry, R. J. M., Staffeldt, E., and Christopher, J. P., Comparative enhancing effects of phenobarbital, amobarbital, diphenylhydantoin, and dichlorodiphenyltrichloroethane on 2-acetylaminofluorene-induced hepatic tumorigenesis in the rat, *Cancer Res.*, 35, 2884, 1975.
25. Goerttler, K. and Loehrke, H., Diaplacental carcinogenesis: initiation with the carcinogens dimethylbenzanthracene (DMBA) and urethane during fetal life and postnatal promotion with the phorbol ester TPA in a modified 2-stage Berenblum/Mottram experiment, *Virchows Arch. A Pathol. Anat. Physiol.*, 372, 29, 1976.
26. Hicks, R. M. and Chowaniew, J., The importance of synergy between weak carcinogens in the induction of bladder cancer in experimental animals and humans, *Cancer Res.*, 37, 2943, 1977.
27. Chang, C. C., Trosko, J. E., and Warren, S. T., *In vitro* assay for tumor promoters and anti-promoters, *J. Environ. Pathol. Toxicol.*, 2, 43, 1978.
28. Van Duuren, B. L. and Goldschmidt, B. M., Cocarcinogenic and tumor-promoting agents in tobacco carcinogenesis, *J. Nat. Cancer. Inst.*, 56, 1237, 1976.
29. Mulvihill, J. J., Miller, R. W., and Fraumeni, J. F., *Genetics of Human Cancer*, Raven Press, New York, 1977.
30. Knudson, A. G., Jr., Heredity and cancer in man, *Prog. Med. Genet.*, 9, 113, 1973.
31. Mulvihill, J. J., Congenital and genetic diseases, in *Persons at High Risk of Cancer*, Fraumeni, J. F., Ed., Academic Press, New York, 1975, 3.
32. Croce, C. M., Huebner, K., Giradi, A. J., and Koprowski, H., Genetics of cell transformation by Simian virus 40, *Cold Spring Harbor Symp. Quant. Biol.*, 42, 335, 1974.
33. Rowley, J. D., A new consistent chromosomal abnormality in chronic myelogenous leukaemia identified by quinacrine fluorescence and giemsa staining, *Nature (London)*, 243, 290, 1973.
34. Zankl, H. and Zang, K. D., Cytological and cytogenetical studies on brain tumors. IV. Identification of the missing G chromosome in human meningiomas as No. 22 by fluorescence technique, *Humangenetik*, 14, 167, 1972.
35. Manolov, G. and Manolova, Y., Marker band in one chromosome 14 from Burkitt Lymphomas, *Nature (London)*, 237, 33, 1972.
36. Wilson, M. G., Towner, J. W., and Fujimoto, A., Retinoblastoma and D-chromosome deletions, *Amer. J. Human Genet.*, 25, 57, 1973.
37. Trosko, J. E., Chang, C. C., and Glover, T., Analysis of experimental evidence of the relation between mutagenesis and carcinogenesis. Role of DNA repair in carcinogenesis, *Colloq. Int. C.N.R.S.*, 256, 353, 1977.
38. Setlow, R. B., The wavelengths in sunlight effective in producing skin cancer: a theoretical analysis, *Proc. Nat. Acad. Sci. U.S.A.*, 71, 3363, 1974.
39. Okuda, T., Vesell, E. S., Plotkin, E., Tarone, R., Bast, R. C., and Gelboin, H. V., Interindividual and intraindividual variations in aryl hydrocarbon hydroxylase in monocytes from monozygotic and dizygotic twins, *Cancer Res.*, 37, 3904, 1977.
40. Paigen, B., Gurtoo, H., Minowada, J., Houten, L., Vincent, R., Paigen, K., Parker, N., Ward, E., and Hayner, N., Questionable relation of aryl hydrocarbon hydroxylase to lung-cancer risk, *N. Engl. J. Med.*, 297, 346, 1977.
41. Thorgeirsson, S. S. and Nebert, D. W., The Ah locus and the metabolism of chemical carcinogens and other foreign compounds, *Adv. Cancer Res.*, 25, 149, 1977.

42. Cleaver, J. E., Bootsma, D., and Friedberg, E., Human diseases with genetically altered DNA repair processes, *Genetics*, 79, 225, 1975.

43. Poon, P. K., O'Brien, R. L., and Parker, J. N., Defective DNA repair in Fanconi's anaemia, *Nature (London)*, 250, 223, 1974.

44. Fujiwara, Y. and Tatsumi, M., Repair of mitomycin C damage to DNA in mammalian cells and its impairment in Fanconi's anemia cells, *Biochem. Biophys. Res. Commun.*, 66, 592, 1975.

45. Paterson, M. C., Smith, B. P., Lohman, P. H. M., Anderson, A. K., and Fishman, L., Defective excision repair of X-ray-damaged DNA in human (ataxia telangiectasia) fibroblasts, *Nature (London)*, 26, 444, 1976.

46. Epstein, J., Williams, J. R., and Little, J., Deficient DNA repair in human progeroid cells, *Proc. Nat. Acad. Sci., U.S.A.*, 170, 977, 1973.

47. Rainbow, A. J. and Howes, M., Decreased repair of gamma ray damaged DNA in progeria, *Biochem. Biophys. Res. Commun.*, 74, 714, 1977.

48. Schmickel, R. D., Chu, E. H. Y., Trosko, J. E., and Chang, C. C., Cockayne syndrome: a cellular sensitivity to ultraviolet light, *Pediatrics*, 60, 135, 1977.

49. Weichselbaum, R. R., Nove, J., and Little, J. B., Skin fibroblasts from a D-deletion type retinoblastoma patient are abnormally X-ray sensitive, *Nature (London)*, 266, 726, 1977.

50. Burnet, F. M., Intrinsic mutagenesis, an interpretation of the pathogenesis of xeroderma pigmentosum, *Lancet*, 2, 495, 1974.

51. Maher, V. M. and McCormick, J. J., Effect of DNA repair on the cytotoxicity and mutagenicity of UV irradiation and of chemical carcinogens in normal and xeroderma pigmentosum cells, in *Biology of Radiation Carcinogenesis*, Yuhas, J. M., Tennant, R. W., and Regan, J. D., Eds., Raven Press, New York, 1976, 129.

52. Penn, I., Occurrence of cancer in immune deficiencies, *Cancer*, 34, 858, 1974.

53. Segaloff, A., Steroids and carcinogenesis, *J. Steroid Biochem.*, 6, 171, 1975.

54. Jensen, E. V., Some newer endocrine aspects of breast cancer, *N. Engl. J. Med.*, 291, 1251, 1974.

55. Nagao, M., Yahagi, T., Kawachi, T., Sugimura, T., Kosuge, T., Tsuji, K., Wakabayashi, K., Mizusaki, S., and Matsumoto, T., Comutagenic action of norharman and harman, *Proc. Jpn. Acad.*, 53, 95, 1977.

56. Boveri, T., *Zur Frage der Entstehung Maligner Tumoren*, Gustav Fisher, Jena, 1914.

57. Trosko, J. E. and Chang, C. C., The role of mutagenesis in carcinogenesis, in *Photochemical and Photobiological Reviews*, Vol. 3, Smith, K. C., Ed., Plenum Press, New York, 1978, 135.

58. McCann, J., Choi, E., Yamasaki, E., and Ames, B. N., Detection of carcinogens as mutagens in the Salmonella/microsome test: assay of 300 chemicals, *Proc. Nat. Acad. Sci. U.S.A.*, 72, 5135, 1975.

59. Pitot, H. C. and Heidelberger, C., Metabolic regulatory circuits and carcinogenesis, *Cancer Res.*, 23, 1694, 1963.

60. Sasaki, M. S., DNA repair capacity and susceptibility to chromosome breakage in xeroderma pigmentosum cells, *Mutat. Res.*, 20, 291, 1973.

61. Knudson, A. G., Jr., Mutations and childhood cancer: a probabilistic model for the incidence of retinoblastoma, *Proc. Nat. Acad. Sci. U.S.A.*, 72, 5116, 1975.

62. Hart, R. W. and Setlow, R. B., Direct evidence that pyrimidine dimers in DNA result in neoplastic transformation, in *Molecular Mechanisms*, Part B, Hanawalt, P. C. and Setlow, R. B., Eds., Plenum Press, New York, 1975, 719.

63. Baird, W. M. and Boutwell, R. K., Tumor-promoting activity of phorbol and four diesters of phorbol in mouse skin, *Cancer Res.*, 31, 1074, 1971.

64. Trosko, J. E., Yager, J. D., Bowden, G. T., and Butcher, F. R., The effects of several croton oil constituents on types of DNA repair and cyclic nucleotide levels in mammalian cells *in vitro*, *Chem. Biol. Interact.*, 11, 191, 1975.

65. Huberman, E., and Sachs, L., Mutability of different genetic loci in mammalian cells by metabolically activated carcinogenic polycyclic hydrocarbons, *Proc. Nat. Acad. Sci. U.S.A.*, 73, 188, 1976.

66. Kihlman, B. A., Sturelid, S., Hartley-Asp, B., and Nilsson, K., Caffeine, caffeine derivatives and chromosome aberrations, *Mutat. Res.*, 17, 271, 1973.

67. Trosko, J. E. and Chu, E. H. Y., Inhibition of repair of UV-damaged DNA by caffeine and mutation induction on Chinese hamster cells, *Chem. Biol. Interact.*, 397, 1973.

68. Roberts, J. J. and Sturrock, J. E., Enhancement by caffeine of N-methyl-N-nitrosourea induced mutations and chromosome aberrations in Chinese hamster cells, *Mutat. Res.*, 20, 243, 1973.

69. Fox, M., The effect of post-treatment with caffeine on survival and UV-induced mutation frequencies in Chinese hamster and mouse lymphoma cells *in vitro*, *Mutat. Res.*, 24, 187, 1974.

70. Maher, V. M., Ouellette, L. M., Curren, R. D., and McCormick, J. J., Caffeine enhancement of the cytotoxic and mutagenic effect of ultraviolet irradiation in a xeroderma pigmentosum variant strain of human cells, *Biochem. Biophys. Res. Commun.*, 71, 228, 1976.

71. Donovan, P. J. and DiPaolo, J., Caffeine enhancement of chemical carcinogen-induced transformation of cultured Syrian hamster cells, *Cancer Res.*, 34, 2730, 1974.

72. Ide, T., Anzai, K., and Andoh, T., Enhancement of SV_{40} transformation by treatment of C3H2K cells with UV light and caffeine, *Virology*, 66, 568, 1975.

73. Chang, C. C., Philipps, C., Trosko, J. E., and Hart, R. W., Mutagenic and epigenetic influence of caffeine on the frequencies of UV-induced ouabain-resistant Chinese hamster cells, *Mutat. Res.*, 45, 125, 1977.

74. Kakunaga, T., Caffeine inhibits cell transformation by 4-nitroquinoline-1-oxide, *Nature (London)*, 258, 248, 1975.

75. Webb, O., Braun, W., and Plescia, O., Antitumor effects of polynucleotides and theophylline, *Cancer Res.*, 32, 1814, 1972.

76. Zajdela, F. and Latarjet, R., Effect inhibiteur de la cafeine sur induction de cancers cutanes par les rayons ultraviolet chez la souris, *C. R. Acad. Sci. Ser. D*, 277, 1073, 1973.

77. Rothwell, K., Dose related inhibition of chemical carcinogenesis in mouse skin by caffeine, *Nature (London)*, 252, 69, 1974.

78. Belman, S. and Troll, W., Phorbol-12-myristate-13-acetate effect on cyclic adenosine 3',5'-monophosphate levels in mouse skin and inhibition of phorbol-myristate-acetate-promoted tumorigenesis, *Cancer Res.*, 34, 3446, 1974.

79. Nomura, T., Diminution of tumorigenesis initiated by 4-nitroquinoline-1-oxide by posttreatment with caffeine in mice, *Nature (London)*, 260, 547, 1976.

80. Belman, S. and Troll, W., The inhibition of croton oil-promoted mouse skin tumorigenesis by steroid hormones, *Cancer Res.*, 32, 450, 1972.

81. Schwarz, J. A., Viaje, A., and Slaga, T. J., Fluocinolone acetonide; a potent inhibitor of mouse skin tumor promotion and epidermal DNA synthesis, *Chem. Biol. Interact.*, 17, 331, 1977.

82. Viaje, A., Slaga, T. J., Wigler, M., and Weinstein, I. B., Effects of antiinflammatory agents in mouse skin tumor promotion, epidermal DNA synthesis phorbol ester induced cellular proliferation, and production of plasminogen activator, *Cancer Res.*, 37, 1530, 1977.

83. Wigler, M., Ford, J. P., and Weinstein, I. B., Glucocorticoid inhibition of the fibrinolytic activity of tumor cells, in *Proteases and Biological Control*, Reich, E., Rifkin, D. B., and Shaw, E., Eds., Cold Spring Harbor Laboratory, New York, 1975, 849.

84. Bern, H. A., Jones, L. A., Mills, K. T., Kohrman, A., and Mori, T., Studying long-term effects of early exposure to hormones and other agents, *J. Toxicol. Environ. Health*, Suppl. 1, 103, 1976.

85. Cohen, S., O'Malley, B. W., and Stastny, M., Estrogenic induction of ornithine decarboxylase *in vivo* and *in vitro*, *Science*, 170, 336, 1970.

86. Sporn, M. B., Dunlop, N. M., Newton, D. L., and Smith, J. M., Prevention of chemical carcinogenesis by vitamin A and its synthetic analogs (retinoids), *Fed. Proc. Fed. Am. Soc. Exp. Biol.*, 35, 1332, 1976.

87. Verma, A. K., and Boutwell, R. K., Vitamin A acid; a potent inhibitor of 12-O-tetradecanoyl-phorbol-13-acetate-induced ornithine decarboxylase activity in mouse epidermis, *Cancer Res.*, 37, 2196, 1977.

88. Kensler, T. W., Kajiwara, K., and Mueller, G. C., Retinoid effects on the phorbol ester-mediated mitogenic response of bovine lymphocytes, *Proc. Am. Assoc. Cancer Res.*, 18, 74, 1977.

89. Wigler, M. and Weinstein, I. B., Tumor promoter induces plasminogen activator, *Nature (London)*, 259, 232, 1976.

90. O'Brien, T. G., Simsiman, R. C., and Boutwell, R. K., Induction of the polyamine-biosynthetic enzymes in mouse epidermis by tumor-promoting agents, *Cancer Res.*, 35, 1662, 1975.

91. O'Brien, T. G. and Diamond, L., Ornithine decarboxylase induction and DNA synthesis in hamster embryo cell culture treated with tumor-promoting phorbol diesters, *Cancer Res.*, 37, 3895, 1977.

92. Yuspa, S. H., Lichti, U., Ben, T., Patterson, E., Hennings, H., Slaga, T. J., Colburn, N., and Kelsey, W., Phorbol esters stimulate DNA synthesis and ornithine decarboxylase activity in mouse epidermal cell cultures, *Nature (London)*, 262, 402, 1976.

93. Mufson, R. A., Astrup, E. G., Simsiman, R., and Boutwell, R. K., Dissociation of increases in level of 3':5'-cyclic AMP and 3':5'-cyclic GMP from the induction of ornithine decarboxylase by the tumor promoter 12-O-tetradecanoyl phorbol-13-acetate in mouse epidermis *in vivo*, *Proc. Nat. Acad. Sci. U.S.A.*, 74, 657, 1977.

94. Chan, L. and O'Malley, B. W., Mechanism of action of the sex steroid hormones, *N. Engl. J. Med.*, 294, 1322, 1976; 294, 1372, 1976; 294, 1430, 1976.

95. Voorhees, J. J., Colburn, N. H., Stawiski, M., Duell, E. A., Haddox, M., and Goldberg, N. D., Imbalanced cyclic AMP and cyclic GMP levels in rapidly dividing, incompletely differentiated epidermis of psoriasis, in *Control of Proliferation of Animal Cells*, Clarkson, B. and Baserga, R., Eds., Cold Spring Harbor Laboratory, New York, 1974, 635.

96. Estensen, R. D., Hadden, J. W., Hadden, E. M., Touraine, F., Touraine, J. L., Haddox, M. K., and Goldberg, N. D., Phorbol myristate acetate: effects of a tumor promoter on intracellular C-GMP in mouse fibroblasts and as a mutagen in human lymphocytes, in *Control of Proliferation in Animal Cells,* Clarkson, B. and Baserga, R., Cold Spring Harbor Laboratory, New York, 1974, 627.

97. Beavo, J. A., Rogers, N. L., Crofford, O. B., Hardman, J. G., Sutherland, E. W., and Newman, E. V., Effects of xanthine derivatives on lipolysis and adenosine 3′,5′-monophosphate phosphodiesterase activity, *Mol. Pharmacol.,* 6, 597, 1970.

98. Goldberg, M. L., Cyclic AMP mediates the activity of steroid hormones, *Med. Hypoth.,* 1, 6, 1975.

99. Dixon-Shanies, D. and Knittle, J. L., Effect of hormones on cyclic AMP levels in cultured human cells, *Biochem. Biophys. Res. Commun.,* 69, 982, 1976.

100. Lee, T. P. and Reed, C. E., Effects of steroids on the regulation of the levels of cyclic AMP in human lympocytes, *Biochem. Biophys. Res. Commun.,* 78, 998, 1977.

101. Mott, D. M., Fabisch, P. and Sorof, S., Cyclic AMP phosphodiesterase inhibitors depress production of plasminogen activator by Chinese hamster ovary cells, *Biochem. Biophys. Res. Commun.,* 70, 1150, 1976.

102. Cho-Chung, Y. S. and Gullino, P. M., *In vivo* inhibition of growth of two hormone-dependent mammary tumors by dibutyryl cyclic AMP, *Science,* 183, 87, 1974.

103. Yasui, T. and Takasugi, N., Prevention by vitamin A of the occurrence of permanent vaginal changes in neonatally estrogen-treated mice, *Cell Tissue Res.,* 179, 475, 1977.

104. Chopra, D. P. and Wilkoff, L. J., β-retinoic acid inhibits and reverses testosterone-induced hyperplasia in mouse prostate organ cultures, *Nature (London),* 265, 339, 1977.

105. Cho-Chung, Y. S., and Redler, B., Dibutyryl cyclic AMP mimics ovarietomy: nuclear protein phosphorylation in mammary tumor regression, *Science,* 197, 272, 1977.

106. Cotzias, G. L. and Tang, L. C., An adenylate cyclase of brain reflects propensity for breast cancer in mice, *Science,* 197, 1094, 1977.

107. Murray, A. W. and Froscio, M., Effect of tumor promoters on the activity of cyclic adenosine 3′:5′-monophosphate-dependent and independent protein kinase from mouse epidermis, *Cancer Res.,* 37, 1360, 1977.

108. Goto, M., Kimura, T., Sato, H., Suzuki, S., and Suzuki, M., Altered growth behavior and phenotypic expression of cells of mouse and hamster cell lines after treatment with polyanions, *Tokoku J. Exp. Med.,* 121, 143, 1977.

109. Moon, R. C., Brubbs, C. V., Sporn, M. B., and Goodman, D. G., Retinyl acetate inhibits mammary carcinogenesis induced by N-methyl-N-nitrosourea, *Nature (London),* 267, 620, 1977.

110. Troll, W., Klassen, A., and Janoff, A., Tumorigenesis in mouse skin: inhibition by synthetic inhibitors of proteases, *Science,* 169, 1211, 1970.

111. McKinnell, R., Deggins, B. A., and Labat, D. D., Transplantation of pluripotential nuclei from triploid frog tumors, *Science,* 165, 394, 1969.

112. Mintz, B. and Illmensee, K., Normal genetically mosiac mice produced from malignant teratocarcinoma cells, *Proc. Nat. Acad. Sci. U.S.A.,* 73, 3585, 1975.

113. Huberman, E., Mager, R., and Sachs, L., Mutagenesis and transformation of normal cells by chemical carcinogens, *Nature (London),* 264, 360, 1976.

114. Bouck, N., and di Mayorca, G., Somatic mutation as the basis for malignant transformation of BHK cells by chemical carcinogens, *Nature (London),* 264, 722, 1976.

115. Stiles, C. D., Desmond, W., Sata, G., and Saier, M., Failure of human cells transformed by simian virus 40 to form tumors in athymic nude mice, *Proc. Nat. Acad. Sci. U.S.A.,* 72, 4971, 1975.

116. Freedman, V. H. and Shin, S., Isolation of human diploid cell variants with enhanced colony-forming efficiency in semisolid medium after a single-step chemical mutagenesis, *J. Nat. Cancer. Inst.,* 58, 1873, 1977.

117. Comings, D. E., A general theory of carcinogenesis, *Proc. Nat. Acad. Sci. U.S.A.,* 70, 3324, 1973.

118. Bonaiti-Pellie, C., Briard-Guillemot, M. L., Feingold, J., and Frezal, J., Mutation theory of carcinogenesis in retinoblastoma, *J. Nat. Cancer Inst.,* 57, 269, 1976.

119. Kondo, S., Misrepair model for mutagenesis and carcinogenesis, in *Fundamentals in Cancer Prevention,* Magee, P. N., Ed., University of Tokyo Press, Tokyo, 1976, 417.

120. Trosko, J. E. and Chang, C. C., Role of DNA repair in mutation and cancer production, in *Aging, Carcinogenesis, and Radiation Biology,* Smith, K. C., Ed., Plenum Press, New York, 1976, 399.

121. Prasad, K. N. and Sinha, P. K., Abnormal regulation of cyclic AMP binding proteins: A critical lesion of malignancy of non-neural cells, *Differentiation,* 6, 59, 1976.

122. Harris, H., Miller, O. J., Klein, G., Worst, P., and Tachibana, T., Suppression of malignancy by cell fusion, *Nature (London),* 223, 363, 1969.

123. Stanbridge, E. J., Suppression of malignancy in human cells, *Nature (London),* 260, 17, 1976.

124. DeLuca, C. and Matheisz, J. S., Glucose-6-phosphate dehydrogenase activity in a hepatoma cell line: preliminary evidence for negative genetic control, *J. Cell Physiol.,* 87, 101, 1975.

125. **Trosko, J. E. and Hart, R. W.**, DNA mutation frequencies in mammals, *Interdiscip. Top. Gerontol.,* 9, 168, 1976.

126. **Duffy, P. E. and Kremzner, L. T.**, Ornithine decarboxylase activity and polyamines in relation to aging of human fibroblasts, *Exp. Cell Res.,* 108, 435, 1977.

127. **Holliday, R., Huschtscha, L. I., Tarrant, G. M., and Kirkwood, T. B. L.**, Testing the commitment theory of cellular aging, *Science,* 198, 366, 1977.

128. **Benditt, E. P.**, The origin of atherosclerosis, *Sci. Am.,* 236, 74, 1977.

129. **Dykhuizen, D.**, Evolution of cell senescence, atherosclerosis, and benign tumors, *Nature (London),* 251, 616, 1974.

130. **Opitz, J. M., Herrmann, J., and Dieker, H.**, The study of malformation syndromes in man, *Birth Defects Orig. Artic. Ser.,* 5, 1, 1969.

131. **Swenberg, J. A., Petzold, G. L., and Harbach, P. R.**, *In vitro* DNA damage/alkaline elution assay for predicting carcinogenic potential, *Biochem. Biophys. Res. Commun.,* 72, 732, 1976.

132. **Sega, G. A.**, Unscheduled DNA synthesis in the germ cells of male mice exposed *in vivo* to the chemical mutagen, ethyl methane-sulfonate, *Proc. Nat. Acad. Sci. U.S.A.,* 71, 4955, 1974.

133. **Masui, Y. and Pederson, R. A.**, Ultraviolet light-induced unscheduled DNA synthesis in mouse oocytes during meiotic maturation, *Nature (London),* 257, 705, 1975.

134. **Beikirch, H.**, Induction of unscheduled DNA synthesis by chemical mutagens in testicular cells of the mouse *in vitro, Arch. Toxicol.,* 37, 195, 1977.

135. **Gori, G. B. and Peters, J. A.**, Etiology and prevention of cancer, *Prev. Med.,* 4, 239, 1975.

INDEX

A

B

C

E

N